If you are living with diabetes or fall into a high-risk
category, what you eat is the key to good health.

Here is the one-stop guide to
lowering risk and managing diabetes.

THE DIABETES CARBOHYDRATE AND CALORIE COUNTER
is a one-of-a-kind book that lists thousands of brand names,
take-out, and restaurant foods, giving reliable counts for
carbohydrates, calories, sugar, and fat—all the information
needed to set up a healthy eating plan. Use the sample
menus and meal planning guides to customize your diet to fit
your food likes and dislikes, your culture, and your life's
demands. Managing diabetes has never been easier!

THE DIABETES CARBOHYDRATE AND CALORIE COUNTER
also includes:

• A thorough discussion of diabetes and
how the body responds to it

• Frequently asked questions—and answers—
from people newly diagnosed with diabetes

Books by Annette B. Natow and Jo-Ann Heslin

The Antioxidant Vitamin Counter
Calcium Counts
Count on a Healthy Pregnancy
The Calorie Counter *(Second Edition)*
The Carbohydrate, Sugar and Fiber Counter
The Cholesterol Counter *(Fifth Edition)*
The Diabetes Carbohydrate and Calorie Counter
(Second Edition)
Eating Out Food Counter
The Fat Attack Plan
The Fat Counter *(Fifth Edition)*
The Food Shopping Counter *(Second Edition)*
Get Skinny the Smart Way
The Healthy Heart Food Counter
Megadoses
The Most Complete Food Counter
No-Nonsense Nutrition for Kids
The Pocket Encyclopedia of Nutrition
The Pocket Fat Counter *(Second Edition)*
The Pocket Protein Counter
The Pregnancy Nutrition Counter
The Protein Counter
The Sodium Counter

Published by POCKET BOOKS

THE
DIABETES
CARBOHYDRATE AND CALORIE COUNTER

SECOND EDITION
Revised and Updated

♦

Annette B. Natow, Ph.D., R.D., *and* Jo-Ann Heslin, M.A., R.D.

POCKET BOOKS
New York   London   Toronto   Sydney

POCKET BOOKS, a division of Simon & Schuster, Inc.
1230 Avenue of the Americas, New York, NY 10020

Copyright © 1991, 2003 by Annette Natow and Jo-Ann Heslin

ISBN: 0-7434-5431-6

First Pocket Books printing of this revised edition
February 2003

20 19 18 17 16 15 14 13 12 11

POCKET and colophon are registered trademarks of
Simon & Schuster, Inc.

For information regarding special discounts for bulk purchases,
please contact Simon & Schuster Special Sales at 1-800-456-6798
or business@simonandschuster.com

Cover design by Lisa Cohen

Printed in the U.S.A.

To our families, who support us through every project:
Harry, Allen, Irene, Sarah, Meryl, Laura, Marty, George,
Emily, Steven, Joe, Kristen, Brian, and Karen.

Acknowledgments

For graciously sharing their knowledge: Martin Lefkowitz, M.D., and Irene E. Rosenberg, M.D.

For reading the book in its many stages of progress: Charles Harvey and Evan Mestman, M.S., R.D., CDN, CDE.

For all her support and help, our agent, Nancy Trichter.

Without the tireless cooperation of Steven Natow, M.D., and Stephen Llano, *The Diabetes Carbohydrate and Calorie Counter,* 2nd edition would never have been completed.

And a special thank you to our editor, Micki Nuding.

"The regulation of the diet is the most important consideration in the treatment of diabetes mellitus."

"While certain general principles in regard to diet for diabetes can be laid down, each patient presents an individual problem. . . ."

Mary Swartz Rose, Ph.D.
Feeding the Family
The MacMillan Company, 1919

Contents

Introduction

Are you overweight?
Do you have any close relatives with diabetes?
Are you over 40?

Rosa R., a 47-year-old who weighed too much, went to the doctor because of a vaginal infection. The doctor treated her problem and found a second one. Rosa was diabetic.

Tom O., whose mother had diabetes at 50, visited the doctor for a checkup after failing the routine eye examination needed to renew his driver's license. After examining his eyes, the doctor suggested that Tom see his family doctor, who told Tom he had diabetes.

Rosa and Tom, like many other people, were unaware of the early warning signs for diabetes. Recurring vaginal infections and vision changes are two of them.

Warning Signs for Diabetes

Increased thirst	Numbness or tingling in arms or legs
Frequent urination	Slow-healing cuts and bruises
Hunger	Diarrhea
Unintended weight loss	Frequent infections, especially in
Blurred vision	the skin, gums, vagina, and
Fatigue and weakness	bladder

People often have one or more of these symptoms but ignore them or simply consider them as part of getting older.

Diabetes, a chronic, incurable condition, is found throughout the world. The World Health Organization (WHO) estimates 120 to 140 million people worldwide have diabetes. The number of people with diabetes in the United States is growing; from 1990 to 1998 the incidence rose 33%, totaling 798,000 new cases a year. One out of every 14 Americans—17 million people—have type 2 diabetes. Many others have diabetes but don't know it. It's one of the leading causes of death in this country.

The risk of getting diabetes increases with age. It is estimated that 18% of the U.S. population over 65 has diabetes. Slightly more women than men are affected. African Americans, Hispanics, Pacific Islanders, American Indians, and natives of Alaska are at greater risk. Half of all Pima Indians have diabetes, making it a major health problem for this group. Lifestyle factors—not eating enough fruits, vegetables, and whole grains; not being active; and weighing too much—can also increase the risk of developing diabetes.

How Diabetes Got Its Name

Writings from ancient Egypt, Greece, Rome, and India described diabetes. People with this disorder passed large amounts of honey-sweet urine, attracting ants and flies. Indian writings blamed overeating, and Egyptians recommended a diet of beer, fruits, grains, and honey.

Romans named the condition *diabetes,* meaning "to flow through," because of frequent thirst and urination. In 1675, a London physician added the term *mellitus,* which is Latin for "honeylike." *Diabetes mellitus* is the correct name for the condition usually called diabetes.

1

Understanding Diabetes

Most people think that a person with diabetes can't eat sugar. That's not true. A person with diabetes cannot efficiently use the energy (calories) found in foods. The foods you eat contain energy in the form of protein, fat, and carbohydrate. After being eaten, foods are broken down in the body and then absorbed by the body's cells. Energy is finally released in the cells, so the breakdown products of food must get inside cells for this to happen. The problem in diabetes is that food, which you need for energy, cannot get into cells.

Energy is carried into cells by the hormone insulin. Insulin is produced in the pancreas, a gland just below and behind the stomach. Some people who have diabetes do not make enough insulin. Others make enough or even too much, but the insulin is not used efficiently by the body.

When a person's pancreas makes too little insulin, needed energy cannot get into cells. For those who make the right amount of insulin or, in some cases, even too much insulin, a different problem occurs: something prevents the body from using insulin. The result of either too little insulin, or insulin that can't be used, is the same: energy doesn't get into cells.

WHAT REALLY HAPPENS

The body uses sugar (glucose) and fat for energy. The way the body changes sugar into energy is very complicated.

Carbohydrates—starches and sugars in milk, fruit, potatoes, breads, and other foods—are easily broken down to sugar. When food starches and sugars are broken down in the body, glucose is formed. Glucose can be used immediately for energy or it can be stored in the liver and muscles for future use. Any glucose not needed for energy, or changed to glycogen and stored in the liver and muscles, is turned into fat and stored in the body. When needed at some future time, this stored fat can be changed back to glucose and used by the body for energy.

Fat is also a source of energy. It's found in butter, margarine, oils, nuts, and meat. When fat is digested, fatty acids are formed. Insulin helps fatty acids enter cells, where they are stored for future use.

Protein, a third source of energy, is found in meat, fish, poultry, cheese, milk, beans, and eggs. When protein is digested, amino acids are formed. Some of these amino acids may be changed into glucose by the liver, but this happens only when there isn't enough glucose from carbohydrates and fatty acids available.

Insulin helps the body use all types of energy. It helps the storage of carbohydrates, fat, and protein by carrying glucose, fatty acids, and amino acids into cells. When energy goes into cells normally, blood sugar (glucose) levels stay normal.

When you eat, your body produces insulin to take care of all these functions. In diabetes, when there is either too little insulin or the insulin does not work well, sugar (glucose) accumulates in the blood.

In hyperglycemia, sugar builds up in the blood and circulates through the body. When the blood sugar rises over 180 milligrams per deciliter (mg/dl), the kidneys cannot handle it. Kidneys try to pass the excess sugar out of the body in urine. So sugar in the urine is a sign that something is wrong.

Hyperglycemia

hyper = too much   *gly* = glucose (sugar)   *emia* = in the blood

Sometimes, in older people, there may be no sugar in the urine even though the blood sugar level is higher than 180. This is because, as we age, the kidneys may work less efficiently. In these cases, diabetes is confirmed through a blood test. This is one reason why your doctor orders a blood test during your annual physical.

2

Types of Diabetes

TYPE 2

There are two main types of diabetes. The most common form, the one that this book focuses on, is type 2 (formerly known as NIDDM, non–insulin-dependent diabetes). The numbers of people with type 2 diabetes, from children to the elderly, is increasing. The risk of developing diabetes increases with age, overweight, and lack of activity. Usually type 2 diabetes occurs in people who are over 40, but during the past decade, diabetes in people in their 30s increased 70%. In the past, children hardly ever had type 2 diabetes, but today 20% of all newly diagnosed cases of diabetes in children are type 2. Researchers blame this spike in type 2 cases on our aging population, the increasing number of people who are overweight, and our lack of physical activity at all ages.

Ninety to 95% of all people with diabetes have type 2. People with this type of diabetes do make some insulin. But their bodies either do not produce enough or their body cells are resistant to insulin's action.

Weighing too much is a major risk factor for type 2 diabetes. Having too many fat cells may prevent the body from using insulin normally. Two thirds of all people with type 2 diabetes are overweight. They are *insulin resistant*.

Many people with type 2 also have high cholesterol, low LDL cholesterol, high triglycerides, and high blood pressure.

The best way to handle type 2 diabetes is to lose weight and become more active. This combination not only lowers blood sugar levels but helps control other problems too, like high blood pressure.

It is recommended that everyone over 40 be routinely tested for type 2 diabetes. But anyone with the following risks should be tested beginning at age 30:

- Having a blood relative with diabetes
- Being overweight
- Having heart disease
- Having high blood pressure (140/90 or higher)
- Having high triglycerides (150 or higher), high LDLs (over 130), or low HDLs (less than 40)
- Having a blood-sugar test higher than 120
- Having diabetes during pregnancy or having a baby that weighs more than 9 pounds

---

You Should Know

You're at greater risk for type 2 diabetes if you watch too much TV and don't get enough sleep. Research has shown that people who watch 40 or more hours of TV a week have triple the risk of developing diabetes. Other studies show that sleeping too little makes controlling diabetes more difficult.

TYPE 1

Type 1 diabetes is the less common form of diabetes, accounting for only 10% of all cases. It was formally known as Insulin Dependent Diabetes Mellitus (IDDM). People with type 1 diabetes do not produce any insulin.

Weight loss is a common early symptom of type 1 diabetes, because the body cannot use energy normally. When there is no insulin, the body starts to burn its own fat for energy. Whenever fat is burned for energy, *ketones* are formed as by-products. Without insulin, ketones build up in the blood resulting in a serious condition called *ketoacidosis*. People with type 1 diabetes must have insulin injections daily to avoid this life-threatening condition. This problem rarely occurs in people with type 2 diabetes.

PREGNANCY DIABETES

Gestational diabetes occurs in 3 to 5% of all pregnancies. Risk factors include being over 30, being overweight, and having a family history of type 2 diabetes.

In the second half of pregnancy, there may be higher than normal levels of sugar in the blood. To prevent problems, all pregnant women are tested for blood sugar levels. If the levels are too high, gestational diabetes is treated by adjusting food intake and monitoring blood sugar levels carefully. In almost all cases, blood sugar levels return to normal when

---

Metabolic Syndrome

More than 40% of adults over 60 have *metabolic syndrome*, also known as *syndrome X*. People with metabolic syndrome are at greater risk for diabetes, stroke, and heart disease. It is diagnosed when a person has three or more of the following:

- insulin resistance
- high blood fats
- low HDL cholesterol
- high blood sugar
- high blood pressure
- extra belly fat (waist measurements over 35 inches in women and over 40 inches in men)

pregnancy ends, but having gestational diabetes increases a woman's risk for type 2 in the future.

INSULIN RESISTANCE

What is insulin resistance? Blood sugar rises after food is eaten. The pancreas responds by pumping out insulin. Insulin helps move glucose out of the blood and into cells, where it's used for energy or stored. When there is insulin resistance, glucose builds up in blood and cannot be used by cells. At the same time, the pancreas keeps pumping out higher than normal amounts of insulin that the body cannot use. Some people have less than the normal amount of insulin receptor sites in their cells. These receptor sites are like doorways. They are the places where insulin hooks up to the cell and lets glucose enter.

According to Gerald Reaven, M.D., professor of medicine, Stanford School of Medicine, about 50% of insulin resistance can be attributed to a person's genetic background and the other 50% is due to lifestyle. Being overweight, inactive, and smoking all increase insulin resistance. Nearly everyone with type 2 diabetes is insulin resistant. Losing weight—as little as 10 pounds—and regular physical activity increase insulin sensitivity.

You Should Know

The American Diabetes Association and the Department of Health and Human Services recommend that people 45 and older who are overweight or have other risk factors for diabetes should be tested for impaired glucose tolerance. Experts believe that when glucose intolerance is detected early, people can make lifestyle changes that could reduce their risk of developing type 2 diabetes by up to 58%.

BLOOD TESTS FOR DIABETES

There are a number of different blood tests that are used to diagnose diabetes or monitor the condition after it has been diagnosed.

You Should Know

Mg (milligrams) and dl (deciliters) are abbreviations used to measure blood sugar.

A milligram is one thousandth of a gram or ¼₀₀₀ of a teaspoon. A deciliter is one tenth of a liter, a little less than half a cup.

BLOOD SUGAR SCREENING requires only a single drop of blood from a finger prick. When the result is more than 126 mg/dl, another test, fasting blood sugar, is given.

RANDOM BLOOD SUGAR TEST is a routine part of a physical exam. Even if you have eaten recently and your blood sugar is at its peak, the level should not be more than 200 mg/dl. If it is, a fasting blood sugar test is given.

FASTING BLOOD SUGAR is done after you have fasted overnight or for at least 8 hours. Blood is drawn from a vein and sent to a lab for evaluation. If your blood sugar measures 126 mg/dl or higher, the test may be repeated. If the result of the second test is 126 mg/dl or higher, the diagnosis is diabetes. If you have pre-diabetes, 110 to 125 mg/dl, your doctor will probably recommend a fasting blood sugar test at least once a year. A normal fasting blood sugar level is 80 to 110 mg/dl. When blood sugar is higher than normal, its called hyperglycemia.

GLUCOSE TOLERANCE TEST requires that after an 8-hour fast, you drink a sugar solution. Your blood sugar is measured before you drink the liquid and then every hour for three hours. If your blood sugar level at the 2-hour point reaches between 140 and 199 mg/dl, you have pre-diabetes. If, at the 2-hour point, your blood sugar is 200 mg/dl or above, you have diabetes.

URINE TESTS showing a high sugar level indicate that you may have diabetes. This test generally is not used to diagnose diabetes. The level of blood sugar that causes sugar in your urine varies from one person to another. You could have high blood sugar without sugar in your urine.

A-1C OR GLYCATED HEMOGLOBIN is a test ordered after you've been diagnosed with diabetes. This test measures your average blood sugar level over the past 2 to 3 months. It is used to monitor your treatment. From the test your doctor finds out how high your blood sugar has been recently. It's an effective way to see how well you're managing your blood sugar. The results of the glycated hemoglobin test help determine your risk of diabetic complications. The higher the reading, the greater your risk of causing damage to other organs in the body, like your eyes or kidneys. The estimated A-1C level is 7 or less.

3

Look at Your Lifestyle Habits

The easiest way to treat type 2 diabetes, or reduce your risk of getting diabetes, is to practice positive lifestyle habits. Take the following quiz to see what changes you need to make.

PRACTICING POSITIVE HABITS

1. I am a normal weight.	YES	NO
2. I am active most days.	YES	NO
3. I usually eat fruits and vegetables.	YES	NO
4. I usually eat whole-grain breads and cereals.	YES	NO
5. I usually eat lowfat and nonfat milk, cheese, yogurt, and ice cream.	YES	NO
6. I eat red meat no more than 2 or 3 times a week.	YES	NO
7. I usually do not eat butter, margarine, salad dressing, and sour cream on most days.	YES	NO
8. I hardly ever eat candy, cookies, and cakes on most days.	YES	NO
9. I usually eat meals at regular times each day.	YES	NO
10. I hardly ever have more than one alcoholic drink a day.	YES	NO

Your goal is to answer *yes* to all the questions. The more yes answers, the easier it will be to control your diabetes.

1. How much did you weigh in your teens and twenties? If you were a normal weight then but have put on some pounds, it's time to seriously consider losing weight. Even a modest weight loss will help lower your blood sugar.

2. If you don't exercise, you should start. Exercising regularly helps control your weight and lower your blood sugar. Find an activity you enjoy—walking, cycling, bowling, dancing. Exercising with someone else can make it more fun, so ask a neighbor or friend to join you. Aim for at least 30 minutes on most days. Your health-care provider can give you advice on getting started. Exercise will help you lose weight, tone your body, help control your diabetes, and lift your spirits.

3. You probably don't eat enough fruits and vegetables. It's recommended that Americans have 5 or more servings a day, but most people eat less. Try to have fruits or vegetables with every meal. Try fresh fruit for breakfast. Raw vegetables—carrots, celery, cherry tomatoes, peppers—are colorful, tasty, low-calorie snacks. Fruits and veggies supply your body with vitamins, minerals, and fiber. They fill you up with few calories, so they won't fill you out.

4. Many people grew up eating white bread. If that describes your relationship with bread, it's time to take a closer look at the variety available. On your next shopping trip, check out different breads. Experts urge us to eat whole grains because they're full of vitamins, minerals, and fiber. Fiber and other important nutrients are lost when the grains are refined to make white bread. Bread labeled "100% whole wheat" contains only whole-wheat flour. But even bread that isn't made

with 100% whole wheat can be nutritious. Pumpernickel, rye, and cornbread are mixtures of white flour with smaller amounts of whole grains. They're healthy, too. Read the ingredients label to find breads that have whole grains. Look for 2 grams of dietary fiber or more per serving.

5. When you choose lowfat or nonfat milk, cheese, yogurt, and ice cream, you get all the vitamins and minerals in the regular variety minus the fat. Sample some of the reduced-fat and fat-free cheeses as well as the wide assortment of lowfat and nonfat yogurts and ice creams.

6. A diet high in red meat, high-fat dairy products, and refined grains increases the risk of type 2 diabetes by over 50% in men. Studies done at Harvard Medical School showed the risk of diabetes was increased even more by a diet heavy in processed meats like bacon, hot dogs, and cold cuts. Combine these food choices with too little activity and being overweight, and the risk climbs even higher. Men who eat more fruits, vegetables, whole grains, fish, and poultry are less likely to develop diabetes.

7. Foods like butter, margarine, salad dressing, and sour cream are loaded with fat and calories. If you are accustomed to spreading butter or margarine on bread, vegetables, and potatoes, you need to pay attention to the *amount* of fat calories you're eating. A tablespoon of butter or margarine adds 100 calories. Four tablespoons of sour cream add 120 calories. Four tablespoons of salad dressing add a whopping 360 calories! How should you handle these calorie-dense toppings? Measure out smaller portions—a teaspoon of butter instead of a tablespoon, 2 tablespoons of sour cream or salad dressing, not 4. Less than that is even better. When cooking,

substitute nonfat cooking spray for oil and consider using reduced-fat products.

8. If you answered "no," you're like many Americans who have a "sweet tooth" and eat an average of 53 teaspoons of sugar a day. That's over 5 times the 10 teaspoons of sugar a day that experts recommend. Though eating too much sugar is not healthy for anyone, you may be surprised to find that a person with diabetes can eat sugar. The American Diabetes Association has changed its position. You can eat moderate amounts of sugar as long as it is counted as part of the total carbohydrate content of your diet. We now know that small amounts of sugar do not raise blood sugar levels in people with type 2 diabetes. But overdoing candy, cookies, and cakes can raise your blood sugar levels and cause weight gain.

9. Try to keep the size and timing of meals and snacks consistent from day to day. This helps you keep your blood sugar from getting too high or too low. It's harder to keep your blood sugar at a healthy level if you eat a big lunch one day and a small lunch the following day.

10. Most experts agree that a moderate amount of alcohol has health benefits. When diabetes is well controlled, alcohol can be used in moderation and enjoyed along with food. Blood sugar levels will not be affected. If alcohol is taken *without* food, low blood sugar can result. Alcohol is a concentrated source of calories with no nutrients. One and a half ounces of liquor contains about 100 calories. Wine and beer contain as many, or even more, calories in a glassful. When you have a drink, alcohol calories should be substituted for fat calories in your diet. The Dietary Guidelines for Americans recommend no more than 2 drinks a day for men and no more than 1 drink

a day for women. This recommendation is good for people with diabetes, as well, but alcohol should be avoided during pregnancy or by those with a history of abuse.

SOFT DRINKS AND HARD DRINKS

Soft drinks by definition include regular carbonated soda, diet and caffeine-free soda, drinks made with juice, sports drinks, and ready-to-drink teas. Some of these beverages are sweetened; the sugar in a 12-ounce can of soda adds up to 150 calories. Diet sodas do not contain any sugar or calories. But some soft drinks do have small amounts of caffeine as a flavor enhancer, about one third of the amount found in coffee.

Hard drinks are beverages that contain alcohol—liquor, beer, or wine. Like soft drinks, these have calories that need to be counted in your total for the day. It is recommended that when you drink alcohol, have it with meals. Your blood sugar may drop too low if you drink alcohol on an empty stomach.

4

Nutrition Basics for Diabetes

The Dietary Guidelines for Americans were last updated in 2000. These guidelines answer the question, "What should Americans do and eat to stay healthy?" Current guidelines emphasize good food plus activity. The focus has been, and still is, on eating a variety of foods to supply nutrients. In the current guidelines, for the first time, the issue of food safety has been included.

The guidelines are recommended for healthy people age 2 and over. The advice is good for people with diabetes, too.

2000 U.S. DIETARY GUIDELINES

Aim for Fitness

- Aim for a healthy weight
- Be physically active each day

Build a Healthy Base

- Let the pyramid guide your food choices
- Eat a variety of grains daily, especially whole grains

- Eat a variety of fruits and vegetables daily
- Keep food safe to eat

Choose Sensibly

- Choose a diet low in saturated fat and cholesterol, and moderate in total fat
- Choose beverages and foods that limit your intake of sugars
- Choose and prepare foods with less salt
- If you drink alcoholic beverages, do so in moderation

CALORIES AND WEIGHT

Americans are getting fatter; 62% weigh too much. And more than 60% of adults aren't physically active. The surgeon general's report, "Call to Action to Prevent and Decrease Overweight and Obesity," found that more than 300,000 deaths a year are linked to being overweight. That is why you should be aware of how many calories you eat each day. You need calories for your body to function normally—breathing, digesting food, repairing damaged tissues, and walking. But too many calories lead to overweight, making it more difficult to handle your diabetes.

You get calories when you eat carbohydrates, fats, and proteins in foods. One gram (about one-quarter teaspoon) of carbohydrate or protein has 4 calories. One gram of fat has 9 calories. Alcohol contains calories, too—7 in a gram.

When you eat more calories than you need, the excess calories are turned to fat and stored for future use. This causes weight gain. When too few calories are eaten, stored fat is used for energy and weight is lost.

You may wonder how many calories you need each day. Your health care provider may have already given you guidelines. If not, it's easy to figure out. First you need to find your target weight. Then you'll figure out your target calorie zone.

Finding Your Target Weight

You probably already have a pretty good idea of what you'd like to weigh and how much you should lose to get there—10 pounds, 25 pounds, maybe even more.

What do you weigh? _____

What do you want to weigh? _____

How much do you need to lose? _____

There are a number of ways to find your target weight. How much did you weigh in your early twenties? If you were a good weight then, that's probably a good weight to maintain throughout your adult life.

Another way to "guesstimate" your target weight is an easy-to-use formula based on your height.

FOR WOMEN: Give yourself 100 pounds for the first 5 feet of your height and add 5 pounds for each additional inch (or subtract 5 pounds for each inch under 5 feet).

For example, if you're 5 feet, 4 inches tall:

100 pounds (for the first 5 feet)
+20 pounds (5 pounds for every inch over 5 feet;
$5 \times 4 = 20$)
120 pounds is a desirable weight

Your target weight is _____

FOR MEN: Give yourself 106 pounds for the first 5 feet of your height and add 6 pounds for each additional inch over 5 feet.

For example, if you're 5 feet, 10 inches tall:

106 pounds (for the first 5 feet)
+60 pounds (6 pounds for every inch over 5 feet;
$\qquad$ $6 \times 10 = 60$)
166 pounds is a desirable weight

Your target weight is: _____

If your target weight and your current weight are very far apart, here is another approach to weight loss: consider a compromise. For example, if your current weight is 200 pounds and your target weight is 150 pounds, make your initial goal 175 to 180 pounds. Any weight loss, even small, makes a positive impact on your diabetes and overall health.

Finding Your Target Calorie Zone

Once you know your target weight, you can find out how many calories you need each day to reach that weight. That's easy to do by following the 2 simple steps below.

1. *Select the calorie factor that best describes you.*

   20 = Very active men
   15 = Moderately active men or very active women
   13 = Inactive men, moderately active women, and all
   people over age 55
   10 = Inactive women, repeat dieters, seriously overweight people

2. *Find your target calorie zone.*

the target weight × calorie factor = your target calorie zone

Your target calorie zone is _____.

For example, if your target weight is 130 pounds and you are a moderately active woman (factor 13), your target calorie zone would be 1600 to 1700 calories a day:

130 pounds (target weight) × 13 (moderately active woman)
= 1690 calories a day

In addition to watching calories, when you have type 2 diabetes, you should track the amount of carbohydrates you eat each day. On the chart "Calories and Carbohydrates Daily," below, find your target calorie zone in the left column. In the right column, find your target carbohydrate amount to eat each day. For example, if you should eat 1800 calories a day, you should also have 225 to 270 grams of carbohydrates a day. The amount of carbohydrates listed on the chart is the daily recommendation of the American Diabetes Association.

CALORIES AND CARBOHYDRATES DAILY

Calories	Carbohydrate grams
1200	150–180
1300	100–195
1400	175–210
1500	190–225
1600	200–240
1700	215–255
1800	225–270
1900	240–285
2000	250–300
2100	265–315
2200	275–330
2300	290–345
2400	300–360
2500	315–375
2600	325–390
2700	340–405

CARBOHYDRATES

Carbohydrates include sugars, starches, and fiber. The sugars and starches are broken down and converted into energy for the body to use. Unused carbohydrates are stored as fat. Fiber cannot be digested and is not used by the body for energy.

Americans get about 55 to 60% of their calories from carbohydrates. People with type 2 diabetes particularly benefit from diets high in carbohydrates. These foods help maintain normal blood sugar levels.

Starch, which is the way energy is stored in plants, is a large sugar complex made up of many simple sugars. Wheat, corn, rice, potatoes, and beans are sources of starch. The starch in foods is broken down into glucose before it is absorbed into cells.

In the past, people with diabetes were told not to eat sugar. That's no longer true. Small amounts of sugar and sweet foods are okay when eaten with other foods, but they need to be counted as part of your total carbohydrates for the day. Fructose is a simple sugar found in fruit. Table sugar is a combination of two simple sugars, glucose and fructose. Most sweeteners—corn syrup, honey, maple syrup—are combinations of simple sugars

The grapefruit and toast you have for breakfast are part of the carbohydrates you need for the day. So is the sugar you put in your coffee. It's best to get your carbohydrates from fruits, vegetables, breads, and cereals. They give you vitamins, minerals, and fiber too. Sugar, jelly, and syrup do not.

Your health care provider may have told you how many grams of carbohydrate to eat each day. If not, see the chart "Calories and Carbohydrates Daily," page 21. When you have diabetes, it's important to count your carbohydrates daily. The total amount of carbohydrates you eat each day is more important than the type you eat.

Fiber

Fiber is the type of carbohydrate that cannot be digested. It's found in foods like whole-wheat bread, beans, fruits, and vegetables. Fiber comes from different parts of plants:

leaves like spinach   roots like carrots
stems like celery   seeds like sunflower
flowers like broccoli   grains like whole wheat
tubers like potatoes

People with diabetes should eat more fiber. Experts recommend 20 to 35 grams of fiber a day, but most Americans eat only 14 grams. Research has shown that fiber is important in the diabetic diet:

- It keeps blood sugar levels from rising quickly after eating
- It helps decrease triglycerides and cholesterol in the blood
- It is bulky, increasing fullness; this helps weight loss

People often experience bloating, diarrhea, and gas when they eat too much fiber too quickly. Gradually increase the amount of high-fiber foods you eat, to give your body time to adjust. Going slowly prevents many of the uncomfortable side effects. When you add high-fiber foods to your diet, be sure to drink plenty of liquids. Constipation can happen when fiber is increased and fluids are not increased at the same time.

ADDING FIBER TO YOUR DIET

- Choose a variety of:
  Whole-grain breads and cereals
  Unpeeled fruits and vegetables
  Dried peas, beans, lentils, and barley
  Start with 1 or 2 servings a day and gradually add more

- Drink 8 to 10 glasses of liquid daily.
- Fiber supplements are not necessary. It's healthier to get your fiber from food.

You Should Know

According to a recent study, eating whole-grain breads and cereals helps reduce the risk of type 2 diabetes and heart disease in overweight adults.

Sugar Substitutes

Sugar substitutes can be used to add sweetness to foods without adding sugar or calories. For all nonnutritive sweeteners, the Food and Drug Administration (FDA) sets an acceptable intake, which is the amount of a sweetener that can be safely eaten daily over a person's lifetime. The FDA has approved 4 calorie-free sweeteners for use in the United States. Each sweetener has a distinctive taste and advantages.

CHEMICAL NAME	BRAND NAMES
saccharin	*Sweet 'n Low, Sugar Twin*
aspartame	*NutraSweet, Equal*
acesulfame K	*Sweet One, Sunette*
sucralose	*Splenda*
neotame	

Because these sugar substitutes are calorie free, they do not need to be counted as part of your calorie or carbohydrate intake for the day.

Polyols are sugar substitutes that have fewer calories than sugar. They have been in use for many years. Mannitol, sorbitol, and xylitol are polyols that are used to replace some or all of the sugar in chewing gum, candy, ice cream, cookies, mouthwashes, and cough syrups. You'll see them on the food labels of sugar-free or reduced-sugar foods. Polyols do not raise blood sugar levels when used in small amounts, but eating large amounts can cause blood sugar to rise and also cause gas and diarrhea. The calories in these sugar substitutes need to be counted as part of your total carbohydrates for the day.

PROTEIN

Protein is part of every cell in the body. It provides the raw material to build the body's tissues. It can also be used for energy when there is not enough energy available from carbohydrates and fat.

Americans eat a lot of protein; most eat more than they need. One problem with this excess is that animal proteins, like steak and cheese, also have a lot of fat. Diets for people with diabetes are usually planned to have 15 to 20% of total calories from protein. Rely on lean protein choices, lowfat cheese and milk, and try to include more vegetable proteins, like beans and soy foods.

FOODS HIGH IN PROTEIN

Cheese	Meat	Seeds
Dried peas & beans	Milk	Soy
Eggs	Nuts	Tofu
Fish	Peanut butter	Veggie burger
Lentils	Poultry	

FAT

Americans eat too much fat. It supplies about 35% of all the calories we eat each day. Fat is a concentrated source of calories; weight for weight, it has more than twice as many calories as carbohydrates or protein. That's why eating a lot of fat can make you fat.

A small amount of fat is needed for good health. Besides calories, fat provides essential fatty acids, which the body can't make. It insulates the body, helping it stay at a constant temperature. Fat protects vital organs, like the kidneys, which are covered with fat. It carries fat-soluble vitamins (A, D, E, and K) into the body. Fat is part of the membranes surrounding every cell. And, just as important, a small amount makes foods taste good.

While it's true we need some fat, too much is unhealthy. High-fat diets raise the levels of fat in the blood, increasing the risk for heart disease and stroke. People with diabetes are at greater risk for heart disease, so lowfat diets should be a priority.

Most of the fats in foods and in the body are triglycerides, which are made up of different fatty acids. Depending on their structure, the fatty acids are either *monounsaturated, polyunsaturated,* or *saturated.*

Monounsaturated fats can lower blood cholesterol when they are used in place of saturated fats. "Monos" lower the "bad" form of cholesterol (LDLs) and do not reduce the good form of cholesterol (HDLs). That's why it is recommended that one third of your daily fat come from foods high in monounsaturated fat. For people with type 2 diabetes, replacing some carbohydrates with monounsaturated fats can help them lose weight and better control their diabetes. Your health care provider may have already recommended some of the following foods to you.

FOODS HIGH IN MONOUNSATURATED FATS

Almonds	Macadamia nuts	Pine nuts (pignolia)
Canola oil	Olive oil	Pistachio nuts
Cashews	Olives	Sesame oil
Chicken fat	Peanut butter	Soybean oil
Filberts	Peanut oil	Soybean oil margarine
Hazelnuts	Peanuts	

Nuts are rich in monounsaturated oil, similar to heart-healthy olive oil. Research has shown that eating moderate amounts of nuts could reduce your risk for heart disease. Nuts are great snacks, but many calories come packaged in a small serving.

MEASURE, DON'T GRAB

Nuts	Calories in 1/4 cup
Almonds	170
Cashews	170
Peanuts	170
Pine nuts	140
Pistachios	160
Walnuts	170

Polyunsaturated fats may help lower your cholesterol, but too much may not be good. Fish contains polyunsaturated fats called *omega-3 fatty acids* or fish oils. These oils are found in fatty, cold-water fish like salmon. Studies have shown that fish oils may reduce the risk for heart disease and high blood pressure.

FOODS HIGH IN POLYUNSATURATED FATS

Bluefish*	Safflower oil	Tub margarine
Corn oil	Salad dressing	Tuna
Cottonseed oil	Salmon*	Vegetable oil
Herring*	Sardines*	Walnut oil
Mackerel*	Sesame oil	Walnuts
Mayonnaise	Soybean oil	Wheat germ
Rainbow trout*	Squid*	Whitefish*
Sablefish	Sunflower oil	

*High in omega-3 fatty acids, fish oil.

Saturated fat is in animal foods: meat, chicken, milk, cheese, and butter. But some vegetable foods—cocoa butter and coconut, palm and palm kernel oils—are high in saturated fat, too. When vegetable oils, like corn oil, are hardened (hydrogenated) to make margarine, they become more saturated. Some but not all saturated fats raise cholesterol.

Experts recommend eating less than 7% of your fat calories as saturated fat each day. Foods high in saturated fat are often high in total fat, too. By eating less saturated fat, you'll benefit twice—you reduce saturated fat and total fat.

FOODS HIGH IN SATURATED FATS

Beef	Cream cheese	Palm oil
Butter	Deli meats	Pork
Cheese	Duck	Sausage
Chicken (skin, dark meat)	Half & half	Sour cream
Chocolate	Hot dogs	Veal
Coconut	Ice cream	Whipped cream
Coconut oil	Lamb	Whole milk
Cream	Palm kernel oil	

A Word About Cholesterol

Cholesterol is needed in the body. Hormones, nerve coverings, vitamin D, bile, and the substance that keeps your skin soft are all made from cholesterol. When the amount in the body gets too high, however, cholesterol increases your risk for heart disease.

All animal foods—meat, poultry, fish, eggs, yogurt, cheese, milk, and butter—contain cholesterol. There's no cholesterol in plant foods like fruits, vegetables, grains, beans, peanut butter, and nuts. It's recommended that healthy adults eat no more than 200 milligrams of cholesterol a day.

VITAMINS AND MINERALS

Vitamins help regulate body functions. You can't live without them because they help turn the food you eat into energy. They also help the body work normally and make new tissues. Though their jobs are important, you need very little of any given vitamin to get the work done. You get most of your vitamins from food, although a very small amount of some vitamins are made in the body.

Minerals, like vitamins, act as regulators in the body and have no calories. They become part of your body, like calcium in bones, or they float in body fluids, like blood and tears. They are needed in even smaller amounts than vitamins and you get all of them from food. Minerals are not made in the body.

Taking too many minerals and vitamins can cause trouble. Overloads of some can be excreted by your body, but the excess of others is stored and can cause damage. It's rare to get too much of a vitamin or mineral in food, but it is easy to take too much as a supplement. People on low-calorie diets and those who eat too few fruits and vegetables may not get all the vitamins and minerals they need from food. Taking a daily multi-vitamin/mineral supplement is a good idea. Select one with no more than 100% of the RDA (Recommended Daily Allowance). You can find this out by reading the label.

5

Individualizing Your Eating Plan

The American Diabetes Association (ADA), in January 2002, released new guidelines for people with diabetes. For the first time, the guidelines included information on weight control and exercise. The new approach to handling and preventing diabetes is to:

> Lose weight, if overweight
> Become more active
> Eat a healthy diet

The ADA also recommended that people with diabetes see a health care provider, a registered dietitian (RD), or a certified diabetes educator (CDE). These professionals can help you individualize your lifestyle changes, taking into consideration:

> Your life's circumstances
> Your culture
> Your heritage
> Your food likes and dislikes
> Your ability to make changes

HEALTHY RECOMMENDATIONS FOR DIABETES

Carbohydrates

- Include whole-grain breads and cereals, fruits and vegetables, and lowfat milk in your daily meals and snacks
- It's important to keep track of the total amount of carbohydrates you eat each day
     Carbohydrate calories should equal 50 to 60% of your daily calorie intake
     Carbohydrate foods should be eaten at every meal and snack
- It's less important to keep track of the type of carbohydrate you eat
- It's okay to use small amounts of low-calorie and no-calorie sweeteners
- It's okay to eat sugar and foods containing sugar if you:
     Eat small amounts
     Count the sugar and sugary foods you eat as part of your day's total carbohydrate Intake
     Eat sweets with other foods

Fat

- A reduced-fat eating plan will help you lose weight, and it improves blood fat values (LDLs, HDLs, cholesterol)
- It is helpful to keep track of the fat you eat each day
     Fat calories should equal 30 to 35% of your total calories each day
     Eat more of the foods that contain monounsaturated fat (olive oil, canola oil, nuts)
     Use moderate amounts of foods that contain polyunsaturated fat (margarine, corn oil, vegetable oil, salad dressing)
     Eat less of the foods that contain saturated fat (meat, whole milk, butter, cheese)

Being Active

- Build activity into every day
  Aim to be active for 30 minutes each day; you can accumulate this in short periods (10 or more minutes) throughout the day
- Weight loss is easier if you are active every day—try walking

Taking Care of Your Family

- Other members of your family may be at risk for type 2 diabetes
  Encourage regular medical checkups
  Encourage daily activity
  If overweight, encourage weight loss
  Select whole-grain breads and cereals, vegetables and fruits, lowfat milk
  Select moderate to lowfat meals and snacks
  Eat well but don't overeat

GETTING STARTED

Regular Serving Sizes

The easiest way to keep meals a normal size is to eat regular serving sizes. Often the amount of food you make at home or are served in restaurants is too much. A recent government survey showed that the usual restaurant serving of potatoes is 2½ times larger than a standard serving, and a pasta serving is up to 4 times the standard amount.

Use measuring cups, measuring spoons, or a kitchen scale to get familiar with regular serving sizes of different foods. To get you started, use the following table, "What Is a Serving?"

WHAT IS A SERVING?

FOOD	SERVING SIZE
Breads, Cereals, High-Carb Foods	
bread	1 slice
cereal	½ cup cooked
	¾ cup ready-to-eat
rice, cooked	⅓ cup
green peas, cooked	½ cup
dried beans, cooked	½ cup
potato	1 small
pasta, cooked	1 cup
Vegetables and Fruits	
raw or cooked vegetables	½ cup
raw or cooked leafy greens	1 cup
raw fruit	1 small
dried fruit	2 tablespoons
canned fruit	½ cup
juice	½ cup
Milk, Yogurt, Cheese	
nonfat or lowfat milk	1 cup
nonfat or lowfat yogurt*	1 cup
cheese	1 ounce or 1 slice
cottage cheese	½ cup
Meat, Poultry, Fish	
cooked	3–4 ounces
egg, cooked	1
Fats	
butter or margarine	1 teaspoon
cream cheese	2 tablespoons
salad dressing	2 tablespoons
oil	1 tablespoon
Sugar	
sugar	1 teaspoon
honey	1 teaspoon
syrup	2 tablespoons

*Flavored and fruit yogurts are often high in calories, sugar, and carbohydrate. Check the labels of your favorites.

Meal Planning

At first, the idea of planning all of your meals and snacks can seem overwhelming. Relax; it isn't that hard. Start slowly. Become accustomed to regular serving sizes and stick with these as often as you can. Next, work on spacing meals and snacks at regular intervals throughout each day. Then work on making the best selections each time you eat. Finally, if you need to be even more careful, you can count calories and carbohydrates. Not all people with type 2 diabetes count calories and carbohydrates. Your health care provider will help you determine the right approach for you.

Meal Planning Hints

Do: Eat regular meals; aim for the same amount of food at about the same time each day
Choose regular serving sizes of all foods
Eat moderate-size meals
Choose foods with carbohydrate and fiber at each meal and each snack
Choose foods low in fat
Bring food with you so that you don't miss a meal or snack

Go easy: On foods containing sugar
On foods containing saturated fat
On alcohol

Don't: Skip meals or snacks
Overeat

Counting Calories

If you need to lose weight or if you're having trouble sticking with a certain amount of food each day, your health care provider may recommend that you count calories. Your overall health and diabetes control will benefit from calorie counting because you'll be able to drop pounds and lower your blood sugar. On page 20, you found your target calorie zone. Use this as a guide.

You Should Know

Don't forget to count sugar. 1 teaspoon sugar = 4 grams carbohydrate

---

Counting Carbohydrates

Foods containing carbohydrates—breads, cereals, vegetables, fruits, lowfat dairy foods—are important to your healthy eating plan. When you have type 2 diabetes, you may need to count carbohydrates. Your health care provider will give you a daily carbohydrate recommendation or you can use the table "Calories and Carbohydrates Daily," page 21, Next, you will learn how many carbohydrate servings to choose at meals and snacks. The following suggestions may be helpful to get you started:

Women: 2 to 3 carbohydrate choices a meal

Men: 3 to 4 carbohydrate choices a meal

Snacks: 1 or more carbohydrate choices a snack

Keep records: Count carbs and calories daily, until you are familiar with the amounts you should be eating each day

> ### One Carbohydrate Choice = 15 grams carbohydrate
>
> | | |
> |---|---|
> | 1 slice bread | ½ cup cooked cereal |
> | ⅓ cup cooked rice | 1 cup milk |
> | 1 small fruit | ½ cup green peas |
> | ½ cup potato | ½ cup corn |

Timing Meals and Snacks

You should try to eat your meals and snacks at the same time each day. This timing helps your body deal with carbs and keeps your blood sugar normal.

Meals: Eat 3 meals at about the same time each day

Snacks: Eat a mid-afternoon and evening snack each day
Eat a midmorning snack when breakfast and lunch are spaced far apart

Choose a wide variety of foods for your meals and snacks. This ensures that you'll get a good complement of vitamins, minerals, and fiber, as well as enjoy tasty and interesting meals. A healthy day's meal plan should include:

SERVINGS PER DAY	FOODS
2 servings	lowfat milk
5 or more servings	fruits and vegetables
2 servings	meat, fish, poultry, or vegetable proteins
___ servings	carbohydrates (as directed by your health care provider

Dividing Calories and Carbs

It is not easy to plan a day's worth of meals that meet an exact number of calories and carbs. Your health care provider will tell you how may calories and carbs to eat each day and then will help you begin to plan menus.

The following table, "Calories and Carbs Divided Throughout the Day," can be used as a guide. Try to come as close as possible to the carb and calorie goals for each meal and snack. You may not be able to hit the goals exactly, but come as close as you can.

For example, if you've been told to eat 1800 calories a day, find the column headed 1800 at the top of the chart. Follow that column down, and you'll find the calorie and carb goals for each meal and snack throughout the day.

CALORIES AND CARBS DIVIDED THROUGHOUT THE DAY

Calories per Day	1200	1300	1400	1500	1600
Breakfast					
Calories	250	300	300	325	350
Carbs	34	41	41	45	48
Snack					
Calories	—	—	—	—	—
Carbs	—	—	—	—	—
Lunch					
Calories	350	350	400	425	450
Carbs	48	48	55	58	62
Snack					
Calories	100	100	100	100	100
Carbs	14	14	14	14	14
Dinner					
Calories	400	450	500	550	600
Carbs	55	62	69	76	82
Snack					
Calories	100	100	100	100	100
Carbs	14	14	14	14	14

(continued)

CALORIES AND CARBS DIVIDED THROUGHOUT THE DAY (cont.)

Calories per Day	1700	1800	1900	2000	2100
Breakfast					
Calories	400	400	400	450	450
Carbs	55	55	55	62	62
Snack					
Calories	—	—	—	—	—
Carbs	—	—	—	—	—
Lunch					
Calories	450	500	550	600	600
Carbs	62	69	76	82	82
Snack					
Calories	100	100	100	125	125
Carbs	14	14	14	17	17
Dinner					
Calories	650	700	750	750	800
Carbs	89	96	103	103	110
Snack					
Calories	100	100	100	125	125
Carbs	14	14	14	17	17

Following are examples of a typical day's eating plan at two different calorie levels, 1800 and 1200.

1800 CALORIE MEAL PLAN

The 1800 calorie level is a weight maintenance eating plan for some women and most men with type 2 diabetes. You'll notice that the actual carbohydrates and calories for each meal and snack may not always meet the goal. The carbohydrate goal is the most important, because that helps to keep your blood sugar normal throughout the day. Some foods have only a trace of carbohydrate. This value does not need to be counted.

CALORIES AND CARBS DIVIDED THROUGHOUT THE DAY (cont.)

Calories per Day	2200	2300	2400	2500	2600	2700
Breakfast						
Calories	450	500	500	500	500	500
Carbs	62	69	69	69	69	69
Snack						
Calories	—	—	100	150	150	150
Carbs	—	—	14	21	21	21
Lunch						
Calories	650	650	650	650	650	700
Carbs	89	89	89	89	89	96
Snack						
Calories	150	150	150	150	150	200
Carbs	21	21	21	21	21	28
Dinner						
Calories	800	850	850	900	950	950
Carbs	110	117	117	124	131	131
Snack						
Calories	150	150	150	150	200	200
Carbs	21	21	21	21	28	28

Many of you may not keep such detailed records of the foods you eat. But once in a while, you should keep track of one day to see how you're doing.

DIABETIC MEAL PLAN WORKSHEET
SAMPLE 1800 CALORIE MEAL PLAN
CARBOHYDRATES: 225–270 GRAMS

FOOD	PORTION	CALORIES	CARBS
Breakfast Goals		**400**	**55**
Pink grapefruit sections	1 cup	69	18
Cottage cheese, 2%	½ cup	101	4
Bran flakes	¾ cup	90	22
Nonfat milk	1 cup	86	12
Coffee + sugar substitute	as desired	0	0
Breakfast Subtotals		**346**	**56**
Morning Snack Goals		—	—
(this snack is usually not included on 1800 calorie meal plan)			
Morning Snack Subtotals		—	—
Lunch Goals		**500**	**69**
Tuna salad	½ cup	192	10
Rye bread	2 slices	130	24
Swiss cheese	1 ounce	107	1
Tomato, sliced	1 medium	24	5
Lettuce	1 leaf	3	tr
Diet cola	1 can	0	0
Lunch Subtotals		**561**	**67**
Afternoon Snack Goals		**100**	**14**
Graham crackers	3 squares	90	15
Tea + sugar substitute	as desired	0	0
Afternoon Snack Subtotals		**90**	**15**
Dinner Goals		**700**	**96**
Roast chicken w/skin	½ breast	142	0
Baked potato w/ skin	1 medium	220	51
Cracked pepper	sprinkle	0	0
Butter	1 tablespoon	108	tr

FOOD	PORTION	CALORIES	CARBS
Dinner Goals (cont.)			
Broccoli, cooked	1 cup	46	8
Orange sherbet	¾ cup	180	39
Sparkling water	as desired	0	0
Dinner Subtotals		**696**	**98**
Evening Snack Goals		**100**	**14**
Nonfat milk	1 cup	86	12
Evening Snack Subtotals		**86**	**12**
Day's Totals		**1779**	**248**

1200 CALORIE MEAL PLAN

A 1200 calorie eating plan is usually used to speed up initial weight loss. Because food is limited, it's best to stay at this calorie level for one month only. You'll be rewarded by a quick weight loss and then you can add more calories to your meal plan.

DIABETIC MEAL PLAN WORKSHEET
SAMPLE 1200 CALORIE MEAL PLAN
CARBOHYDRATES: 150–180 GRAMS

FOOD	PORTION	CALORIES	CARBS
Breakfast Goals		**250**	**34**
Pink grapefruit sections	½ cup	35	9
Whole wheat toast	1 slice	70	13
Margarine	2 teaspoons	68	0
Nonfat milk	1 cup	86	12
Coffee + sugar substitute	as desired	0	0
Breakfast Subtotals		**259**	**34**

(continued)

DIABETIC MEAL PLAN WORKSHEET
SAMPLE 1200 CALORIE MEAL PLAN
CARBOHYDRATES: 150–180 GRAMS

FOOD	PORTION	CALORIES	CARBS
Morning Snack Goals		—	—
(this snack is usually not included on a 1200 calorie eating plan)			
Morning Snack Subtotals		—	—
Lunch Goals		**350**	**48**
Turkey breast	4 slices	92	0
Rye bread	2 slices	130	24
Reduced-calorie mayonnaise	1 tablespoon	34	2
Lettuce	1 leaf	3	tr
Grapes	20	72	18
Diet cola	1 can	0	0
Lunch Subtotals		**331**	**44**
Afternoon Snack Goals		**100**	**14**
Graham crackers	3 squares	90	15
Tea + sugar substitute	as desired	0	0
Afternoon Snack Subtotals		**90**	**15**
Dinner Goals		**400**	**55**
Flounder, broiled	4 ounces	132	0
Peas, cooked	½ cup	59	11
Corn on the cob	1 ear	83	19
Margarine	1 teaspoon	34	0
Cantaloupe, cubed	1 cup	57	13
Nonfat milk	1 cup	86	12
Dinner Subtotals		**451**	**55**
Evening Snack Goals		**100**	**14**
Popcorn, air popped	3 cups	90	18
Evening Snack Subtotals		**90**	**18**
Day's Totals		**1221**	**166**

YOUR MEAL PLAN

Following is a blank worksheet that you can use to set up your day's eating plan. What is your daily calorie target? Find that on the table "Calories and Carbs Divided Throughout the Day," on page 37. Next, write in your carb goals for each meal and snack on the worksheet. Now you are ready to plan your meals and snacks for the day by listing the food, portion, calories, and carbs on the worksheet. Add up the subtotals for each meal and snack. Do they meet the goals for each meal and snack? Finally, add up all the subtotals for the entire day to see if they match the total calorie and carb goals for your eating plan.

Another way to use the worksheet is simply to keep track of the amount of calories and carbs you eat at each meal and snack on any given day and then check your daily totals against the recommendations on the table, page 21. This method is simply a check to see how you're doing. Everyone with type 2 diabetes should do this once in a while. Meeting daily calorie and carb goals is the key to controlling type 2 diabetes, and helps protect you from complications.

DIABETIC MEAL PLAN WORKSHEET
_____ CALORIE EATING PLAN
_____ CARBOHYDRATES GRAMS

FOOD	PORTION	CALORIES	CARBS
Breakfast Goals		_____	____
Breakfast Subtotals		_____	____
Morning Snack Goals		_____	____
Morning Snack Subtotals		_____	____
Lunch Goals		_____	____
Lunch Subtotals		_____	____
Afternoon Snack Goals		_____	____
Afternoon Snack Subtotals		_____	____

FOOD	PORTION	CALORIES	CARBS
Dinner Goals		_____	____
Dinner Subtotals		_____	____
Evening Snack Goals		_____	____
Evening Snack Subtotals		_____	____
Day's Totals		_____	____

6

When You Want to Know More

How can I enjoy eating out and still eat healthy?

You can enjoy eating out and still balance your restaurant meals with the rest of your food choices for the day. Plan to dine out at approximately the same time as your usual meals. If that's not possible, check your blood sugar more often and carry along a small snack to prevent a drop in your blood sugar.

Read the restaurant menu thoroughly so you can match your food choices and portion sizes to your usual meal plan. If the portion sizes you receive are larger than what you would normally eat, ask the waitperson to pack up part of your food to take home for another meal. You may find that an appetizer, instead of a main dish, is just the right amount. You can use the listings of more than 450 take-out foods found in Part 2 to estimate the calorie and carbohydrate values of the menu items you ordered.

Remember to ask questions about how the restaurant prepares the food. Grilled or broiled foods have fewer calories and less fat than fried foods. Ask that dressings, gravies, and sauces be served on the side. Choose baked potatoes instead of fried, top with cracked pepper or salsa instead of butter, and order fresh fruit for dessert. After you've selected a choice from the bread basket, ask that the bread be removed from the table, so you don't overdo carbs.

At a party where there's lots of food, you can avoid overeating by having a snack before you go. A banana or crackers and cheese can take the edge off your appetite. If you do eat too much, adjust your food choices at your next meal.

I'm a vegetarian; how will that affect my diabetes?
Changing to a diet based on more plant foods has advantages for people with diabetes. Vegetarian diets are naturally high in carbohydrates, and diets high in carbohydrates increase insulin sensitivity. If you eat eggs, milk, and cheese, your diet will be similar to any other diabetic meal plan, minus meat, fish, and poultry. If you exclude dairy choices, you'll need to rely on vegetable proteins, like tofu, seitan, and soy milk, which offer a good amount of protein with a small amount of carbohydrate. Eating more fruits, vegetables, leafy greens, whole wheat, nuts, seeds, and beans is a healthy diet for both vegetarians and people with diabetes.

My doctor wants me to exercise regularly; why?
Regular exercise helps control blood sugar. A study of type 2 diabetes found that subjects who had low levels of fitness and were physically inactive had higher death rates than those who were active and fit. Researchers from this study recommended that doctors encourage all their patients with type 2 diabetes to become more active. Another study found that people with diabetes who included strength training as part of their regular exercise program achieved better control of their blood sugar. Weight training builds muscle, and active muscle uses up to 80% of the glucose circulating in the blood. And, just as important, regular exercise is an excellent way to help you lose weight or maintain your target weight.

Does eating too much sugar cause diabetes?

No, it does not, but eating large amounts of sugar can cause an abnormally high rise in blood sugar. For many years, people with diabetes were told to avoid sugar. It was assumed that candy and other sweets would raise blood sugar faster and higher than fruits, vegetables, and milk, all of which contain natural sugars. Many studies have shown there is no difference in blood sugar response between natural sugars and sugars added to food.

People with diabetes can eat any food, in moderation, that is part of a carefully planned diet. All carbohydrates, including sugar, affect blood sugar the same way. Eat sweets with other foods and count them as carbohydrates. The total amount of carbohydrates you eat, not their source, is what affects blood sugar.

While there's no problem eating sugar and foods containing sugar in moderate amounts, large amounts can increase blood sugar and cause you to gain weight. Cookies, candy, cake, ice cream, and soda have few vitamins and minerals, but most are loaded with calories. Stick with snack-size versions whenever available, and don't eat these foods between meals. In Part 2, you'll find sugar values listed for many foods. You don't need to count sugar, because you are already counting carbohydrates, but these values will alert you to those foods that are very high in sugar.

Can taking magnesium help control my diabetes?

Researchers are currently exploring magnesium's role in insulin resistance. But at this time, the American Diabetes Association still does not advise magnesium supplements for people with diabetes. Magnesium is found in many foods: whole grains, spinach, potatoes, almonds, beans, tofu, and seafood. Even chocolate and tap water can be sources.

What does my diabetes medicine do?

For many people with type 2 diabetes, changing your diet and adding regular exercise may be enough to control your condition. For others, medication may be needed. There are now several types of medications that can be used to treat high blood sugar. Your doctor will prescribe the one that is best for you.

Sulfonylureas (Diabinese, Glucotrol) and meglitinides (Prandin) help the pancreas release insulin.

Biguanides (Glucophage) and thiazolidinediones (Actos, Avandia) decrease insulin resistance.

Alpha glucosidase inhibitors (Precose, Glyset) slow down absorption of sugar into the blood stream.

These drugs can also be combined to improve blood glucose control, so you may be taking more than one. It has been estimated that 40 to 60% of people with type 2 diabetes will, at some point, need insulin to control blood sugar levels. Some experts disagree with this estimate and believe the need for insulin can be forestalled by those who carefully manage their diabetes.

Why is it important to control my diabetes?

If you have type 2 diabetes, it can cause some problems after you've had the disease for many years. These complications can affect your eyes, kidneys, nerves, and blood vessels. Problems are more likely if your diabetes hasn't been well controlled. Keeping blood sugar as close to normal as possible will reduce your risks of long-term complications. Even though we understand that some of the long-term consequences of diabetes can be minimized with good control, only one third of people with diabetes self-monitor their blood sugar.

Where can I get more information about diabetes?

There are a number of reliable resources that offer information to people with diabetes.

The American Diabetes Association
National Service Center
1701 North Beauregard Street
Alexandria, VA 22311
1-800-DIABETES (1-800-342-2383)
www.diabetes.org

National Diabetes Information Clearinghouse (NDIC)
1 Information Way
Bethesda, MD 20892-3560
1-800-860-8747
www.niddk.nih.gov/health/diabetes/diabetes.htm

National Diabetes Education Program (NDEP)
31 Center Drive, Building 31, Room 9A04
Bethesda, MD 20892
1-800-438-5383
www.ndep.nih.gov

Diabetes Action Resource and Education Foundation
426 C Street, NE
Washington, DC 20002
202-333-4520
www.diabetesaction.org

Diabetes Exercise and Sports Association (DESA)
1647 West Bethany Home Road, #B
Phoenix, AZ 85015
1-800-898-4322
www.diabetes-exercise.org

Canadian Diabetes Association (CDA)
National Office
15 Toronto, ON M5C 2E3
Canada
1-800-226-8464
www.diabetes.ca

International Diabetes Institute (IDI)
260 Kooyoung Road
Victoria 3162
Australia
061-03-9258-5050
www.diabetes.com.au *or* www.diabetes.org.au

7

Using the Counter Section of *The Diabetes Carbohydrate and Calorie Counter*

The Diabetes Carbohydrate and Calorie Counter lists the calorie, carbohydrate, sugar, and fat content of more than 10,000 foods. Now you can check and compare the values in your favorite foods and, when necessary, choose substitutes before you go out to shop or eat. This will help you make the right choices when you are deciding what to buy.

The counter section of the book is divided into two parts: Part 1: Brand-Name, Nonbranded, and Take-Out Foods; and Part 2: Restaurant Chains.

In Part 1, all foods are listed alphabetically, from ABALONE to ZUCCHINI. For each category, you will first find nonbranded (generic) foods listed in alphabetical order, followed by an alphabetical listing of brand-name foods. The nonbranded listing will help you determine calorie, carbohydrate, sugar, and fat values for foods when you aren't able to find your favorite brand. They will also help you to evaluate store brands. Large categories are often divided into subcategories such as canned, fresh, frozen, and ready-to-eat, to make it easier to find what you're looking for.

Because we all eat out so often, there are more than 450 take-out foods listed in Part 1. These are found in the take-out subcategory in many categories throughout this section of the book. Look there for foods you take out or order in, because these choices are not nutrition labeled.

In some cases, foods are grouped by category. For example, chow mein is found under the category ASIAN FOOD. Group categories include:

Asian Food   Page 61
    includes all types of Asian foods
    except egg rolls and sushi, which
    are found in separate categories

Deli Meats/Cold Cuts   Page 178
    includes all sandwich meats
    except chicken, ham, and turkey,
    which are found in separate
    categories

Dinner   Page 180
    Includes all by brand name

Liquor/Liqueur   Page 247
    includes all alcoholic beverages
    except beer, champagne, and
    wine, which are found in separate
    categories

Nutrition Supplements   Page 270
    includes all meal replacers and
    diet drinks, except energy bars,
    energy drinks, and sports drinks,
    which are found in separate
    categories

In Part 2, Restaurant Chains, there are 59 national and
regional restaurant, doughnut, ice cream, candy, and coffee
chains listed.

DEFINITIONS

as prep (as prepared): refers to food that has been prepared
according to package directions

lean and fat: describes meat with some fat on its edges that
is not cut away before cooking, or poultry prepared with
skin and fat as purchased

lean only: refers to lean meat that is trimmed of all visible fat,
or poultry without skin

shelf stable: refers to prepared products found on the super-
market shelf that are ready-to-eat or are to be heated and
do not require refrigeration

take-out: describes prepared dishes that you purchase ready-
to-eat; those included serve as a guide to the calorie, carbohydrate, sugar, and fat values of similar products you
may purchase

ABBREVIATIONS

avg	=	average
diam	=	diameter
fl	=	fluid
frzn	=	frozen
g	=	gram
in	=	inch
lb	=	pound
lg	=	large
med	=	medium
mg	=	milligram
oz	=	ounce
pkg	=	package
pt	=	pint
prep	=	prepared
qt	=	quart
reg	=	regular
sec	=	second
serv	=	serving
sm	=	small
sq	=	square
tbsp	=	tablespoon
tr	=	trace
tsp	=	teaspoon
w/	=	with
w/o	=	without
<	=	less than

NOTES

Carb = Carbohydrate.

All carbohydrate, sugar, and fat values are given in grams (g).

tr (trace) = less than 1 gram of carbohydrate, sugar, or fat.

— means values are not available.

Discrepancies in figures are due to rounding, product reformulation, and reevaluation. Labeling law allows rounding of values. Because much of the data is analysis data, obtained directly from manufacturers, not from labels, in some cases our values may not be exactly the same as label information because they have not been rounded.

Part 1

Brand-Name, Nonbranded (Generic) and Take-Out Foods

FOOD	PORTION	CAL	FAT	CARB	SUG
ABALONE					
fresh fried	3 oz	161	6	9	—
ACEROLA					
fresh	1	2	tr	tr	—
ACEROLA JUICE					
juice	1 cup	51	1	12	—
ADZUKI BEANS					
canned sweetened	1 cup	702	tr	163	—
dried cooked	1 cup	294	tr	57	—
AKEE					
fresh	3.5 oz	223	20	5	—
ALE					
(see BEER AND ALE, and MALT)					
ALFALFA					
sprouts	1 tbsp	1	tr	tr	—
ALLIGATOR					
cooked	3 oz	126	2	0	0
ALLSPICE					
ground	1 tsp	5	tr	1	—
ALMONDS					
almond butter w/ salt	1 tbsp	101	9	3	—
almond paste	1 oz	127	8	12	—
jordan almonds	10 (1.4 oz)	190	7	28	24
praline	17 pieces (1.4 oz)	210	12	21	17
Lance					
Smoked	1 pkg (0.8 oz)	130	10	4	0
Planters					
Almonds	1 oz	170	15	5	1
Gold Measure Slivered	1 pkg (2 oz)	340	31	11	2

FOOD	PORTION	CAL	FAT	CARB	SUG
Honey Roasted	1 oz	160	14	7	4
ANCHOVY					
canned in oil	5	42	2	0	0
fresh fillets	3 (0.4 oz)	21	1	tr	—
ANISE					
seed	1 tsp	7	tr	1	—
ANTELOPE					
roasted	3 oz	127	2	0	0
APPLE					
canned					
Del Monte					
Fruit Pleasures Pie Spiced Apples	½ cup (4 oz)	70	0	18	17
Luck's					
Fried Apples	½ cup (4.7 oz)	130	0	33	20
dried					
Sonoma					
Pieces	10–12 pieces (1.4 oz)	110	0	29	25
fresh					
Chiquita					
Apple	1 med (5.4 oz)	80	0	22	16
Tastee					
Candy Apple	1 (3 oz)	160	5	26	16
Caramel Apple	1 (3 oz)	160	5	26	16
frozen					
Stouffer's					
Escalloped	1 cup (6 oz)	180	3	37	30
take-out					
baked	1 (5.3 oz)	126	tr	33	29
baked no sugar	1 (5.9 oz)	82	1	21	18

FOOD	PORTION	CAL	FAT	CARB	SUG
APPLE JUICE					
Apple & Eve					
100% Juice	8 fl oz	110	0	26	22
Cider	8 fl oz	110	0	27	24
Hansen's					
Junior Juice 100%	1 box (4.23 oz)	60	0	15	14
Mott's					
100% Juice	8 fl oz	120	0	29	23
Ocean Spray					
100% Juice	8 oz	110	0	28	28
Swiss Miss					
Hot Apple Cider Mix	1 serv	84	tr	20	19
Hot Apple Cider Mix Low Calorie	1 serv	14	0	3	tr
Turkey Hill					
Herbal Cider w/ Chamomile & Lemongrass	1 cup	100	0	24	24
APPLESAUCE					
White House					
Applesauce	½ cup (4.4 oz)	90	0	23	18
APRICOT JUICE					
nectar	1 cup	141	tr	36	—
APRICOTS					
canned					
juice pack w/ skin	3 halves	40	tr	10	—
dried					
halves	10	83	tr	22	—
fresh					
Chiquita					
Apricots	3 med (4 oz)	60	1	11	11

FOOD	PORTION	CAL	FAT	CARB	SUG
ARROWHEAD					
fresh boiled	1 med (⅕ oz)	9	tr	2	—
ARROWROOT					
flour	1 cup (4.5 oz)	457	tr	113	—
ARTICHOKE					
canned					
Progresso					
Hearts	2 pieces (2.9 oz)	30	0	6	1
Hearts Marinated	2 pieces (1.1 oz)	170	5	2	0
fresh					
boiled	1 med (4 oz)	60	tr	13	—
hearts cooked	½ cup	42	tr	9	—
ARUGULA					
raw	½ cup	2	tr	tr	—
ASIAN FOOD					
canned					
Chun King					
Beef Pepper Oriental BiPack	1 cup (8.8 oz)	98	2	13	0
Chow Mein Beef BiPack	1 cup (8.6 oz)	78	1	11	3
Chow Mein BiPack Chicken	1 cup (8.8 oz)	98	3	11	2
Chow Mein Pork BiPack	1 cup (8.6 oz)	78	2	9	0
Hot & Spicy Chicken BiPack	1 cup (8.6 oz)	98	3	11	0
Sweet & Sour Chicken BiPack	1 cup (8.9 oz)	161	2	29	26
La Choy					
Beef Pepper Oriental BiPack	1 cup (8.8 oz)	98	2	13	0

FOOD	PORTION	CAL	FAT	CARB	SUG
Chow Mein Beef BiPack	1 cup (8.6 oz)	78	1	11	3
Chow Mein Chicken PiBack	1 cup (8.9 oz)	98	3	11	2
Chow Mein Shrimp BiPack	1 cup (8.6 oz)	52	1	9	0
Main Entree Chow Mein Chicken	1 cup (9.3 oz)	80	4	6	2
Oriental Beef w/ Noodles BiPack	1 cup (8.8 oz)	156	3	18	2
Oriental Chicken w/ Noodles BiPack	1 cup (8.7 oz)	154	4	18	3
Sweet & Sour Chicken BiPack	1 cup (8.9 oz)	161	2	29	26
Teriyaki Chicken BiPack	1 cup (8.6 oz)	109	3	15	5
frozen					
Banquet					
Fried Rice w/ Chicken & Egg Rolls	1 meal (8.5 oz)	330	9	51	3
Birds Eye					
Easy Recipe Creations Oriental Lo Mein as prep	2¼ cups (8.7 oz)	230	4	40	11
Easy Recipe Creations Sesame Ginger Teriyaki as prep	2¼ cups (8.7 oz)	140	2	24	15
Easy Recipe Creations Spicy Szechuan Cashews	2¼ cups (8.7 oz)	180	5	29	18
Green Giant					
Create A Meal LoMein Stir Fry as prep	1¼ cups (10 oz)	320	70	35	9
Create A Meal Sweet & Sour Stir Fry as prep	1¼ cups (10 oz)	290	7	29	16

FOOD	PORTION	CAL	FAT	CARB	SUG
Create A Meal Szechuan Stir Fry as prep	1¼ cups (10 oz)	340	15	22	10
Create A Meal Teriyaki Stir Fry as prep	1¼ cups (10 oz)	240	6	18	10
La Choy					
Beef Pepper Oriental	1 cup (7.1 oz)	151	1	30	7
Chow Mein Vegetable	1 cup (8.9 oz)	108	2	20	3
Lean Cuisine					
Everyday Favorites Oriental Style Dumplings	1 pkg (9 oz)	300	6	51	14
Everyday Favorites Teriyaki StirFry	1 pkg (10 oz)	290	4	45	9
Tyson					
Chicken Fried Rice Kit w/ Sauce	1 pkg (14 oz)	440	6	69	15
Weight Watchers					
Smart Ones Chicken Chow Mein	1 pkg (9 oz)	200	2	34	5
Smart Ones Hunan Style Rice & Vegetables	1 pkg (10.34 oz)	280	0	45	4
Smart Ones King Pao Noodles & Vegetables	1 pkg (10 oz)	250	8	37	12
Smart Ones Spicy Szechaun Style Vegetables & Chicken	1 pkg (9 oz)	220	2	39	1
take-out					
buddha's delight w/ cellophane noodles fat choi jai	1 serv (7.6 oz)	211	4	44	3

FOOD	PORTION	CAL	FAT	CARB	SUG
cha siu bao steamed buns w/ chicken filling	1 (2.3 oz)	160	3	26	4
chicken teriyaki w/ rice	1 serv (11 oz)	430	6	77	10
chop suey w/ beef & pork	1 cup	300	17	13	—
chop suey w/ pork	1 cup	375	29	29	—
chow mein chicken	1 cup	255	10	10	—
chow mein pork	1 cup	425	24	21	—
chow mein shrimp	1 cup	221	10	21	—
chow mein vegetable	1 serv (8 oz)	90	3	15	2
filipino chicken adobo	1 serv (15 oz)	555	26	45	tr
fried rice	6.6 oz	249	6	48	—
fried rice w/ egg	6.7 oz	395	20	49	—
phad thai	1 serv (9.2 oz)	232	9	30	2
sesame seed paste bun	1 (2.5 oz)	220	6	39	12
shrimp chips	1¼ cups (1 oz)	140	6	19	1
shu mai chicken & vegetable dumplings	6 (3.6 oz)	160	5	18	6
spring roll	1 (3.5 oz)	112	2	37	—
sweet & sour pork	1 serv (8 oz)	250	8	37	30
sweet red bean bun	1 (2.5 oz)	130	1	38	17
szechuan chicken w/ lo mein	1 cup (5.3 oz)	190	1	35	3
wonton fried	½ cup (1 oz)	111	8	8	—
wonton soup	1 cup	205	3	26	—

ASPARAGUS
canned

Green Giant

Cut Spears	½ cup (4.2 oz)	20	0	3	tr
Spears	4.5 oz	20	0	3	tr

FOOD	PORTION	CAL	FAT	CARB	SUG
fresh					
cooked	4 spears	14	tr	3	—
frozen					
Green Giant					
Harvest Fresh Cuts	⅔ cup (3 oz)	25	0	4	tr
ATEMOYA					
fresh	½ cup	94	1	24	—
AVOCADO					
Chiquita					
Fresh	⅛ med (1 oz)	55	5	3	0
take-out					
guacamole	1 serv (2.2 oz)	105	10	5	1
BACON					
gammon lean & fat grilled	4.2 oz	274	15	0	0
Black Label					
Cooked	2 slices (0.5 oz)	80	7	0	0
Hormel					
Bacon Bits	1 tbsp (7 g)	30	2	0	0
Microwave cooked	2 slices (0.5 oz)	70	5	0	0
Old Smokehouse					
Cooked	2 slices (0.5 oz)	80	7	0	0
Oscar Mayer					
Bacon Bits	1 tbsp (0.2 oz)	25	2	0	0
Center Cut oooked	2 slices (0.4 oz)	70	5	0	0
Range Brand					
Cooked	2 slices (0.7 oz)	100	9	0	0
Red Label					
Cooked	2 slices (0.5 oz)	80	7	0	0

FOOD	PORTION	CAL	FAT	CARB	SUG
BACON SUBSTITUTES					
Bac-Os					
Chips or Bits	1½ tbsp (7 g)	30	2	2	0
Lightlife					
Fakin' Bacon Bits	1 tsp	45	1	1	0
Smart Bacon	2 strips (0.8 oz)	45	2	2	0
Louis Rich					
Turkey Bacon	1 slice (0.5 oz)	35	3	0	0
Morningstar Farms					
Breakfast Strips	2 (0.5 oz)	60	5	2	0
Worthington					
Stripples	2 strips (0.5 oz)	60	5	2	0
BAGEL					
fresh					
Pepperidge Farm					
Plain	1 (3.5 oz)	290	1	60	6
Thomas'					
Everything	1 (3.6 oz)	300	4	56	7
Multi-Grain	1 (3.6 oz)	280	2	55	7
Plain	1 (3.6 oz)	280	2	56	7
Wonder					
Blueberry	1 (3 oz)	210	1	43	9
Cinnamon Raisin	1 (3 oz)	210	1	42	9
Onion	1 (3 oz)	210	1	43	5
Rye	1 (3 oz)	220	1	42	1
Wheat	1 (3 oz)	210	1	43	5
frozen					
Amy's Organic					
Cinnamon Raisin	1 (3.5 oz)	240	2	52	9
Plain	1 (3.5 oz)	230	2	48	2

FOOD	PORTION	CAL	FAT	CARB	SUG
Poppy Seed	1 (3.5 oz)	230	2	48	2
Sesame	1 (3.5 oz)	240	2	48	2
Otis Spunkmeyer					
Barnstormin' Blueberry	1 (3.6 oz)	250	3	50	6
Barnstormin' Cinnamon Raisin	1 (3.6 oz)	230	2	47	6
Barnstormin' Onion	1 (3.6 oz)	230	2	47	6
Barnstormin' Plain	1 (3.6 oz)	240	3	49	5
Sara Lee					
Blueberry	1 (2.8 oz)	210	1	41	5
Cinnamon Raisin	1 (2.8 oz)	220	1	45	12
Egg	1 (2.8 oz)	210	1	44	7
Plain	1 (2.8 oz)	210	1	43	3
Poppy Seed	1 (2.8 oz)	210	1	41	5
Sesame Seed	1 (2.8 oz)	210	2	42	5

BAKING POWDER
Calumet

Baking Powder	¼ tsp (1 g)	0	0	0	0

BAKING SODA

baking soda	1 tsp	0	0	0	0

BALSAM PEAR

leafy tips cooked	½ cup	10	tr	2	—
pods cooked	½ cup	12	tr	3	—

BAMBOO SHOOTS

fresh cooked	½ cup	15	tr	2	—
Chun King					
Bamboo Shoots	2 tbsp (0.8 oz)	3	tr	1	tr
La Choy					
Bamboo Shoots	2 tbsp (0.8 oz)	3	tr	1	tr

FOOD	PORTION	CAL	FAT	CARB	SUG
BANANA					
banana chips	1 oz	147	10	17	—
powder	1 tbsp	21	tr	5	—
Chiquita					
Fresh	1 med (4.4 oz)	110	0	29	21
Rainforest Farms					
Slices Dried	5 slices (1.3 oz)	60	0	12	10
BARBECUE SAUCE					
Healthy Choice					
Hickory	2 tbsp (1.1 oz)	26	0	6	2
Hot & Spicy	2 tbsp (1.1 oz)	25	0	6	2
Original	2 tbsp (1.1 oz)	25	0	6	2
House Of Tsang					
Hong Kong	1 tbsp (0.6 oz)	10	0	2	1
Hunt's					
Bold Hickory	2 tbsp (1.2 oz)	47	tr	11	9
Bold Original	2 tbsp (1.2 oz)	46	tr	11	10
Hickory & Brown Sugar	2 tbsp (1.3 oz)	75	tr	18	16
Honey Hickory	2 tbsp (1.2 oz)	54	tr	12	12
Honey Mustard	2 tbsp (1.2 oz)	48	tr	12	4
Hot & Spicy	2 tbsp (1.2 oz)	48	tr	12	4
Light Original	2 tbsp (1.2 oz)	23	tr	6	5
Open Range Original	2 tbsp (1.2 oz)	39	tr	9	8
Original	2 tbsp (1.2 oz)	40	tr	9	8
Teriyaki	2 tbsp (1.2 oz)	46	tr	11	10
Kraft					
Char-Grill	2 tbsp (1.3 oz)	60	0	13	11
Hickory Smoke	2 tbsp (1.2 oz)	40	0	9	7
Honey	2 tbsp (1.3 oz)	50	0	13	11
Honey Mustard	2 tbsp (1.3 oz)	60	0	13	12
Hot	2 tbsp (1.2 oz)	40	0	9	7

FOOD	PORTION	CAL	FAT	CARB	SUG
Kansas City Style	2 tbsp (1.2 oz)	50	0	11	9
Mesquite Smoke	2 tbsp (1.2 oz)	40	0	9	7
Molasses	2 tbsp (1.3 oz)	70	0	16	14
Original	2 tbsp (1.2 oz)	40	0	9	7
Thick'N Spicy Brown Sugar	2 tbsp (1.2 oz)	60	0	15	13
Thick'N Spicy Hickory Bacon	2 tbsp (1.2 oz)	60	1	13	11
Thick'N Spicy Hickory Smoke	2 tbsp (1.2 oz)	50	0	12	10
Thick'N Spicy Honey Mustard	2 tbsp (1.3 oz)	60	0	14	12
McIlhenny					
Sauce	2 tbsp (1.1 oz)	70	5	6	3
Muir Glen					
Garlic Mesquite	2 tbsp (1.3 oz)	40	0	6	6
Hot & Smoky	2 tbsp (1.2 oz)	40	0	6	6
Original	2 tbsp (1.2 oz)	40	0	6	6
BARLEY					
flour	1 cup (5.2 oz)	511	2	110	—
malt flour	1 cup (5.7 oz)	585	3	127	—
pearled cooked	1 cup (5.5 oz)	193	1	44	—
BARRACUDA					
fresh	3 oz	122	8	0	0
BASIL					
fresh chopped	2 tbsp	1	tr	tr	—
ground	1 tsp	4	tr	1	—
BASS					
freshwater raw	3 oz	97	3	0	0
sea cooked	3 oz	105	2	0	0
striped baked	3 oz	105	3	0	0

FOOD	PORTION	CAL	FAT	CARB	SUG
BAY LEAF					
crumbled	1 tsp	2	tr	tr	—
BEANS					
(see also individual names)					
canned					
B&M					
99% Fat Free	½ cup (4.6 oz)	160	1	31	8
Baked Beans					
Baked With Honey	½ cup (4.7 oz)	170	2	30	7
Barbeque Baked Beans	½ cup (4.6 oz)	210	1	42	19
Brick Oven Baked	½ cup (4.6 oz)	180	2	32	10
Bush's					
Barbecue	½ cup (4.6 oz)	150	1	32	13
Vegetarian	½ cup (4.6 oz)	130	0	24	4
Chi-Chi's					
Refried	½ cup (4.2 oz)	100	1	18	1
Refried Beans	½ cup (4.2 oz)	120	0	17	1
Fat Free					
Eden					
Organic Baked w/ Sweet Sorghum & Orangic Mustard	½ cup (4.6 oz)	150	0	27	6
Friend's					
Original Baked	½ cup (4.6 oz)	170	1	32	10
Gebhardt					
Chili	½ cup (4.6 oz)	134	1	31	1
Refried No Fat	½ cup (4.5 oz)	92	tr	20	2
Refried Traditional	½ cup (4.5 oz)	109	3	20	2
Green Giant					
Pork And Beans w/ Tomato Sauce	½ cup (4.5 oz)	120	1	23	4

FOOD	PORTION	CAL	FAT	CARB	SUG
Spicy Chili	½ cup (4.5 oz)	110	1	20	1
Three Bean Salad	½ cup (4.2 oz)	90	0	20	10
Health Valley					
Honey Baked	½ cup	110	0	25	11
Heartland					
Iron Kettle Baked	½ cup (4.6 oz)	150	1	29	13
Hormel					
Beans & Wieners	1 can (7.5 oz)	290	12	34	12
Hunt's					
Homestyle Country Kettle	½ cup (4.6 oz)	152	2	31	11
Mix & Serve	½ cup (4.7 oz)	125	3	30	16
Pork & Beans	½ cup (4.6 oz)	157	5	27	11
Kid's Kitchen					
Microwave Meals Beans & Weiners	1 cup (7.5 oz)	310	13	37	13
Old El Paso					
Mexe-Beans	½ cup (4.6 oz)	110	1	19	0
Refried	½ cup (4.2 oz)	110	2	17	1
Refried Fat Free	½ cup (4.4 oz)	110	0	20	1
Refried Vegetarian	½ cup (4.1 oz)	100	1	16	2
Open Range					
Ranch	½ cup (4.4 oz)	124	3	23	5
Pringles					
Vegetarian	1 cup (7.9 oz)	250	1	48	24
Rosarita					
3 Bean Recipe Bacon & Jalapeno	½ cup (4.6 oz)	117	2	22	1
3 Bean Recipe Chiles & Chicken	½ cup (4.6 oz)	115	1	22	3
Fiesta Beans Bacon & Jalapenos	½ cup (4.6 oz)	117	2	22	1

FOOD	PORTION	CAL	FAT	CARB	SUG
Fiesta Beans Chilies & Chorizo	½ cup (4.6 oz)	110	2	19	3
Fiesta Beans Onions & Peppers	½ cup (4.6 oz)	104	1	20	2
Refried Bacon	½ cup (4.5 oz)	116	3	19	2
Refried Low Fat Black	½ cup (4.5 oz)	107	1	23	tr
Refried Nacho Cheese	½ cup (4.5 oz)	108	2	19	1
Refried No Fat	½ cup (4.5 oz)	120	0	28	1
Refried Onion	½ cup (4.5 oz)	114	3	21	2
Refried Traditional	½ cup (4.5 oz)	108	1	19	1
Refried Vegetarian	½ cup (4.5 oz)	237	5	42	6
S&W					
Barbecue Beans Ranch Recipe	½ cup (4.5 oz)	100	2	25	9
Taco Bell					
Home Originals Fat Free Refried Beans	½ cup (4.6 oz)	110	0	21	1
Home Originals Refried Beans	½ cup (4.7 oz)	140	3	23	1
Van Camp					
Baked Fat Free	½ cup (4.6 oz)	132	tr	29	11
Baked Original	½ cup (4.7 oz)	143	1	29	11
Beanee Weenee Baked	1 cup (9.1 oz)	410	14	58	25
Beanee Weenee Original	1 cup (9.1 oz)	320	14	35	10
Brown Sugar	½ cup (4.6 oz)	170	3	31	13
Pork And Beans	½ cup (4.6 oz)	110	2	23	7
Vegetarian	½ cup (4.6 oz)	110	1	23	7
frozen					
Natural Touch					
Nine Bean Loaf	1 in slice (3 oz)	160	8	13	tr

FOOD	PORTION	CAL	FAT	CARB	SUG
mix					
Melting Pot					
Terrazza Napoli Mixed Beans	1 cup	200	2	41	7
BEAR					
simmered	3 oz	220	11	0	0
BEAVER					
roasted	3 oz	140	6	0	0
BEECHNUTS					
dried	1 oz	164	14	10	—
BEEF					
canned					
Armour					
Chopped Beef	2 oz	170	15	2	2
Corned Beef	2 oz	120	7	1	1
Potted Meat	1 can (3 oz)	120	7	0	0
Tripe	3 oz	90	2	0	0
Hormel					
Cubed Beef	½ cup (4.9 oz)	130	3	0	0
Treet					
Luncheon Loaf	2 oz	130	11	3	3
Luncheon Loaf 50% Less Fat	2 oz	110	8	4	2
dried					
Armour					
Sliced	7 slices (1 oz)	60	2	2	2
fresh					
bottom round lean & fat trim 0 in Choice roasted	3 oz	172	8	0	0

FOOD	PORTION	CAL	FAT	CARB	SUG
bottom round lean & fat trim ¼ in Choice braised	3 oz	241	15	0	0
bottom round lean & fat trim ¼ in Choice roasted	3 oz	221	14	0	0
brisket flat half lean & fat trim ¼ in braised	3 oz	309	24	0	0
brisket whole lean & fat trim ¼ in braised	3 oz	327	27	0	0
chuck arm pot roast lean & fat trim ¼ in braised	3 oz	282	20	0	0
chuck blade roast lean & fat trim ¼ in braised	3 oz	293	22	0	0
corned beef brisket cooked	3 oz	213	16	tr	—
eye of round lean & fat trim ¼ in Choice roasted	3 oz	205	12	0	0
ground extra lean broiled medium	3 oz	217	14	0	0
ground extra lean broiled well done	3 oz	225	14	0	0
ground extra lean fried medium	3 oz	216	14	0	0
ground extra lean fried well done	3 oz	224	14	0	0
ground lean broiled medium	3 oz	231	16	0	0
ground lean broiled well done	3 oz	238	15	0	0

FOOD	PORTION	CAL	FAT	CARB	SUG
ground regular broiled medium	3 oz	246	18	0	0
ground regular broiled well done	3 oz	248	17	0	0
porterhouse steak lean & fat trim ¼ in Choice broiled	3 oz	260	19	0	0
porterhouse steak lean only trim ¼ in Prime broiled	3 oz	185	9	0	0
rib large end lean & fat trim ¼ in broiled	3 oz	295	24	0	0
rib large end lean & fat trim ¼ in roasted	3 oz	310	25	0	0
rib small end lean & fat trim ¼ in broiled	3 oz	285	22	0	0
rib small end lean & fat trim ¼ in roasted	3 oz	295	24	0	0
rib whole lean & fat trim ¼ in Choice broiled	3 oz	306	25	0	0
rib whole lean & fat trim ¼ in Choice roasted	3 oz	320	27	0	0
rib whole lean & fat trim ¼ in Prime roasted	3 oz	348	30	0	0
shank crosscut lean & fat trim ¼ in Choice simmered	3 oz	224	12	0	0

FOOD	PORTION	CAL	FAT	CARB	SUG
short loin top loin lean & fat trim ¼ in Choice braised	3 oz	253	18	0	0
short loin top loin lean & fat trim ¼ in Choice broiled	1 steak (6.3 oz)	536	38	0	0
short loin top loin lean & fat trim ¼ in Prime broiled	1 steak (6.3 oz)	582	43	0	0
short loin top loin lean only trim ¼ in Choice broiled	1 steak (5.2 oz)	314	15	0	0
shortribs lean & fat Choice braised	3 oz	400	36	0	0
t-bone steak lean & fat trim ¼ in Choice broiled	3 oz	253	18	0	0
t-bone steak lean only trim ¼ in Choice broiled	3 oz	182	9	0	0
tenderloin lean & fat trim ¼ in Choice broiled	3 oz	259	19	0	0
tenderloin lean & fat trim ¼ in Choice roasted	3 oz	288	22	0	0
tenderloin lean & fat trim ¼ in Choice broiled	3 oz	208	12	0	0
tenderloin lean & fat trim ¼ in Prime broiled	3 oz	270	20	0	0

FOOD	PORTION	CAL	FAT	CARB	SUG
tenderloin lean only trim ¼ in Choice broiled	3 oz	188	10	0	0
tip round lean & fat trim ¼ in Choice roasted	3 oz	210	13	0	0
tip round lean & fat trim ¼ in Prime roasted	3 oz	233	15	0	0
top round lean & fat trim ¼ in Choice braised	3 oz	221	11	0	0
top round lean & fat trim ¼ in Choice broiled	3 oz	190	9	0	0
top round lean & fat trim ¼ in Choice fried	3 oz	235	13	0	0
top round lean & fat trim ¼ in Prime broiled	3 oz	195	9	0	0
top sirloin lean & fat trim ¼ in Choice broiled	3 oz	228	14	0	0
top sirloin lean & fat trim ¼ in Choice fried	3 oz	277	19	0	0
tripe raw	4 oz	111	4	0	0
Healthy Choice					
Ground Extra Lean	4 oz	130	4	2	0
Organic Valley					
Extra Lean Ground	3 oz	130	6	0	0
Extra Lean Patties	1 (3.2 oz)	130	6	0	0

FOOD	PORTION	CAL	FAT	CARB	SUG
ready-to-eat					
Alpine Lace					
Roast Beef 97% Fat Free	2 oz	70	2	1	0
Boar's Head					
Corned Beef Brisket	2 oz	80	4	0	0
Eye Round Pepper Seasoned	2 oz	90	3	0	0
Italian Style Oven Roasted Top Round	2 oz	80	2	2	0
Roast Beef Cajun	2 oz	80	3	0	0
Top Round Deluxe	2 oz	90	3	0	0
Healthy Choice					
Deli-Thin Roast Beef	6 slices (2 oz)	60	2	1	1
Fresh-Trak Roast Beef	1 slice (1 oz)	30	1	0	0
Thomas E. Wilson					
Roast Beef In Brown Gravy	1 serv + gravy (3.5 oz)	160	6	3	1
Tyson					
Beef Strips Seasoned	1 serv (3 oz)	140	6	1	1
BEEF DISHES **canned**					
Armour					
Corned Beef Hash	1 cup (8.3 oz)	440	30	23	1
Roast Beef Hash	1 cup (8.4 oz)	400	25	23	0
Roast Beef In Gravy	½ cup (4.6 oz)	150	4	3	0
Stew	1 cup (8.6 oz)	220	12	21	0
Dinty Moore					
Meatball Stew	1 cup (8.4 oz)	250	15	17	3
Sliced Potatoes & Beef	1 can (7.5 oz)	230	9	28	1

FOOD	PORTION	CAL	FAT	CARB	SUG
Stew	1 cup (8.3 oz)	230	14	16	3
Hormel					
Beef Goulash	1 can (7.5 oz)	230	11	19	6
Roast Beef With Gravy	2 oz	60	2	1	0
Mary Kitchen					
Corned Beef Hash	1 cup (8.3 oz)	410	27	22	1
Corned Beef Hash 50% Reduced Fat	1 cup (8.3 oz)	280	12	25	1
Roast Beef Hash	1 cup (8.3 oz)	390	24	22	1
Sausage Hash	1 cup (8.3 oz)	410	27	23	1
frozen					
Banquet					
Sandwich Toppers Creamed Chipped Beef	1 pkg (4 oz)	120	6	8	4
Sandwich Toppers Gravy & Salisbury Steak	1 pkg (5 oz)	210	16	8	5
Sandwich Toppers Gravy & Sliced Beef	1 pkg (4 oz)	70	2	5	1
mix					
Hamburger Helper					
BBQ Beef as prep	1 cup	320	10	37	8
Beef Pasta as prep	1 cup	270	10	26	2
Beef Stew as prep	1 cup	260	10	26	6
Beef Taco as prep	1 cup	280	10	31	6
Beef Teriyaki as prep	1 cup	290	10	34	5
Cheddar Melt as prep	1 cup	310	12	31	8
Cheeseburger Macaroni as prep	1 cup	360	16	33	9
Cheesy Hashbrowns as prep	1 cup	400	19	39	5
Cheesy Italian as prep	1 cup	320	14	28	7

FOOD	PORTION	CAL	FAT	CARB	SUG
Chili Macaroni as prep	1 cup	290	10	30	5
Fettuccine Alfredo as prep	1 cup	300	13	26	5
Four Cheese Lasagne as prep	1 cup	330	14	31	6
Lasagne as prep	1 cup	270	10	29	7
Meat Loaf as prep	⅛ loaf	270	14	11	3
Meaty Spaghetti & Cheese as prep	1 cup	290	10	30	5
Mushroom & Wild Rice as prep	1 cup	310	12	30	4
Nacho Cheese as prep	1 cup	320	13	30	5
Pizzabake as prep	⅛ pie	270	10	28	4
Potatoes Au Gratin as prep	1 cup	280	13	25	5
Potatoes Stroganoff as prep	1 cup	250	11	23	5
Rice Oriental as prep	1 cup	280	10	32	2
Salisbury as prep	1 cup	270	10	26	4
Spaghetti as prep	1 cup	270	10	27	6
Stroganoff as prep	1 cup	320	13	30	7
Swedish Meatballs as prep	1 cup	290	14	25	3
Three Cheeses as prep	1 cup	340	15	32	5
Zesty Italian as prep	1 cup	300	10	32	8
Zesty Mexican as prep	1 cup	280	10	31	8
shelf-stable					
Dinty Moore					
Microwave Cup Corned Beef Hash	1 pkg (7.5 oz)	350	22	19	1
Microwave Cup Hearty Burger Stew	1 pkg (7.5 oz)	240	13	19	5

FOOD	PORTION	CAL	FAT	CARB	SUG
Microwave Cup Stew	1 pkg (7.5 oz)	190	10	15	2
Lunch Bucket					
Beef Stew	1 pkg (7.5 oz)	170	9	17	0
take-out					
beef bouriguignon	1 serv (7 oz)	254	16	3	—
bubble & squeak	5 oz	186	13	16	—
bulgoghi korean grilled beef	1 serv (5.2 oz)	256	15	5	3
cornish pasty	1 (8 oz)	847	52	79	—
greek moussaka	1 serv (8.5 oz)	450	33	12	4
irish stew	1 cup (7 oz)	280	16	10	—
kebab indian	1 (5.4 oz)	553	40	2	—
kheena	6.7 oz	781	71	1	—
koftas	5	280	22	3	—
samosa	2 (4 oz)	652	62	20	—
shepherds pie	1 serv (7 oz)	282	16	20	—
steak & kidney pie w/ top crust	1 slice (5 oz)	400	26	23	—
stew	6 oz	208	13	6	—
stew w/ vegetables	1 cup	220	11	15	—
stroganoff	¾ cup	260	19	43	—
swiss steak	4.6 oz	214	9	10	—
toad in the hole	1 (4.7 oz)	383	29	23	—
BEEFALO					
roasted	3 oz	160	5	0	0
BEER AND ALE					
alcohol free beer	7 fl oz	50	tr	11	5
ale brown	10 oz	77	0	8	—
ale pale	10 oz	88	0	12	—

FOOD	PORTION	CAL	FAT	CARB	SUG
beer light	12 oz can	100	0	5	—
beer regular	12 oz can	146	0	13	—
lager	10 oz	80	0	4	—
stout	10 oz	102	0	6	—

BEET JUICE
juice	7 oz	72	0	16	—

BEETS
canned
Green Giant
Harvard	⅓ cup (3.1 oz)	60	0	15	10
Sliced	½ cup (4.2 oz)	35	0	8	5
Whole	½ cup (4.2 oz)	35	0	8	5

fresh
greens cooked	½ cup	20	tr	4	—
sliced cooked	½ cup (3 oz)	38	tr	9	—
whole cooked	2 (3.5 oz)	44	tr	10	—

BEVERAGES
(*see* BEER AND ALE, CHAMPAGNE, COFFEE, DRINK MIXERS, ENERGY DRINKS, FRUIT DRINKS, ICED TEA, LIQUOR/LIQUEUR, MALT, MILKSHAKES, SODA, SPORTS DRINKS, TEA/HERBAL TEA, WATER, WINE, WINE COOLER)

BISCUIT
mix
Bisquick
Buttermilk	½ cup	150	6	21	1
Cheese Garlic	½ cup	160	7	22	2
Cinnamon Swirl	½ cup	150	4	30	6
Mix	⅓ cup (1.4 oz)	160	6	25	1
Reduced Fat	⅓ cup	140	3	27	2
Kentucky Kernel					
Biscuit	¼ cup (1 oz)	171	5	28	1

FOOD	PORTION	CAL	FAT	CARB	SUG
refrigerated					
1869 Brand					
Buttermilk	1 (1.1 oz)	100	5	12	1
Hungry Jack					
Butter Tastin' Flaky	1 (1.2 oz)	100	5	14	2
Cinnamon & Sugar	1 (1.2 oz)	110	4	17	5
Flaky	1 (1.2 oz)	100	5	14	2
Pillsbury					
Big Country Butter Tastin'	1 (1.2 oz)	100	4	13	2
Big Country Buttermilk	1 (1.2 oz)	100	4	14	2
Big Country Southern Style	1 (1.2 oz)	100	4	14	2
Buttermilk	1 (2.2 oz)	150	2	29	3
Grands Blueberry	1 (2.1 oz)	210	9	29	10
Grands Butter Tastin'	1 (2.1 oz)	200	10	24	5
Grands Buttermilk	1 (2.1 oz)	200	10	24	5
Grands Buttermilk Reduced Fat	1 (2.1 oz)	190	7	27	5
Southern Style Flakey	1 (1.2 oz)	100	5	14	2
Tender Layer Buttermilk	1 (2.2 oz)	160	5	27	3
take-out					
tea biscuit	1 (3 oz)	210	3	30	12
w/ egg	1 (4.8 oz)	316	20	24	—
w/ egg & bacon	1 (5.2 oz)	458	31	29	—
w/ egg & ham	1 (6.7 oz)	442	27	30	—
w/ egg & sausage	1 (6.3 oz)	581	39	41	—
w/ egg & steak	1 (5.2 oz)	410	28	21	—
w/ egg cheese & bacon	1 (5.1 oz)	477	31	33	—
w/ ham	1 (4 oz)	386	18	44	—
w/ sausage	1 (4.4 oz)	485	32	40	—
w/ steak	1 (4.9 oz)	455	26	44	—

FOOD	PORTION	CAL	FAT	CARB	SUG
BISON					
roasted	3 oz	122	2	0	0
BLACK BEANS					
canned					
Eden					
Organic w/ Ginger & Lemon	½ cup (4.6 oz)	120	0	21	1
Green Giant					
Black Beans	½ cup (4.5 oz)	50	0	18	tr
Old El Paso					
Black Beans	½ cup (4.6 oz)	100	1	17	0
Refried	½ cup (4.2 oz)	120	2	18	2
Progresso					
Black Beans	½ cup (4.6 oz)	110	1	17	0
dried					
cooked	1 cup	227	1	41	—
BLACKBERRIES					
canned in heavy syrup	½ cup	118	tr	30	—
fresh	½ cup	37	tr	9	—
unsweetened frzn	1 cup	97	1	24	—
BLACKBERRY JUICE					
Clear Fruit					
Blackberry Rush	8 oz	90	0	23	23
BLACKEYE PEAS					
canned					
Green Giant					
Blackeye Peas	½ cup (4.4 oz)	90	0	16	tr
dried					
cooked	1 cup	198	1	36	—

FOOD	PORTION	CAL	FAT	CARB	SUG
Hurst					
HamBeens California w/ Ham	1 serv	120	1	22	1
frozen					
Birds Eye					
Blackeye Peas	½ cup (2.8 oz)	110	1	21	1
BLINTZE					
Golden					
Cheese	1 (2.1 oz)	80	2	13	5
take-out					
cheese	1 (2.7 oz)	160	9	15	4
BLUEBERRIES					
canned in heavy syrup	1 cup	225	1	56	—
fresh	1 cup	82	1	20	—
unsweetened frzn	1 cup	78	1	19	—
Sonoma					
Dried	¼ cup (1.3 oz)	140	0	33	17
BLUEBERRY JUICE					
After The Fall					
Maine Coast	1 cup (8 oz)	90	0	25	19
BLUEFISH					
fresh baked	3 oz	135	5	0	0
BOAR					
wild roasted	3 oz	136	4	0	0
BOK CHOY					
(*see* CABBAGE)					
BONITO					
fresh	3 oz	117	4	0	0

FOOD	PORTION	CAL	FAT	CARB	SUG
BORAGE					
fresh chopped cooked	3½ oz	25	1	4	—
raw chopped	½ cup	9	tr	1	—
BOTTLED WATER					
(see WATER)					
BOYSENBERRIES					
in heavy syrup	1 cup	226	tr	57	—
unsweetened frzn	1 cup	66	tr	16	—
BRAINS					
beef pan-fried	3 oz	167	13	0	0
beef simmered	3 oz	136	11	0	0
lamb braised	3 oz	124	9	0	0
pork braised	3 oz	117	8	0	0
veal braised	3 oz	115	8	0	0
Armour					
Pork Brains In Milk Gravy	⅖ cup (5.5 oz)	150	5	10	0
BRAN					
Hodgson Mill					
Oat	¼ cup (1.4 oz)	120	3	23	0
Quaker					
Oat	½ cup (1.4 oz)	150	3	25	1
BRAZIL NUTS					
dried	1 oz	186	19	4	—
BREAD					
canned					
B&M					
Brown Bread	½ in slice (2 oz)	130	1	29	9

FOOD	PORTION	CAL	FAT	CARB	SUG
frozen					
Marie Callender's					
Cornbread & Honey Butter	1 piece + butter	210	11	28	2
Original Garlic	1 piece	190	8	23	5
New York					
Garlic	1 slice (2 oz)	190	8	27	1
Garlic Reduced Fat	1 slice (2 oz)	160	4	29	1
Texas Garlic Toast	1 in slice (1.4 oz)	160	9	17	1
Pepperidge Farm					
Garlic	1 slice (1.8 oz)	170	10	15	2
Garlic Sourdough 30% Reduced Fat	1 slice (1.8 oz)	170	7	22	2
Mozzeralla Garlic Cheese	1 slice (2 oz)	201	10	21	2
mix					
Hodgson Mill					
European Cheese & Herb	¼ cup (1.2 oz)	130	1	21	3
Honey Whole Wheat	¼ cup (1.2 oz)	120	1	22	2
ready-to-eat					
baguette whole wheat	2 oz	140	0	29	tr
challah	1 slice (2 oz)	160	3	29	5
navajo fry	1 (5 in diam)	296	9	48	—
white toasted	1 slice	67	1	13	—
white cubed	1 cup	80	1	15	—
Arnold					
Country Buttermilk	1 slice (1.3 oz)	110	2	20	4
Country Wheat	1 slice (1.3 oz)	100	2	10	4
Bread Du Jour					
French	3 in slice (2 oz)	140	1	26	3

FOOD	PORTION	CAL	FAT	CARB	SUG
Damascus					
Mountain Shepard Lahvash	⅛ loaf (2 oz)	135	0	28	0
Pita	1 (2 oz)	130	0	29	0
Pita Whole Wheat	1 (2 oz)	160	0	32	0
Wraps Honey Wheat	½ wrap (2 oz)	130	0	28	3
Wraps Plain	½ wrap (2 oz)	130	0	29	tr
Wraps Spinach	1 (2 oz)	280	0	56	tr
Wraps Tomato	1 12-inch (4 oz)	240	0	58	1
Home Pride					
Wheat	1 slice (1 oz)	80	1	14	2
La Mexicana					
Wraps Chocolate	1 (1.3 oz)	120	3	18	1
Wraps Spinach	1 (1.3 oz)	120	4	18	1
Wraps Tomato Basil	1 (1.3 oz)	120	4	18	1
Meditarranean Magic					
Focaccia	⅛ loaf (1.8 oz)	140	2	27	2
Milton's					
Healthy Multi-Grain	1 slice (1.4 oz)	110	1	24	6
Pepperidge Farm					
Apple Cinammon	1 slice (1 oz)	80	2	15	4
Deli Swirl Rye & Pump	1 slice (1.1 oz)	80	1	15	tr
Farmhouse Sourdough	1 slice (1.5 oz)	110	2	20	2
Natural Whole Grain Whole Wheat	1 slice (1.2 oz)	90	1	16	2
Sandwich Pocket Wheat	1 (2 oz)	160	1	30	2
Sandwich Pocket White	1 (2 oz)	150	1	30	2
Swirl Cinnamon	1 slice (1 oz)	90	3	15	tr
Stroehmann					
100% Whole Wheat	1 slice (1.3 oz)	90	1	17	3

FOOD	PORTION	CAL	FAT	CARB	SUG
D'Italiano Italian Seeded	1 slice (1 oz)	80	1	15	tr
Family White	1 slice (0.8 oz)	65	1	13	1
Homestyle Split Top Wheat	1 slice (0.8 oz)	60	0	13	2
Homestyle Split Top White	1 slice (0.8 oz)	65	1	12	1
Honey Cracked Wheat	1 slice (1.2 oz)	80	1	16	2
Potato	1 slice (1.2 oz)	100	2	19	3
Rye	1 slice (1.1 oz)	80	1	15	tr
Twelve Grain	1 slice (1.2 oz)	90	1	17	3
Valley Lahvosh					
Valley Wraps	1 (1 oz)	100	1	19	3
refrigerated					
Pillsbury					
Crusty French Loaf	⅛ loaf (2.2 oz)	150	2	27	3
Grands Wheat	1 (2.1 oz)	200	8	27	6
take-out					
chapatis as prep w/ fat	1 bread (1.6 oz)	95	2	18	1
chapatis as prep w/o fat	1 (2½ oz)	141	1	31	—
cornstick	1 (1.3 oz)	101	4	13	—
focaccia onion	1 piece (4.6 oz)	282	10	43	2
focaccia rosemary	1 piece (3.5 oz)	251	7	40	1
focaccia tomato olive	1 piece (4.7 oz)	270	8	42	1
garlic bread	2 slices (2 oz)	190	8	27	1
naan	1 bread (3.5 oz)	286	9	43	3
papadums fried	2 (1.5 oz)	81	4	9	—
paratha	1 bread (2.1 oz)	201	10	23	1

BREAD COATING

Don's Chuck Wagon

Chicken Baking Mix	¼ cup (1 oz)	95	0	21	0

FOOD	PORTION	CAL	FAT	CARB	SUG
Fish & Chips Mix	¼ cup (1 oz)	100	0	21	0
Mushroom Batter Mix	¼ cup (1 oz)	95	0	21	0
Onion Ring Mix	¼ cup (1 oz)	100	0	21	0
Seafood Bake & Fry Mix	¼ cup (1 oz)	95	0	21	0
Luzianne					
Cajun Chicken Coating Mix	2 tbsp (1 oz)	100	1	20	2
Oven Fry					
Extra Crispy For Chicken	⅛ pkg (0.5 oz)	60	1	10	2
Extra Crispy For Pork	⅛ pkg (0.5 oz)	60	2	11	1
Shake 'N Bake					
Buffalo Wings	¹⁄₁₀ pkg (0.4 oz)	40	1	8	3
Classic Italian Chicken or Pork	⅛ pkg (0.4 oz)	40	1	7	tr
Country Mild Recipe	⅛ pkg (0.3 oz)	35	2	5	0
Glazes Barbecue Chicken Or Pork	⅛ pkg (0.4 oz)	45	1	9	5
Glazes Honey Mustard Chicken Or Pork	⅛ pkg (0.4 oz)	45	1	9	6
Glazes Tangy Honey Chicken Or Pork	⅛ pkg (0.4 oz)	45	1	9	6
Home Style Flour Recipe For Chicken	⅛ pkg (0.4 oz)	40	1	7	0
Hot & Spicy Chicken Or Pork	⅛ pkg (0.4 oz)	40	1	7	tr
Original For Chicken	⅛ pkg (0.4 oz)	40	1	7	tr
Original For Fish	¼ pkg (0.7 oz)	80	2	14	tr
Original For Pork	⅛ pkg (0.4 oz)	45	1	8	tr

BREAD MACHINE MIX

Fleischmann's

FOOD	PORTION	CAL	FAT	CARB	SUG
Apple Cinnamon	⅛ loaf	160	1	32	12

FOOD	PORTION	CAL	FAT	CARB	SUG
Cinnamon Raisin	⅛ loaf	160	1	33	4
Country White	⅛ loaf (1.6 oz)	170	3	31	4
Cranberry Orange	⅛ loaf	150	2	33	4
Honey Oatmeal	⅛ loaf	160	1	33	5
Italian Herb	⅛ loaf	160	2	29	2
Sourdough	⅛ loaf	150	2	29	3
Stoneground Wheat	⅛ loaf	160	1	32	4
Sassafras					
Apricot Oatmeal	1 slice (1.4 oz)	140	1	29	3
BREADCRUMBS					
fresh	⅔ cup	76	1	14	—
Progresso					
Garlic & Herb	¼ cup (1 oz)	100	2	18	1
Italian Style	¼ cup (1 oz)	110	2	20	1
Parmesan	¼ cup (1 oz)	100	2	17	1
Plain	¼ cup (1 oz)	110	2	19	1
BREADFRUIT					
fresh	¼ small	99	tr	26	—
seeds cooked	1 oz	48	1	9	—
seeds roasted	1 oz	59	tr	11	—
BREADNUTTREE SEEDS					
dried	1 oz	104	tr	23	—
BREADSTICKS					
Bread Du Jour					
Original	1 (1.9 oz)	130	1	25	3
Sourdough	1 (1.9 oz)	130	1	25	1
New York					
Garlic Soft	1 (1.5 oz)	140	4	23	1
Pillsbury					
Soft	1 (1.4 oz)	110	2	19	2

FOOD	PORTION	CAL	FAT	CARB	SUG
Stella D'Oro					
Garlic	1 (0.4 oz)	40	1	7	tr
Grissini Style Fat Free	3 (0.5 oz)	60	0	12	1
Original	1 (0.4 oz)	45	1	7	0
Roasted Garlic	1 (0.4 oz)	45	1	8	tr
Sesame	1 (0.4 oz)	50	3	7	tr
Snack Stix Cracked Pepper	4 (0.5 oz)	70	2	11	tr
Snack Stix Salted	4 (0.5 oz)	70	2	11	tr
Wheat	1 (0.3 oz)	40	1	6	tr

BREAKFAST BARS

(*see* CEREAL BARS, ENERGY BARS)

BREAKFAST DRINKS

FOOD	PORTION	CAL	FAT	CARB	SUG
Carnation					
Instant Breakfast Vanilla as prep w/ skim milk	1 serv	220	1	39	—

BROAD BEANS

FOOD	PORTION	CAL	FAT	CARB	SUG
dried cooked	1 cup	186	1	33	—

BROCCOFLOWER

FOOD	PORTION	CAL	FAT	CARB	SUG
fresh raw	½ cup (1.8 oz)	16	tr	3	—

BROCCOLI
fresh

FOOD	PORTION	CAL	FAT	CARB	SUG
chinese broccoli (gai lan) cooked	1 cup (3.1 oz)	19	1	3	—
chopped cooked	½ cup	22	tr	4	—

frozen

FOOD	PORTION	CAL	FAT	CARB	SUG
Amy's Organic					
Pocket Sandwich Broccoli & Cheese	1 (4.5 oz)	270	10	37	4

FOOD	PORTION	CAL	FAT	CARB	SUG
Birds Eye					
Florets	1 cup (3 oz)	25	0	4	1
In Cheese Sauce	½ cup (4 oz)	70	4	7	3
Green Giant					
Butter Sauce	4 oz	50	2	7	2
Cheese Sauce	⅔ cup (3.9 oz)	70	3	9	5
Harvest Fresh Cut	⅔ cup (3.2 oz)	25	0	4	tr
Harvest Fresh Spears	3.5 oz	25	0	4	1
Select Florets	1⅛ cups (2.9 oz)	25	0	4	1
Select Spears	3 oz	25	0	4	2
Health Is Wealth					
Broccoli Munchees	2 (1 oz)	60	2	10	0
Stouffer's					
Au Gratin	1 serv (4 oz)	100	4	10	3

BROWNIE
frozen

Greenfield

Fat Free Homestyle	1 (1.3 oz)	110	0	27	19
Otis Spunkmeyer					
Blue Yonder w/ Walnuts	1 (2 oz)	230	10	34	22
Weight Watchers					
Brownie A La Mode	1 (0.14 oz)	190	4	33	15
Double Fudge Brownie Parfait	1 (5.3 oz)	190	3	39	20

mix

Betty Crocker

Chocolate Chunk as prep	1	180	9	25	18
Dark Chocolate Fudge as prep	1	170	7	24	17
Fudge as prep	1	170	7	23	17
Hot Fudge as prep	1	170	8	23	16

FOOD	PORTION	CAL	FAT	CARB	SUG
Original as prep	1	180	6	27	19
Peanut Butter as prep	1	180	8	23	17
Stir'n Bake w/ Mini Kisses as prep	1 serv	220	7	38	27
Turtle w/ Caramel & Pecans as prep	1	170	8	25	16
Walnut as prep	1	180	9	23	15
Estee					
Brownie Mix as prep	2	100	4	23	10
No Pudge!					
Fudge	1	100	0	21	13
Sweet Rewards					
Low Fat Fudge as prep	1	130	3	27	18
Reduced Fat Supreme as prep	1	140	3	27	19
ready-to-eat					
Dolly Madison					
Fudge	1 (3 oz)	330	11	54	11
Entenmann's					
Little Bites	3 (2.2 oz)	290	16	37	26
Ultimate Fudge	1 (1.6 oz)	220	13	27	18
Greenfield					
Blondie Fat Free Apple Spice	1 (1.3 oz)	110	0	26	19
Health Valley					
Bar w/ Fudge Filling	1 bar	110	0	26	17
Hostess					
Brownie Bites	3 (1.3 oz)	170	9	21	17
Fudge	1 (3 oz)	330	11	54	11
Light	1 (1.4 oz)	140	3	28	19
Lance					
Fudge Nut	1 (2.25 oz)	340	13	56	26

FOOD	PORTION	CAL	FAT	CARB	SUG
Little Debbie					
Brownie Lights	1 (2 oz)	190	3	39	27
Fudge	1 pkg (2.1 oz)	270	13	39	24
Tastykake					
Fudge Walnut	1 (3 oz)	370	17	52	37
Tom's					
Fudge Nut	1 pkg (2.5 oz)	300	13	45	19
BRUSSELS SPROUTS					
fresh					
cooked	1 sprout	8	tr	2	—
frozen					
Birds Eye					
Brussels Sprouts	11 sprouts	35	0	7	2
Green Giant					
Butter Sauce	⅔ cup (3.6 oz)	60	2	9	3
BUCKWHEAT					
groats roasted cooked	1 cup (5.9 oz)	647	1	34	—
BUFFALO					
water buffalo roasted	3 oz	111	2	0	0
BULGUR					
cooked	1 cup (6.3 oz)	151	tr	34	—
BURBOT (FISH)					
fresh baked	3 oz	98	1	0	0
BURDOCK ROOT					
cooked	1 cup	110	tr	26	—
BUTTER					
clarified butter	3½ oz	876	99	0	0
stick	1 stick (4 oz)	813	92	tr	—

FOOD	PORTION	CAL	FAT	CARB	SUG
stick	1 pat (5 g)	36	4	tr	—
whipped	1 pat (4 g)	27	3	tr	—
Breakstone's					
Salted	1 tbsp (0.5 oz)	100	11	0	0
Hotel Bar					
Stick	1 tbsp (0.5 oz)	100	11	0	0
Keller's					
European	1 tbsp (0.5 oz)	100	11	0	0
Land O Lakes					
Salted	1 tbsp (0.5 oz)	100	11	0	0
Organic Valley					
Butter	1 tbsp (0.5 oz)	100	11	0	0

BUTTER BEANS
canned

FOOD	PORTION	CAL	FAT	CARB	SUG
Green Giant					
Butter Beans	½ cup (4.5 oz)	90	0	16	1
Van Camp					
Butter Beans	½ cup (4.6 oz)	110	1	22	0
frozen					
Birds Eye					
Speckled	½ cup (2.7 oz)	100	0	20	1

BUTTER BLENDS

FOOD	PORTION	CAL	FAT	CARB	SUG
Brummel & Brown					
Spread Make With Yogurt	1 tbsp (0.5 oz)	50	5	0	0

BUTTER SUBSTITUTES

FOOD	PORTION	CAL	FAT	CARB	SUG
Molly McButter					
Natural Butter	1 tsp	5	0	1	—
Mrs. Bateman's					
Butterlike Baking Butter	1 tbsp (0.5 oz)	36	1	8	0

FOOD	PORTION	CAL	FAT	CARB	SUG
BUTTERBUR					
canned fuki chopped	1 cup	3	tr	tr	—
fresh fuki	1 cup	13	tr	3	—
BUTTERFISH					
baked	3 oz	159	9	0	0
BUTTERNUTS					
dried	1 oz	174	16	3	—
BUTTERSCOTCH					
Nestle					
Morsels	1 tbsp	80	4	9	9
CABBAGE					
chinese bok choy shredded cooked	½ cup	10	tr	2	—
chinese pak-choi raw shredded	½ cup	5	tr	1	—
chinese pe-tsai raw shredded	1 cup	12	tr	2	—
chinese pe-tsai shredded cooked	1 cup	16	tr	3	—
danish raw shredded	½ cup (1.2 oz)	9	tr	2	—
danish shredded cooked	½ cup (2.6 oz)	17	tr	3	—
green raw shredded	½ cup (1.2 oz)	9	tr	2	—
green shredded cooked	½ cup (2.6 oz)	17	tr	3	—
napa cooked	1 cup (3.8 oz)	13	tr	2	—
red raw shredded	½ cup	10	tr	2	—
red shredded cooked	½ cup	16	tr	3	—
savoy raw shredded	½ cup	10	tr	2	—
savoy shredded cooked	½ cup	18	tr	4	—

FOOD	PORTION	CAL	FAT	CARB	SUG
take-out					
korean kimchee	½ cup	22	tr	4	—
stuffed cabbage	1 (6 oz)	373	22	18	—
sweet & sour red cabbage	4 oz	61	3	8	—
CACTUS					
napoles fresh sliced	½ cup (1.5 oz)	7	tr	1	—
pricklypear fresh	1 cup (5.3 oz)	56	1	13	—
CAKE					
Baby Watson					
Cheesecake	1 slice (3 oz)	260	18	19	15
Entenmann's					
Apple Puffs	1 (3 oz)	270	13	37	20
Hostess					
Crumb Cake	1 (1 oz)	100	2	18	11
Light					
Jell-O					
Dessert Delights Cheesecake	1 bar (1.4 oz)	160	7	20	13
Dessert Delights Chocolate Fudge Pudding	1 bar (1.4 oz)	150	6	23	15
Marie Callender's					
Cobbler Apple	1 serv (4.25 oz)	370	20	45	31
Cobbler Cherry	1 serv (4.25 oz)	380	19	50	32
Cobbler Peach	1 serv (4.25 oz)	380	18	47	24
Natural Touch					
Toaster Square Blueberry	1 (2.8 oz)	180	2	33	12
Sara Lee					
Cheesecake Cherry Cream	¼ cake (4.7 oz)	350	12	55	35

FOOD	PORTION	CAL	FAT	CARB	SUG
Cheesecake Chocolate Chip	¼ cake (4.2 oz)	410	21	47	43
Cheesecake French	⅙ cake (3.9 oz)	350	21	24	22
Coffee Cake Crumb	⅛ cake (2 oz)	220	9	32	17
Coffee Cake Pecan	⅙ cake (1.9 oz)	230	12	24	9
Coffee Cake Raspberry	⅙ cake (1.9 oz)	220	8	27	13
Coffee Cake Reduced Fat Cheese	⅙ cake (1.9 oz)	180	6	28	11
Layer Cake Coconut	⅛ cake (2.8 oz)	260	14	33	25
Layer Cake Double Chocolate	⅛ cake (2.8 oz)	260	13	33	24
Layer Cake Fudge Golden	⅛ cake (2.8 oz)	260	13	34	23
Layer Cake German Chocolate	⅛ cake (2.9 oz)	280	14	35	26
Layer Cake Vanilla	⅛ cake (2.8 oz)	260	14	32	22
Original Cheesecake	¼ cake (4.2 oz)	350	18	39	30
Pound Cake All Butter	¼ cake (2.7 oz)	320	16	38	21
Pound Cake Chocolate Swirl	¼ cake (2.9 oz)	330	16	42	31
Pound Cake Reduced Fat	¼ cake (2.7 oz)	280	11	42	26
Strawberry Shortcake	⅛ cake (2.5 oz)	180	7	27	15
take-out					
angelfood	1/12 cake (1 oz)	73	tr	16	—
apple crisp	½ cup (5 oz)	230	5	46	—
baklava	1 oz	126	9	10	—
boston cream pie	⅙ cake (3.3 oz)	293	12	43	—
carrot w/ cream cheese icing	1/12 cake (3.9 oz)	484	29	52	—
cheesecake w/ cherry topping	1/12 cake (5 oz)	359	23	33	—

FOOD	PORTION	CAL	FAT	CARB	SUG
chocolate w/ chocolate frosting	⅛ cake (2.2 oz)	235	11	35	—
coffeecake cheese	⅙ cake (2.7 oz)	258	12	38	—
coffeecake crumb topped cheese	⅙ cake (2.7 oz)	258	12	38	—
coffeecake crumb topped cinnamon	⅑ cake (2.2 oz)	263	15	29	—
cream puff w/ custard filling	1 (4.6 oz)	336	20	30	—
french apple tart	1 (3.5 oz)	302	15	37	15
fruitcake	1/36 cake (2.9 oz)	302	10	54	—
gingerbread	⅑ cake (2.6 oz)	264	12	36	—
panettone	1/12 cake (2.9 oz)	300	12	43	21
petit fours	2 (0.9 oz)	120	7	15	12
pineapple upside down	⅑ cake (4 oz)	367	14	58	—
pound fat free	1 oz	80	tr	17	—
pound cake	1 slice (1 oz)	120	5	15	—
sacher torte	1 slice (2.2 oz)	240	11	30	11
sheet cake w/ white frosting	⅑ cake	445	14	77	—
strudel apple	1 piece (2½ oz)	195	8	29	—
tiramisu	1 piece (5.1 oz)	409	30	31	17
trifle w/ cream	6 oz	291	16	34	—
yellow w/ vanilla frosting	⅛ cake (2.2 oz)	239	9	38	—

CAKE ICING

Betty Crocker

FOOD	PORTION	CAL	FAT	CARB	SUG
HomeStyle Mix Coconut Pecan as prep	2 tbsp	160	2	21	17
HomeStyle Mix White Fluffy as prep	6 tbsp	100	0	24	23

FOOD	PORTION	CAL	FAT	CARB	SUG
Party Frosting Chocolate w/ Stars	2 tbsp (1.2 oz)	140	5	22	20
Rich & Creamy Butter Cream	2 tbsp (1.3 oz)	140	5	23	20
Rich & Creamy Cherry	2 tbsp (1.2 oz)	140	5	23	20
Rich & Creamy Chocolate	2 tbsp (1.2 oz)	130	5	21	17
Rich & Creamy Cream Cheese	2 tbsp (1.2 oz)	140	5	23	20
Rich & Creamy Vanilla	2 tbsp (1.2 oz)	140	5	23	20
Toppers Milk Chocolate	2 tbsp (1.2 oz)	130	5	22	18
Toppers Vanilla	2 tbsp (1.2 oz)	140	5	24	20
Sweet Rewards					
Ready-To-Spread Reduced Fat Chocolate	2 tbsp (1.2 oz)	120	2	24	22
Ready-To-Spread Reduced Fat Vanilla	2 tbsp (1.2 oz)	130	2	27	25
CAKE MIX					
Betty Crocker					
Angel Food Fat Free	1/12 cake	140	0	32	24
Cheesecake Chocolate Chip as prep	1/8 cake	410	28	32	23
Cheesecake Original as prep	1/8 cake	400	27	30	20
Cheesecake Strawberry Swirl as prep	1/8 cake	380	25	32	21
Pineapple Upside Down as prep	1/8 cake	420	14	64	43

FOOD	PORTION	CAL	FAT	CARB	SUG
Quick Bread Banana	1/12 cake	170	7	25	13
Quick Bread Cinnamon Streusel as prep	1/14 cake	180	7	26	15
Quick Bread Cranberry Orange as prep	1/12 cake	170	6	29	16
Quick Bread Lemon Poppy Seed as prep	1/12 cake	170	7	25	12
Stir'n Bake Carrot Cake w/ Cream Cheese Frosting as prep	1/6 cake	260	7	46	32
Stir'n Bake Coffee Cake w/Cinnamon Streusel as prep	1/6 cake	230	2	36	20
Stir'n Bake Devils Food w/ Chocolate Frosting as prep	1/6 cake	240	7	42	27
Stir'n Bake Yellow w/ Chocolate Frosting as prep	1/6 cake	240	7	43	26
SuperMoist Butter Pecan as prep	1/12 cake	240	10	35	20
SuperMoist Butter Yellow as prep	1/12 cake	260	11	36	20
SuperMoist Carrot as prep	1/10 cake	320	15	42	24
SuperMoist Cherry Chip	1/10 cake	300	13	41	23
SuperMoist Chocolate Fudge as prep	1/12 cake	270	12	35	21
SuperMoist Golden Vanilla as prep	1/12 cake	240	10	35	20
SuperMoist Lemon as prep	1/12 cake	240	10	35	20

FOOD	PORTION	CAL	FAT	CARB	SUG
SuperMoist Milk Chocolate as prep	½2 cake	240	10	34	20
SuperMoist Pineapple as prep	½2 cake	250	7	25	20
SuperMoist Spice as prep	½2 cake	240	10	36	20
SuperMoist Strawberry as prep	½2 cake	250	10	35	21
SuperMoist White as prep	½2 cake	230	14	34	18
SuperMoist White Light as prep	½0 cake	210	3	43	24
Bisquick					
Mix	⅓ cup (1.4 oz)	160	6	25	1
Reduced Fat	⅓ cup (1.4 oz)	140	3	27	3
Hodgson Mill					
Gingerbread Whole Wheat	¼ cup (1 oz)	110	0	24	10
Sweet Rewards					
Reduced Fat White as prep	½2 cake	180	3	36	20
Reduced Fat Yellow as prep	½2 cake	200	5	37	21

CALABAZA
fresh	⅓ cup	32	tr	8	—

CALZONE
take-out
cheese	1 (12 oz)	1020	54	86	26

CANADIAN BACON
Boar's Head
Canadian Bacon	2 oz	70	3	1	1

FOOD	PORTION	CAL	FAT	CARB	SUG
Hormel					
Sandwich Style	3 slices (2 oz)	70	3	0	0
Oscar Mayer					
Canandian Bacon	2 slices (1.6 oz)	50	2	0	0
CANADIAN BACON SUBSTITUTES					
Yves					
Canadian Veggie Bacon	1 serv (2 oz)	80	1	1	1
CANDY					
candied cherries	1 (4 g)	12	tr	3	—
candied citron	1 oz	89	tr	23	—
candied lemon peel	1 oz	90	tr	23	—
candied orange peel	1 oz	90	tr	23	—
candied pineapple slice	1 slice (2 oz)	179	tr	45	—
candy corn	1 oz	105	0	27	—
crisped rice bar chocolate chip	1 bar (1 oz)	115	4	21	9
milk chocolate w/ almonds	1 bar (1.45 oz)	215	14	22	20
peanuts chocolate covered	10 (1.4 oz)	208	13	20	—
pretzels chocolate covered	1 (0.4 oz)	50	2	8	—
sesame crunch	20 pieces (1.2 oz)	181	12	18	—
100 Grand					
Bar	1 bar (1.5 oz)	200	8	30	27
Andes					
Chocolate Covered Mint Patties	1 (0.5 oz)	60	1	13	12
Baby Ruth					
Bar	1 bar (2.1 oz)	270	13	36	27
Fun Size	1 bar (1 oz)	130	6	17	13

FOOD	PORTION	CAL	FAT	CARB	SUG
Barricini					
Dark Chocolate Raspberry Creme Shells	1 piece (0.3 oz)	47	3	5	4
Bittyfinger					
Bars	2	170	7	27	18
Body Smarts					
Chocolate Peanut Crunch	2 bars (1.8 oz)	210	6	34	20
Butterfinger					
BB's	1 pkg (1.7 oz)	230	9	33	25
Bar	1 (2.1 oz)	270	11	42	29
Fun Size	1 bar	100	4	15	10
Cape Cod Provisions					
Cranberry Bog Frogs	3 pieces (1.9 oz)	250	12	34	27
Charms					
Blow Pop	1 (0.6 oz)	70	0	17	14
Lollipop Sour	1 (0.6 oz)	70	0	18	17
Lollipop Sweet	1 (0.6 oz)	70	0	18	17
Chunky					
Bar	1 (1.4 oz)	210	11	24	21
Crunch					
Fun Size	4 bars	210	11	26	22
Del Monte					
Radical Raizins Cinnamon	1 pkg (0.7 oz)	70	0	18	16
Radical Raizins Rainbow	1 pkg (0.7 oz)	70	0	18	16
Estee					
Caramels Vanilla & Chocolate	5	115	5	26	3

FOOD	PORTION	CAL	FAT	CARB	SUG
Dark Chocolate	½ bar (1.4 oz)	200	14	23	15
Milk Chocolate	½ bar (1.4 oz)	230	17	17	15
Milk Chocolate w/ Almonds	½ bar (1.4 oz)	230	17	16	14
Milk Chocolate w/ Crisp Rice	½ bar (1.2 oz)	370	26	29	24
Milk Chocolate w/ Fruit & Nuts	½ bar (1.4 oz)	220	16	18	15
Mint Chocolate	½ bar (1.4 oz)	200	14	23	15
Peanut Brittle	⅓ box (1.3 oz)	160	9	28	1
Peanut Butter Cups	5	200	12	19	13
Sugar Free Assorted Fruit	5	30	0	16	0
Sugar Free Assorted Mint	5	30	0	16	0
Sugar Free Butterscotch	2	25	0	12	0
Sugar Free Fruit Gum Drops	23	80	0	36	0
Sugar Free Gourmet Jelly Beans	26	70	0	24	0
Sugar Free Gummy Bears Assorted Fruit	17	100	0	30	0
Sugar Free Licorice Gum Drops	11	90	0	36	0
Sugar Free Peppermint Swirl	3	30	0	14	0
Sugar Free Sour Citrus Slices	9	60	0	30	0
Sugar Free Toffee	5	30	0	16	0
Sugar Free Tropical Fruit	5	30	0	16	0

FOOD	PORTION	CAL	FAT	CARB	SUG
Favorite Brands					
Candy Corn	24 pieces (1.4 oz)	150	0	37	34
Circus Peanuts	5 pieces (1.6 oz)	160	0	39	33
Gummi Bears	18 pieces (1.4 oz)	130	0	30	19
Jelly Beans	13 (1.4 oz)	150	0	37	28
Marshmallow Eggs	3 (1.3 oz)	140	0	34	32
Godiva					
Chocolatier Dark Chocolate w/ Raspberry	1 bar (1.5 oz)	220	11	28	22
Chocolatier Milk Chocolate	1 bar (1.5 ox)	230	13	26	25
Mochaccino Mousse	2 pieces (1.25 oz)	210	15	17	14
Truffles Assorted	2 pieces (1.5 oz)	220	13	24	20
Goetze's					
Cow Tales	1 pkg (1 oz)	110	3	20	11
Goobers					
Peanuts	1 pkg (1.38 oz)	210	13	20	17
Haviland					
Chocolate Covered Thin Mints	6 (1.5 oz)	170	5	33	32
Hershey					
Amazin'Fruit Gummy Candy	1 snack pkg (0.7 oz)	60	0	15	10
Bar	1 (0.6 oz)	100	6	9	—
Kisses	1	25	2	3	—
Milk Chocolate	1 bar (0.6 oz)	90	5	10	—
Milk Chocolate w/ Almonds	1 bar (0.6 oz)	100	6	9	—
PayDay Snack Size	1 (0.66 oz)	90	5	11	8
ReeseSticks Snack Size	2 pieces (1.2 oz)	190	11	19	14

FOOD	PORTION	CAL	FAT	CARB	SUG
Sweet Escapes Triple Chocolate Wafer	1 bar (0.7 oz)	80	3	14	12
Jolly Rancher					
Lollipops All Flavors	1 (0.6 oz)	60	0	16	12
Junior Mints					
Snack Size	1 pkg (0.7 oz)	75	1	16	16
Just Born					
Hot Tamales	1 pkg (2.1 oz)	220	0	55	34
Mike and Ike Original	1 pkg (1.2 oz)	220	0	55	34
Super Hot Tamales	1 pkg (2.1 oz)	220	0	55	34
Teenee Beanee Assorted Fruits	36 pieces (1.4 oz)	150	0	36	23
Kit Kat					
Bar	1 (0.56 oz)	80	4	10	—
Krackel					
Bar	1 (0.6 oz)	90	5	11	—
Lance					
Chocolaty Peanut Bar	1 (2 oz)	290	15	32	23
Cinnamon Chews	1 pkg (1.06 oz)	120	1	28	22
Fruit Chews	1 pkg (1.06 oz)	120	1	28	22
Gum Ball Pops	1 (0.45 oz)	45	0	12	12
Mint Chews	1 pkg (1.06 oz)	120	1	28	22
Peanut Bar	1 (1.75 oz)	270	15	23	15
Pop-A-Lance	1 piece (0.42 oz)	45	0	11	10
Popcorn'n'Carmel	1 bar (0.75 oz)	90	0	20	14
Strawberry Chews	1 pkg (1.06 oz)	120	1	28	22
Suckers	3 pieces (0.5 oz)	50	0	13	10
Whistle Pop	1 (0.67 oz)	70	0	19	17
Lifesavers					
Gummi Shapes	1 pkg (0.8 oz)	70	0	18	13
Barnum's Animals					

FOOD	PORTION	CAL	FAT	CARB	SUG
Lindt					
Truffles Milk Chocolate	3 pieces (1.3 oz)	210	17	15	15
Milk Duds					
Snack Size	4 boxes (1.3 oz)	160	6	26	18
Mounds					
Bar	1 (0.68 oz)	90	5	11	—
Mr. Goodbar					
Miniature	1 (0.3 oz)	45	3	4	—
Necco					
Bridge Mix	¼ cup (1.5 oz)	180	9	27	23
Chocolate Covered Raisins	30 pieces (1.5 oz)	170	7	30	27
Malted Milk Balls	11 pieces (1.5 oz)	180	6	28	25
SkyBar	1 bar (1.5 oz)	190	9	28	25
Nestle					
Crunch	1 bar (1.55 oz)	230	12	29	24
Milk Chocolate	1 bar (1.45 oz)	220	13	26	24
Treasures Butterfinger	3 pieces	180	9	24	19
Treasures Crunch	4 pieces (1.4 oz)	210	11	26	21
Treasures Peanut Butter	4 pieces	250	17	23	21
Turtles	2 pieces (1.2 oz)	160	9	20	15
Turtles Bite Size	1 piece (0.4 oz)	50	2	6	5
White Crunch	1 bar (1.4 oz)	220	13	23	20
Newman's Own					
Organic Peanut Butter Cups Dark Chocolate	3 pieces (1.2 oz)	180	12	18	14
Organic Peanut Butter Cups Milk Chocolate	3 pieces (1.2 oz)	180	12	18	14
Organic Peppermint Cups	3 pieces (1.2 oz)	180	12	20	18

FOOD	PORTION	CAL	FAT	CARB	SUG
Nips					
Butter Rum	2 pieces	60	2	11	7
Caramel	2 pieces	60	2	11	7
Chocolate	2 pieces	60	2	11	7
Coffee	2 pieces	50	2	10	7
Oh Henry!					
Bar	1 (1.8 oz)	120	5	16	12
Palmer					
Milk Chocolate Lollipop	1 (0.9 oz)	130	7	16	15
Pearson's					
Irish Cream Parfait	2 pieces	60	2	10	6
Mint Patties	5 (1.3 oz)	150	3	31	27
Pez					
Candy	1 roll (0.3 oz)	35	0	9	9
Candy Sugar Free	1 roll (0.3 oz)	30	0	8	0
Raisinets					
Candy	1 pkg (1.58 oz)	200	8	31	28
Fun Size	3 pkg (1.7 oz)	200	8	43	29
Reese's					
FastBreak	1 bar (2 oz)	270	13	34	30
ResseSticks Peanut Butter	2 pieces (1.2 oz)	190	11	19	14
Rokeach					
Cotton Candy	2 cups (1 oz)	110	0	28	28
Russell Stover					
Peanut Butter & Grape Jelly	1 piece (0.8 oz)	100	6	10	8
Pecan Delights	1 pkg (1.8 oz)	250	17	22	14
Pecan Roll	1 (1.75 oz)	260	18	23	19
S'mores	3 (1.4 oz)	210	12	22	18

FOOD	PORTION	CAL	FAT	CARB	SUG
Simply Lite					
Sugar Free Lil'l Bits Chocolately	36 pieces (1.4 oz)	130	5	28	0
Sugar Free Lil'l Bits Peanut Buttery	36 pieces (1.4 oz)	140	5	26	0
Sugar Free Patteez	5 pieces (1.3 oz)	110	3	29	0
Smucker's					
Fruit Fillers Strawberry	1 pkg (0.9 oz)	80	0	19	13
Snickers					
Cruncher	3 fun size (1.4 oz)	230	13	25	18
Sno Caps					
Candies	1 pkg (2.3 oz)	300	13	48	38
Steel's					
Salt Water Taffy Assorted	3 pieces (1 oz)	90	1	22	16
Swedish Fish					
Original	19 pieces (1.4 oz)	160	0	39	24
Sweet'N Low					
Sugar Free Cinnamon	1 piece	7	0	4	—
Sugar Free Fruit Flavors	1 piece	7	0	4	—
Tobler					
Orange Dark Chocolate	5 pieces (1.5 oz)	210	13	28	25
Tom's					
Cherry Sours	1 pkg (2.25 oz)	210	0	53	38
Jelly Beans	1 pkg (2.25 oz)	230	0	58	44
Twix					
Caramel	1 fun size (0.5 oz)	80	4	10	8
York					
Chocolate Covered Peppermint Bites	15 pieces (1 oz)	150	3	31	29
Peppermint Patty	1 (0.49 oz)	50	1	11	8

FOOD	PORTION	CAL	FAT	CARB	SUG
CANTALOUPE					
dried	3.5 pieces (1.4 oz)	140	0	34	32
Chiquita					
Wedge	¼ med (4.7 oz)	50	0	12	11
CARAWAY					
seed	1 tsp	7	tr	1	—
CARDAMON					
ground	1 tsp	6	tr	1	—
CARDOON					
fresh cooked	3½ oz	22	tr	5	—
CARIBOU					
roasted	3 oz	142	4	0	0
CARISSA					
fresh	1	12	tr	3	—
CAROB					
flour	1 tbsp	14	tr	7	—
CARP					
fresh cooked	3 oz	138	6	0	0
roe raw	1 oz	37	tr	tr	—
CARROT JUICE					
canned	6 oz	73	tr	17	—
CARROTS					
canned					
Green Giant					
Sliced	½ cup (4.2 oz)	25	0	6	3
LeSueur					
Baby Whole	½ cup (4.2 oz)	35	0	8	5
fresh					
baby raw	1 (½ oz)	6	tr	1	—
raw	1 (2.5 oz)	31	tr	7	—

FOOD	PORTION	CAL	FAT	CARB	SUG
raw shredded	½ cup	24	tr	6	—
slices cooked	½ cup	35	tr	8	—
Dole					
Shredded	1 cup (3 oz)	40	0	9	5
frozen					
Green Giant					
Harvest Fresh Baby	⅔ cup (3 oz)	20	0	5	3
Select Baby Cut	¾ cup (2.8 oz)	30	0	7	3
CASABA					
cubed	1 cup	45	tr	11	—
fresh	⅒	43	tr	10	—
CASHEWS					
Frito Lay					
Salted	1 oz	180	15	7	2
Lance					
Cashews	1 pkg (1⅛ oz)	200	16	8	3
Planters					
Fancy Oil Roasted	1 oz	170	14	8	tr
Halves Lightly Salted Oil Roasted	1 oz	160	13	9	0
Honey Roasted	1 oz	150	12	11	5
Munch'N Go Honey Roasted	1 pkg (2 oz)	310	24	23	7
Munch'N Go Singles Oil Roasted	1 pkg (2 oz)	330	28	16	1
CASSAVA					
raw	3½ oz	120	tr	27	—
CATFISH					
channel breaded & fried	3 oz	194	11	7	—

FOOD	PORTION	CAL	FAT	CARB	SUG
CATSUP					
(*see* KETCHUP)					
CAULIFLOWER					
fresh					
cooked	½ cup (2.2 oz)	14	tr	3	—
flowerets cooked	3 (2 oz)	12	tr	2	—
flowerets raw	3 (2 oz)	14	tr	3	—
green cooked	1½ cup (3.2 oz)	29	tr	6	—
green raw floweret	1 (0.9 oz)	8	tr	2	—
frozen					
Green Giant					
Cheese Sauce	½ cup (3.5 oz)	60	3	8	4
Florets	1 cup (2.8 oz)	25	0	4	1
CAVIAR					
black	1 tbsp	40	3	1	—
red	1 tbsp	40	3	1	—
CELERIAC					
fresh cooked	3½ oz	25	tr	6	—
raw	½ cup	31	tr	7	—
CELERY					
diced cooked	½ cup	13	tr	3	—
fresh	1 stalk (1.3 oz)	6	tr	1	—
raw diced	½ cup	10	tr	2	—
seed	1 tsp	8	tr	1	—
CELTUCE					
raw	3½ oz	22	tr	4	—
CEREAL					
Albers					
Hominy Quick Grits uncooked	¼ cup	140	1	31	0

FOOD	PORTION	CAL	FAT	CARB	SUG
Alpen					
Corn Flakes	1 serv (1 oz)	110	tr	25	0
No Salt No Sugar	1 serv (2 oz)	200	3	34	10
Regular	1 serv (2 oz)	200	3	37	17
Barbara's					
Shredded Spoonfuls	¾ cup (1.1 oz)	120	2	23	5
Barbara's Bakery					
Bite Size Shredded Oats	1¼ cups (2 oz)	220	3	46	12
Cinnamon Puffins	1¼ cup (2 oz)	100	1	26	6
Cocoa Crunch Stars	1 cup (1 oz)	110	1	26	8
Frosted Corn Flakes	1 cup (1 oz)	110	1	27	8
Fruit Juice Sweetened Breakfast O's	1 cup (1 oz)	120	2	22	2
Fruit Juice Sweetened Brown Rice Crisps	1 cup (1 oz)	120	1	25	2
Fruit Juice Sweetened Corn Flakes	1 cup (1 oz)	110	0	26	3
GrainShop	⅔ cup (1 oz)	90	1	24	5
Honey Crunch Stars	1 cup (1 oz)	110	0	26	8
Honey Nut Toasted O's	¾ cup	120	2	23	11
Organic Fruity Punch	1 cup (1 oz)	110	1	26	8
Organic Soy Essence	¾ cup (1 oz)	100	1	25	5
Puffins	¾ cup (0.9 oz)	90	1	23	5
Shredded Spoonfuls	¾ cup (1.1 oz)	110	2	23	5
Shredded Wheat	2 biscuits (1.4 oz)	140	1	31	0
General Mills					
Basic 4	1 cup (1.9 oz)	200	2	42	14
Boo Berry	1 cup (1 oz)	120	1	27	14
Cheerios	1 cup (1 oz)	110	2	22	1
Cheerios Apple Cinnamon	¾ cup (1 oz)	120	2	25	13

FOOD	PORTION	CAL	FAT	CARB	SUG
Cheerios Frosted	1 cup (1 oz)	120	1	25	13
Cheerios Honey Nut	1 cup (1 oz)	120	2	24	11
Cheerios Multi Grain	1 cup (1 oz)	110	1	24	8
Cheerios Team	1 cup (1 oz)	120	1	25	11
Chex Corn	1 cup (1 oz)	110	0	26	3
Chex Honey Nut	¾ cup	120	1	26	9
Chex Morning Mix Cinnamon	1 pkg (1.1 oz)	130	4	24	8
Chex Morning Mix Fruit & Nut	1 pkg (1.1 oz)	180	4	24	8
Chex Morning Mix Honey Nut	1 pkg (1.1 oz)	130	4	24	8
Chex Multi-Bran	1 cup (2 oz)	200	2	49	12
Chex Rice	1¼ cup (1.1 oz)	120	0	27	2
Cinnamon Grahams	¾ cup (1 oz)	120	1	26	11
Cinnamon Toast Crunch	¾ cup (1 oz)	130	4	24	10
Cocoa Puffs	1 cup (1 oz)	120	1	26	14
Cookie Crisp	1 cup (1 oz)	120	1	26	13
Count Chocula	1 cup (1 oz)	120	1	26	14
Country Corn Flakes	1 cup (1 oz)	120	0	26	2
Fiber One	½ cup (1 oz)	60	1	24	0
Franken Berry	1 cup (1 oz)	120	1	27	14
French Toast Crunch	¾ cup (1 oz)	120	1	26	12
Gold Medal Raisin Bran	1⅓ cups (1.9 oz)	170	2	41	12
Golden Grahams	¾ cup (1 oz)	120	1	25	10
Harmony	1¼ cups (1.9 oz)	200	4	44	13
Honey Nut Clusters	1 cup (1.9 oz)	210	3	46	17
Kaboom	1¼ cup (1 oz)	120	1	24	8
Kix	1⅓ cup (1 oz)	120	1	26	3
Kix Berry Berry	¾ cup (1 oz)	120	2	26	9

FOOD	PORTION	CAL	FAT	CARB	SUG
Lucky Charms	1 cup (1 oz)	120	1	25	13
Nature Valley Low Fat Fruit Granola	⅔ cup (1.9 oz)	210	3	44	19
Newquick	¾ cup (1 oz)	120	2	25	12
Oatmeal Crisp Almond	1 cup (1.9 oz)	220	5	42	16
Oatmeal Crisp Apple Cinnamon	1 cup (1.9 oz)	210	2	45	19
Oatmeal Crisp Raisin	1 cup (1.9 oz)	210	2	44	18
Para Su Familia Cinnamon Stars	1 cup (1 oz)	120	1	28	6
Para Su Familia Fruitis	1 cup (1 oz)	120	1	25	6
Para Su Familia Raisin Bran	1¼ cups (2 oz)	170	2	41	12
Raisin Nut Bran	¾ cup (1.9 oz)	200	4	41	18
Reese's Puffs	¾ cup	130	3	23	13
Snack'N Dash Cinnamon Toast Crunch	1 pkg (1.2 oz)	140	4	27	12
Snack'N Dash Honey Nut Cheerios	1 pkg (1 oz)	110	1	23	10
Snack'N Dash Lucky Charms	1 pkg (1 oz)	110	1	24	12
Sunrise Organic	¾ cup (1 oz)	110	1	25	10
Total Brown Sugar & Oat	¾ cup (1 oz)	110	1	23	9
Total Corn Flakes	1⅓ cup (1 oz)	110	0	24	4
Total Raisin Bran	1 cup (1.9 oz)	170	1	41	20
Total Whole Grain	¾ cup (1 oz)	110	1	23	5
Trix	1 cup (1 oz)	120	1	27	13
Wheaties	1 cup (1 oz)	110	1	24	4
Wheaties Energy Crunch	1 cup (1.9 oz)	210	3	42	13

FOOD	PORTION	CAL	FAT	CARB	SUG
Wheaties Frosted	¾ cup (1 oz)	110	1	27	12
Wheaties Raisin Bran	1 cup (1.9 oz)	180	1	45	18
Grainfield's					
Brown Rice	1 serv (1 oz)	110	1	24	1
Crisp Rice	1 serv (1 oz)	112	tr	25	0
Raisin Bran	1 serv (1 oz)	90	2	20	tr
Wheat Flakes	1 serv (1 oz)	100	1	20	tr
Health Valley					
Golden Flax	½ cup	190	3	38	8
Granola 98% Fat Free Date Almond	⅔ cup	180	1	43	10
Healthy Crunches & Flakes Almond	¾ cup	130	0	31	4
Organic Bran w/ Raisin	¾ cup	160	0	40	10
Organic Fiber 7 Flakes	¾ cup	100	0	24	4
Organic Oat Bran Flakes	¾ cup	100	0	24	4
Real Oat Bran	½ cup	200	3	34	9
Hodgson Mill					
Cracked Wheat	¼ cup (1.4 oz)	110	1	26	0
Multi Grain w/ Flaxseed & Soy	⅓ cup (1.4 oz)	160	3	25	1
Kashi					
Breakfast Pilaf as prep	½ cup (4.9 oz)	170	3	30	0
Go Apple Spice	½ cup (4.9 oz)	270	3	56	10
Go Banana Almond	½ cup (4.9 oz)	280	4	57	11
Go Berry Tart	½ cup (4.9 oz)	260	3	55	8
Go Blueberry Bliss	½ cup (4.9 oz)	260	3	55	8
Go Cherry Vanilla	½ cup (4.9 oz)	260	3	54	15

FOOD	PORTION	CAL	FAT	CARB	SUG
Go Just Peachy	½ cup (4.9 oz)	260	3	54	17
GoLean	¾ cup (1.4 oz)	120	1	28	7
Good Friends	¾ cup (1 oz)	90	1	24	6
Honey Puffed	1 cup (1 oz)	120	1	25	7
Medley	½ cup (1 oz)	100	1	20	5
Pillows Apple	¾ cup (1.9 oz)	200	1	45	19
Pillows Chocolate	¾ cup (1.9 oz)	200	1	45	19
Pillows Strawberry Crisp	¾ cup (1.9 oz)	200	1	46	19
Puffed	1 cup (0.9 oz)	70	tr	13	0
Kellogg's					
All-Bran	½ cup (1.1 oz)	80	1	24	6
Apple Jacks	1 cup (1.2 oz)	120	0	30	16
Cocoa Krispies	¾ cup (1.1 oz)	120	1	27	13
Corn Flakes	1 cup (1 oz)	100	0	24	2
Cracklin' Oat Bran	¾ cup (1.7 oz)	190	7	35	15
Crispix	1 cup (1 oz)	110	0	25	3
Frosted Flakes	¾ cup (1.1 oz)	120	0	28	13
Granola Low Fat	½ cup (1.7 oz)	190	3	39	14
Mini-Wheat Frosted	1 cup (1.8 oz)	180	1	41	10
Product 19	1 cup (1 oz)	100	0	25	4
Raisin Bran	1 cup (2.1 oz)	200	2	47	18
Rice Krispies	1¼ cup (1.2 oz)	120	0	29	3
Smart Start	1 cup (1.8 oz)	180	1	43	15
Special K	1 cup (1.1 oz)	110	0	21	4
Lundberg					
Purely Organic Hot'n Creamy Rice	⅓ cup	190	2	43	0
Nabisco					
100% Bran	⅓ cup (1 oz)	80	1	23	7
Cream Of Wheat Quick as prep	1 cup	120	0	25	0

FOOD	PORTION	CAL	FAT	CARB	SUG
Original Shredded Wheat	2 biscuits (1.6 oz)	160	1	38	0
Original Shredded Wheat Spoon Size	1 cup (1.7 oz)	170	1	41	0
Nutri-Grain					
Almond Raisin	1¼ cup (2 oz)	200	3	43	8
Golden Wheat	¾ cup (1.1 oz)	100	1	24	0
Post					
Alpha-Bits	1 cup (1 oz)	130	2	27	13
Cocoa Pebbles	¾ cup (1 oz)	120	1	26	13
Grape-Nuts	¾ cup (1 oz)	100	1	24	5
Grape-Nuts Flakes	¾ cup (1 oz)	100	1	24	5
Honey Bunches Of Oats	¾ cup (1 oz)	120	2	25	6
Honeycomb	1⅓ cups (1 oz)	110	1	26	11
Raisin Bran	1 cup (2 oz)	190	1	47	20
Selects Blueberry Morning	¾ cup (1.3 oz)	140	2	30	9
Quaker					
Oatmeal Instant	1 pkg (1 oz)	100	2	19	0
Oatmeal Instant Apples & Cinnamon	1 pkg (1.2 oz)	130	2	27	12
Oatmeal Instant Cinnamon & Spice	1 pkg (1.6 oz)	170	2	35	16
Oatmeal Instant Maple & Brown Sugar	1 pkg (1.5 oz)	160	2	32	13
Oatmeal Nutrition for Women Golden Brown Sugar	1 pkg (1.6 oz)	170	2	33	13
Oats Old Fashion	½ cup (1.4 oz)	150	3	27	1
Oats Quick	½ cup (1.4 oz)	150	3	27	1

FOOD	PORTION	CAL	FAT	CARB	SUG
Sunbelt					
Granola Banana Nut	½ cup (1.9 oz)	250	9	37	13
Granola Cinnamon Raisins	½ cup (1.9 oz)	200	3	42	20
Granola Fruit & Nut	½ cup (1.9 oz)	240	7	40	21
Muesli 5 Whole Grains	½ cup (1.9 oz)	210	2	44	17
Uncle Sam					
Cereal	1 cup (1.9 oz)	190	1	38	tr
Weetabix					
Cereal	2 biscuits (1.2 oz)	100	1	21	2
Wheatena					
Cereal	⅓ cup (1.4 oz)	150	1	33	0

CEREAL BARS

FOOD	PORTION	CAL	FAT	CARB	SUG
Barbara's Bakery					
Nature's Choice Apple Cinnamon	1 bar (1.3 oz)	120	2	27	11
Nature's Choice Blueberry	1 bar (⅓ oz)	120	2	27	11
Nature's Choice Cherry	1 bar (1.3 oz)	120	2	27	11
Nature's Choice Granola Carob Chip	1 bar (0.7 oz)	80	2	16	8
Nature's Choice Granola Cinnamon & Raisin	1 bar (0.7 oz)	80	2	16	7
Nature's Choice Granola Oats 'N Honey	1 bar (0.7 oz)	80	2	15	7
Nature's Choice Granola Peanut Butter	1 bar (0.7 oz)	80	3	14	7
Nature's Choice Raspberry	1 bar (1.3 oz)	120	2	27	11

FOOD	PORTION	CAL	FAT	CARB	SUG
Nature's Choice Strawberry	1 bar (1.3 oz)	120	2	27	11
Nature's Choice Triple Berry	1 bar (1.3 oz)	120	2	27	11
Dolly Madison					
Apple	1 (1.3 oz)	120	2	25	14
Blueberry	1 (1.3 oz)	120	2	25	14
Entenmann's					
Apple Cinnamon	1 (1.3 oz)	140	3	25	15
Blueberry	1 (1.3 oz)	140	3	25	15
Raspberry	1 (1.3 oz)	140	3	27	15
Strawberry	1 (1.3 oz)	140	3	25	15
Estee					
Rice Crunchie Chocolate	1 (0.7 oz)	50	0	15	0
Rice Crunchie Peanut Butter	1 (0.7 oz)	60	1	15	0
Rice Crunchie Vanilla	1 (0.7 oz)	60	0	14	0
General Mills					
Milk 'N Cereal Bars Chex	1 bar (1.6 oz)	160	4	26	13
Milk 'N Cereal Bars Cinnamon Toast Crunch	1 bar (1.6 oz)	180	4	30	19
Hershey's					
Crispy Rice Snacks Peanut Butter	1 bar (0.5 oz)	60	2	9	5
Kellogg's					
Nutri-Grain Apple Cinnamon	1 (1.3 oz)	140	3	27	13
Rice Krispies Treats	1 (0.8 oz)	90	2	18	8

FOOD	PORTION	CAL	FAT	CARB	SUG
Kudos					
Low Fat Blueberry	1 (0.7 oz)	90	2	15	7
Sunbelt					
Apple	1 (1.3 oz)	130	3	28	18
Weight Watchers					
Apple Cinnamon	1 (1 oz)	100	2	21	12
Blueberry	1 (1 oz)	100	2	21	10
Raspberry	1 (1 oz)	100	2	21	12

CHAMPAGNE

sekt german champagne	3.5 fl oz	84	0	5	—

CHAYOTE

fresh cooked	1 cup	38	1	8	—

CHEESE

beaufort	1 oz	115	9	tr	tr
blue crumbled	1 cup (4.7 oz)	477	39	3	—
brie	1 oz	95	8	tr	—
camembert	1 oz	85	7	tr	—
cantal	1 oz	105	9	tr	tr
chabichou	1 oz	95	8	tr	tr
chaource	1 oz	83	7	tr	tr
comte	1 oz	114	9	tr	tr
coulommiers	1 oz	88	7	tr	tr
crottin	1 oz	105	9	tr	tr
edam	1 oz	101	8	tr	—
edam reduced fat	1.4 oz	92	4	tr	—
feta	1 oz	75	6	1	—
goat fresh	1 oz	23	2	tr	tr
gouda	1 oz	101	8	1	—
gruyere	1 oz	117	9	tr	—

FOOD	PORTION	CAL	FAT	CARB	SUG
maroilles	1 oz	97	8	tr	tr
morbier	1 oz	99	8	tr	tr
picodon	1 oz	99	8	tr	tr
pont l'eveque	1 oz	86	7	tr	tr
provolone	1 oz	100	8	1	—
pyrenees	1 oz	101	8	tr	tr
raclette	1 oz	102	8	tr	tr
reblochon	1 oz	88	7	tr	tr
rouy	1 oz	95	8	tr	tr
saint marcellin	1 oz	94	8	tr	tr
saint nectaire	1 oz	97	8	tr	tr
saint paulin	1 oz	85	6	tr	tr
sainte maure	1 oz	99	8	tr	tr
selles sur cher	1 oz	93	8	tr	tr
tome	1 oz	92	7	tr	tr
triple creme	1 oz	113	11	tr	tr
vacherin	1 oz	92	8	tr	tr
whey cheese	1 oz	126	8	9	0
yogurt cheese	1 oz	80	7	0	0
Alouette					
Garlic & Herbs	2 tbsp (0.8 oz)	70	7	1	tr
Alpine Lace					
American Jalapeno Peppers	1 slice (1 oz)	80	6	2	0
American Less Fat Less Sodium White	1 slice (1 oz)	50	6	2	0
American Less Fat Less Sodium Yellow	1 slice (1 oz)	80	6	2	0
Cheddar Reduced Fat	1 slice (1 oz)	70	5	1	0
Colby Reduced Fat	1 slice (1 oz)	80	5	1	0
Fat Free Parmesan	2 tsp (5 g)	10	0	0	0

FOOD	PORTION	CAL	FAT	CARB	SUG
Feta Reduced Fat	1 oz	50	3	1	0
Feta Reduced Fat Sun Dried Tomato & Basil	1 oz	50	3	1	0
Goat Reduced Fat	1 oz	40	3	tr	0
Mozzarella Reduced Fat	1 oz	70	3	1	0
Muenster Reduced Sodium	1 slice (1 oz)	100	9	1	0
Provolone Smoked Reduced Fat	1 slice (1 oz)	70	5	1	0
Swiss Reduced Fat	1 slice (1 oz)	90	6	1	0
Boar's Head					
American	1 oz	100	9	1	0
Baby Swiss	1 oz	110	9	tr	0
Canadian Cheddar	1 oz	110	10	0	0
Havarti	1 oz	110	10	0	0
Lacey Swiss	1 oz	90	6	0	0
Longhorn Colby	1 oz	110	9	tr	0
Monterey Jack	1 oz	100	9	0	0
Monterey Jack w/ Jalapeno	1 oz	100	9	0	0
Mozzarella	1 oz	90	7	tr	0
Muenster	1 oz	100	8	0	0
Muenster Low Sodium	1 oz	100	8	0	0
Provolone Picante Sharp	1 oz	100	8	1	0
Swiss	1 oz	110	8	tr	0
Swiss No Salt Added	1 oz	110	8	tr	0
Cabot					
Cheddar	1 oz	110	9	tr	0
Cheddar Five Peppercorn	1 oz	110	9	tr	0

FOOD	PORTION	CAL	FAT	CARB	SUG
Cheddar Mediterranean	1 oz	110	9	tr	0
Cheddar Sundried Tomato Basil	1 oz	110	9	tr	0
Cheddar Toasted Onion & Chive	1 oz	110	9	tr	0
Cheddar Light 50% Reduced Fat	1 oz	70	5	1	0
Cheddar Light 50% Reduced Fat Jalapeno	1 oz	70	5	1	0
Cheddar Light 50% Reduced Fat Tomato Basil	1 oz	70	5	1	0
Cheddar Light 75% Reduced Fat	1 oz	60	3	1	0
Dehyrdated Cheddar Powder	2 tsp (5 g)	25	2	1	1
Monterey Jack	1 oz	110	9	tr	0
Cedar Grove					
Marble Colby	1 oz	110	9	0	0
Organic Tomato Basil Cheddar	1 oz	110	9	0	0
Cheez Whiz					
Light	2 tbsp (1.2 oz)	80	3	6	3
Cracker Barrel					
Baby Swiss	1 oz	110	9	0	0
Cheddar Extra Sharp	1 oz	120	10	0	0
Cheddar Sharp	1 oz	120	10	0	0
Reduced Fat Cheddar Sharp	1 oz	90	6	tr	0
Di Giorno					
Parmesan Grated	2 tsp (5 g)	25	2	0	0
Romano Grated	2 tsp (5 g)	25	2	0	0

FOOD	PORTION	CAL	FAT	CARB	SUG
Fleurs De France					
Brie	3.5 oz	311	25	tr	0
Friendship					
Farmer	2 tbsp (1 oz)	50	3	0	0
Handi-Snacks					
Mozzarella String Cheese	1 piece (1 oz)	80	6	0	0
Kraft					
Singles American	1 (0.7 oz)	60	5	2	1
Singles Reduced Fat American	1 (0.7 oz)	50	3	2	2
Singles Swiss	1 slice (0.7 oz)	70	5	1	1
Slices Swiss	1 (0.8 oz)	90	7	0	0
Land O Lakes					
American	1 slice (0.7 oz)	80	6	1	0
American Jalapeno	1 slice (0.6 oz)	70	6	1	tr
American Light	1 oz	70	5	2	0
American Reduced Salt	1 oz	110	9	tr	0
American Sharp	2 slices (1 oz)	100	9	1	tr
American & Swiss	1 slice (0.6 oz)	70	5	1	0
Baby Swiss	1 oz	110	0	0	0
Chedarella	1 oz	100	8	0	0
Cheddar	1 oz	100	9	tr	0
Cheddar Extra Sharp	1 oz	110	8	tr	0
Cheddar Sharp	1 oz	110	9	tr	0
Cheese Spread Golden Velvet	1 oz	80	6	2	2
Colby	1 oz	110	9	tr	0
Jalapeno Light	1 oz	70	4	1	0
Monterey Jack	1 oz	110	8	tr	0
Monterey Jack Hot Pepper	1 oz	110	8	tr	0

FOOD	PORTION	CAL	FAT	CARB	SUG
Mozzarella	1 oz	80	6	tr	0
Muenster	1 oz	100	8	0	0
Parmesan Grated	1 tbsp	35	4	0	0
Provolone	1 oz	100	8	tr	0
Swiss	1 oz	110	8	tr	0
Swiss Light	1 oz	80	4	tr	0
Organic Valley					
Aged Swiss Unpasteurized	1 oz	100	8	tr	0
Cheddar Reduced Fat Low Sodium	1 oz	90	6	1	0
Cheddar Sharp & Mild	1 oz	110	9	1	0
Cheddar Sharp & Mild Unpasteurized	1 oz	110	9	1	0
Colby	1 oz	110	9	1	0
Colby Unpasteurized	1 oz	110	9	1	0
Farmer Reduced Fat	1 oz	90	6	1	0
Feta	1 oz	90	7	0	0
Monterey Jack	1 oz	100	8	1	0
Monterey Jack Reduced Fat	1 oz	80	5	1	0
Mozzarella Part Skim	1 oz	80	5	1	0
Muenster	1 oz	100	8	1	0
Pepper Jack	1 oz	110	9	1	0
Provolone	1 oz	100	8	1	0
String Part Skim	1 oz	80	5	1	0
Wisconsin Raw Milk Cheese	1 oz	100	8	1	0
Polly-O					
String Lite	1 piece (1 oz)	60	3	tr	tr
President					
Feta Fat Free	1 oz	30	0	2	tr

FOOD	PORTION	CAL	FAT	CARB	SUG
Sargento					
Blue Crumbled	¼ cup (1 oz)	100	8	1	0
Cheddar	1 slice (1 oz)	110	9	1	1
Cheddar Shredded	¼ cup (1 oz)	110	9	1	tr
Cheese For Nachos & Tacos Shredded	¼ cup (1 oz)	110	9	1	0
Cheese For Pizza Shredded	¼ cup (1 oz)	90	6	0	0
Cheese For Tacos Shredded	¼ cup (1 oz)	110	9	1	0
Colby	1 slice (1 oz)	110	9	0	0
Jarlsberg	1 slice (1.2 oz)	120	9	1	0
Monterey Jack	1 slice (1 oz)	100	9	0	0
Monterey Jack Shredded	¼ cup (1 oz)	100	9	0	0
Mozzarella	1 slice (1.5 oz)	130	9	2	0
Mozzarella Shredded	¼ cup (1 oz)	80	6	1	0
Muenster	1 slice (1 oz)	100	9	tr	0
Parmesan Grated	1 tbsp (5 g)	25	2	0	0
Provolone	1 slice (1 oz)	100	8	0	0
Ricotta Light	¼ cup (2.2 oz)	60	3	3	3
Ricotta Part-Skim	¼ cup (2.2 oz)	80	5	2	3
Swiss	1 slice (0.7 oz)	80	6	0	0
Velveeta					
Light	1 oz	60	3	3	2
Shredded	¼ cup (1.3 oz)	130	9	3	3
Spread	1 oz	90	6	3	2
Weight Watchers					
Cheddar Mild Yellow	1 oz	80	5	1	0
Cheddar Sharp Yellow	1 oz	80	5	1	0
Fat Free Grated Italian Topping	1 tbsp	20	0	2	1

FOOD	PORTION	CAL	FAT	CARB	SUG
CHEESE DISHES					
frozen					
Health Is Wealth					
Mozzarella Sticks	2 (1.3 oz)	120	5	14	0
Stouffer's					
Welsh Rarebit	½ cup (2.5 oz)	120	9	5	2
take-out					
cheese omelette as prep w/ 2 eggs	1 (6.8 oz)	519	44	tr	—
fondue	½ cup (3.8 oz)	247	15	4	—
souffle	1 serv (7 oz)	504	38	18	5
CHEESE SUBSTITUTES					
Yves					
Good Slice American	1 slice (0.7 oz)	35	2	0	0
Good Slice Cheddar	1 slice (0.7 oz)	35	2	1	0
Good Slice Jalapeno Jack	1 slice (0.7 oz)	35	2	0	0
Good Slice Mozzarella	1 slice (0.7 oz)	30	2	0	0
Good Slice Swiss	1 slice (0.7 oz)	35	2	1	0
CHERIMOYA					
fresh	1	515	2	131	—
CHERRIES					
canned					
sour in heavy syrup	½ cup	232	tr	60	—
sour in light syrup	½ cup	189	tr	49	—
sweet in heavy syrup	½ cup	107	tr	27	—
sweet in light syrup	½ cup	85	tr	22	—
dried					
Sonoma					
Pitted	¼ cup (1.4 oz)	140	0	34	25

FOOD	PORTION	CAL	FAT	CARB	SUG
fresh					
Chiquita					
Cherries	21 (1 cup)	90	1	22	19
frozen					
sweet sweetened	1 cup	232	tr	58	—
CHERRY JUICE					
Juicy Juice					
Drink	1 box (4.23 oz)	70	0	17	16
Drink	1 box (8.5 oz)	140	0	34	32
Kool-Aid					
Black Cherry Drink as prep w/ sugar	1 serv (8 oz)	100	0	25	25
Sugar Free Drink Mix as prep	1 serv (8 oz)	5	0	0	0
Veryfine					
Juice-Ups	8 fl oz	130	0	33	33
CHERVIL					
seed	1 tsp	1	tr	tr	—
CHESTNUTS					
chinese cooked	1 oz	44	tr	10	—
chinese dried	1 oz	103	tr	23	—
chinese roasted	1 oz	68	tr	15	—
cooked	1 oz	37	tr	8	—
creme de marrons	1 oz	73	tr	18	10
dried peeled	1 oz	105	1	22	—
japanese cooked	1 oz	16	tr	4	—
japanese dried	1 oz	102	tr	23	—
roasted	2 to 3 (1 oz)	70	1	15	—
CHEWING GUM					
Beech-Nut					
Spearmint	1 stick (3 g)	10	0	2	2

FOOD	PORTION	CAL	FAT	CARB	SUG
Bubble Yum					
Regular	1 piece (0.3 oz)	25	0	6	6
Sugarless	1 piece (0.2 oz)	15	0	3	0
Care*Free					
Sugarless Bubble Gum	1 stick (3 g)	10	0	2	0
Sugarless Cinnamon	1 piece (3 g)	5	0	2	0
Sugarless Peppermint	1 piece (3 g)	5	0	2	0
Sugarless Spearmint	1 piece (3 g)	5	0	2	0
Dentyne					
Ice Peppermint	2 pieces (3 g)	5	0	2	0
Lance					
Big Red Cinnamon	1 piece (3 g)	10	0	2	2
Double Bubble	1 piece (7 g)	25	0	6	5
Double Mint	1 piece (3 g)	10	0	2	2
Winterfresh					
Stick	1 stick (3 g)	10	0	2	2
CHIA SEEDS					
dried	1 oz	134	7	14	—
CHICKEN fresh					
broiler/fryer breast w/ skin batter dipped & fried	½ breast (4.9 oz)	364	18	13	—
broiler/fryer breast w/ skin batter dipped & fried	2.9 oz	218	11	8	—
broiler/fryer breast w/ skin roasted	½ breast (3.4 oz)	193	8	0	0
broiler/fryer breast w/ skin roasted	2 oz	115	5	0	0
broiler/fryer breast w/ skin stewed	½ breast (3.9 oz)	202	8	0	0

FOOD	PORTION	CAL	FAT	CARB	SUG
broiler/fryer breast w/o skin fried	½ breast (3 oz)	161	4	tr	—
broiler/fryer breast w/o skin roasted	½ breast (3 oz)	142	3	0	0
broiler/fryer breast w/o skin stewed	2 oz	86	2	0	0
broiler/fryer drumstick w/ skin batter dipped & fried	1 (2.6 oz)	193	11	6	—
broiler/fryer drumstick w/ skin floured & fried	1 (1.7 oz)	120	7	1	—
broiler/fryer drumstick w/ skin roasted	1 (1.8 oz)	112	6	0	0
broiler/fryer drumstick w/ skin stewed	1 (2 oz)	116	6	0	0
broiler/fryer drumstick w/o skin fried	1 (1.5 oz)	82	3	0	0
broiler/fryer drumstick w/o skin roasted	1 (1.5 oz)	76	2	0	0
broiler/fryer drumstick w/o skin stewed	1 (1.6 oz)	78	3	0	0
broiler/fryer neck w/ skin stewed	1 (1.3 oz)	94	7	0	0
broiler/fryer skin batter dipped & fried	from ½ chicken (6.7 oz)	748	55	44	—
broiler/fryer skin floured & fried	from ½ chicken (2 oz)	281	24	5	—
broiler/fryer skin roasted	from ½ chicken (2 oz)	254	23	0	0
broiler/fryer skin stewed	from ½ chicken (2.5 oz)	261	24	0	0

FOOD	PORTION	CAL	FAT	CARB	SUG
broiler/fryer thigh w/ skin batter dipped & fried	1 (3 oz)	238	14	8	—
broiler/fryer thigh w/ skin floured & fried	1 (2.2 oz)	162	9	2	—
broiler/fryer thigh w/ skin roasted	1 (2.2 oz)	153	10	0	0
broiler/fryer thigh w/ skin stewed	1 (2.4 oz)	158	10	0	0
broiler/fryer thigh w/o skin fried	1 (1.8 oz)	113	5	1	—
broiler/fryer thigh w/o skin roasted	1 (1.8 oz)	109	6	0	0
broiler/fryer thigh w/o skin stewed	1 (1.9 oz)	107	5	0	0
broiler/fryer w/o skin roasted	1 cup (5 oz)	266	10	0	0
broiler/fryer w/o skin stewed	1 cup (5 oz)	248	9	0	0
broiler/fryer wing w/ skin batter dipped & fried	1 (1.7 oz)	159	11	5	—
broiler/fryer wing w/ skin floured & fried	1 (1.1 oz)	103	7	1	—
broiler/fryer wing w/ skin roasted	1 (1.2 oz)	99	7	0	0
broiler/fryer wing w/ skin stewed	1 (1.4 oz)	100	7	0	0
cornish hen w/ skin roasted	1 hen (8 oz)	595	42	0	0
cornish hen w/ skin roasted	½ hen (4 oz)	296	21	0	0

FOOD	PORTION	CAL	FAT	CARB	SUG
Perdue					
Boneless Skinless Breasts Cooked	3 oz	110	2	0	0
Boneless Breast Roasted Garlic Herb	1 piece (3 oz)	90	1	3	—
Breaded Breast Strips Barbecue	3 oz	120	1	16	4
Breaded Breast Strips Hot & Spicy	3 oz	110	1	13	1
Breaded Breast Strips Original	3 oz	120	1	14	1
Burger Cooked	1 (3 oz)	160	10	0	0
Chicken Breast Seasoned Italian Cooked	1 piece (3 oz)	90	1	3	1
Chicken Breast Seasoned Lemon Pepper Cooked	1 piece (3 oz)	90	1	3	—
Chicken Breast Seasoned Teriyaki Cooked	1 piece (3 oz)	90	1	3	1
Ground Cooked	3 oz	170	11	0	0
Ground Breast Cooked	3 oz	80	1	0	0
Honey Rotisserie Dark Meat	3 oz	200	16	1	1
Honey Rotisserie White Meat	3 oz	140	8	1	1
Oven Stuffer Dark Meat Roasted	3 oz	210	15	0	0
Oven Stuffer Drumstick Roasted	1 (3.6 oz)	190	11	0	0
Oven Stuffer White Meat Roasted	3 oz	170	9	0	0

FOOD	PORTION	CAL	FAT	CARB	SUG
Oven Stuffer Wingette Roasted	3 (3.4 oz)	220	15	0	0
Seasoned Roasting Chicken Toasted Garlic Dark Meat	3 oz	190	14	1	—
Seasoned Roasting Chicken Toasted Garlic White Meat	3 oz	160	9	1	—
Seasoned Strips Parmesan Garlic cooked	3 oz	100	2	2	—
Seasoned Strips Savory Classic cooked	3 oz	90	1	1	0
Seasoned Strips Spicy Fiesta cooked	3 oz	140	7	3	1
Split Breast Cooked	1 piece (6.8 oz)	370	20	0	0
Thin Sliced Breast Rosemary Garlic Thyme	1 piece (3 oz)	90	2	1	—
Thin Sliced Breast Tomato Herb	1 piece (3 oz)	90	2	1	—
Whole Dark Meat cooked	3 oz	150	16	0	0
Whole White Meat cooked	3 oz	170	10	0	0
Wings Roasted	2 (3.2 oz)	210	15	0	0
Tyson					
Broth Marinated Breast Filet	1 (4.7 oz)	140	4	0	0
Broth Marinated Drums	2 (4 oz)	140	7	0	0
Broth Marinated Thighs	1 (4.9 oz)	380	34	1	1

FOOD	PORTION	CAL	FAT	CARB	SUG
Broth Marinated Wings	4 pieces (4.2 oz)	240	18	0	0
Chicken Broccoli & Cheese	1 piece (5.9 oz)	320	16	23	3
Chicken Stuffed w/ Wild Rice & Mushroom	1 piece (5.9 oz)	300	12	25	4
Cordon Bleu	1 piece (5.9 oz)	350	17	24	3
Cornish Hen	1 serv (4 oz)	180	12	0	0
Kiev	1 piece (5.9 oz)	460	32	24	3
frozen					
Banquet					
Breast Nuggets	7	280	20	11	2
Breast Patties Grilled Honey BBQ	1	110	5	3	2
Breast Patties Grilled Honey Mustard	1	120	5	5	3
Breast Tenders Our Original	3	250	15	15	1
Breast Tenders Southern	3 pieces	260	16	16	1
Country Fried	1 serv (3 oz)	270	18	13	1
Fat Free Baked Breast Patties	1	100	0	15	3
Fried Our Original	1 serv (3 oz)	280	18	15	1
Honey BBQ Skinless Fried	1 serv (3 oz)	230	13	9	1
Hot 'n Spicy Fried	1 serv (3 oz)	260	18	13	1
Nuggets Our Original	6	270	19	12	2
Nuggets Southern Fried	5	270	18	16	4
Patties Our Orignal	1	190	14	10	2
Patties Southern Fried	1	190	12	10	tr
Skinless Fried	1 serv (3 oz)	220	13	7	1

FOOD	PORTION	CAL	FAT	CARB	SUG
Smokehouse Big Wings	2 (0.6 oz)	200	17	4	3
Southern Fried	1 serv (3 oz)	280	18	15	1
Wings Firehouse Big	2	190	14	1	0
Wings Honey BBQ	4	380	24	15	4
Wings Hot & Spicy	4 pieces	280	20	9	0
Country Skillet					
Bites	5	270	16	18	2
Breast Tenders	3	240	14	16	1
Chunks	5	270	18	18	2
Fried	3 oz	270	18	13	1
Nuggets	10	280	17	16	2
Patties	1	190	12	12	3
Southern Fried Chunks	5	270	18	17	4
Southern Fried Patties	1	190	12	12	3
Health Is Wealth					
Nuggets	4 (3 oz)	150	6	9	0
Patties	1 (3 oz)	150	6	9	0
Tenders	3 (3 oz)	130	3	11	0
Kid Cuisine					
Dino Mite Nuggets	4 pieces	300	23	10	3
Radical Racin' Nuggets w/ Cheese	4 pieces	300	23	12	3
Weaver					
Breast Strips	3 pieces (3.3 oz)	210	11	13	1
Breast Tenders	5 pieces (3 oz)	220	15	8	0
Croquettes	1 serv (3.5 oz)	290	18	22	4
Dutch Frye Nuggets	5 pieces (3.3 oz)	280	20	12	0
Honey Battered Tenders	5 pieces (2.9 oz)	230	15	12	3
Hot Wings Buffalo Style	3 pieces (2.7 oz)	190	13	0	0
Mini Drums Crispy	5 pieces (3.3 oz)	250	16	14	2
Nuggets	4 pieces (2.7 oz)	210	15	9	0

FOOD	PORTION	CAL	FAT	CARB	SUG
Patties	1 (2.6 oz)	180	11	10	1
Rondelet	1 (2.6 oz)	170	10	10	1
Rondelet Dutch Frye	1 (2.6 oz)	230	16	10	1
Rondelet Italian	1 (2.6 oz)	210	14	12	1
ready-to-eat					
Banquet					
Fat Free Baked Breast Tenders	3	120	0	16	0
Boar's Head					
Breast Hickory Smoked	2 oz	60	1	tr	0
Breast Oven Roasted	2 oz	50	1	tr	0
Breast Bar B Q Sauce Basted	2 oz	60	1	3	1
Butterball					
Crispy Baked Breasts Italian Style Herb	1 piece (0.5 oz)	190	6	16	0
Crispy Baked Breasts Lemon Pepper	1 piece (0.5 oz)	200	7	16	2
Crispy Baked Breasts Original	1 piece (0.5 oz)	180	6	16	2
Crispy Baked Breasts Parmesan	1 piece (0.5 oz)	200	7	16	5
Crispy Baked Breasts Southwestern	1 piece (0.5 oz)	170	6	13	0
Tenders Baked Breast	3 pieces	170	6	15	2
Tenders Hickory Smoked Grilled	4 pieces + sauce	160	5	12	9
Tenders Oriental Grilled	4 pieces + sauce	160	5	12	10
Carl Buddig					
Chicken Sliced	1 pkg (2.5 oz)	110	7	1	1
Lean Slices Honey Smoked Breast	1 pkg (2.5 oz)	70	1	3	3

FOOD	PORTION	CAL	FAT	CARB	SUG
Lean Slices Roasted Breast	1 pkg (2.5 oz)	60	1	1	1
Chicken By George					
Cajun	1 breast (4 oz)	130	4	3	0
Caribbean Grill	1 breast (4 oz)	150	4	8	6
Garlic & Herb	1 breast (4 oz)	120	3	3	1
Italian Bleu Cheese	1 breast (4 oz)	130	5	2	0
Lemon Herb	1 breast (4 oz)	120	3	3	2
Lemon Oregano	1 breast (4 oz)	130	4	3	1
Mesquite Barbecue	1 breast (4 oz)	130	3	5	3
Mustard Dill	1 breast (4 oz)	140	5	2	1
Roasted	1 breast (4 oz)	110	3	1	0
Teriyaki	1 breast (4 oz)	130	3	6	4
Tomato Herb With Basil	1 breast (4 oz)	140	5	5	4
Louis Rich					
Carving Board Classic Baked	2 slices (1.6 oz)	45	1	2	0
Carving Board Grilled	2 slices (1.6 oz)	45	1	2	0
Deli-Thin Oven Roasted Breast	4 slices (1.8 oz)	50	1	1	tr
Oven Roasted Deluxe Breast	1 slice (1 oz)	30	1	1	0
Oscar Mayer					
Free Oven Roasted Breast	4 slices (1.8 oz)	45	0	1	tr
Perdue					
Breast Cutlets Homestyle	1 (2.9 oz)	110	1	12	—
Breast Cutlets Italian Style	1 (2.9 oz)	120	2	11	—
Breast Filets In Barbecue Sauce	1 piece + 3 tbsp sauce (5.9 oz)	200	1	24	23

FOOD	PORTION	CAL	FAT	CARB	SUG
Breast Strips In Garlic & Herb Sauce	1 serv (5 oz)	100	1	4	1
Breast Strips In Marinara Sauce	1 serv (5 oz)	120	3	5	1
Breast Strips In Teriyaki Sauce	1 serv (5 oz)	190	1	26	22
Carved Breast Honey Roasted	½ cup (2.5 oz)	100	2	2	1
Carved Breast Original Roasted	½ cup (2.5 oz)	90	2	1	—
Cutlets Cooked	1 (3.5 oz)	220	11	15	—
Nuggets	5 (3.4 oz)	210	11	15	—
Nuggets Chicken & Cheese	5 (3.4 oz)	230	13	15	—
Short Cuts Italian	½ cup (2.5 oz)	100	3	0	0
Short Cuts Lemon Pepper	½ cup (2.5 oz)	100	3	1	—
Short Cuts Southwestern	½ cup (2.5 oz)	100	3	1	—
Tyson					
Breaded Breast Chunks	6 pieces (2.9 oz)	230	16	13	0
Breaded Breast Fillet	2 pieces (2.8 oz)	180	8	15	0
Breaded Breast Pattie	1 (2.6 oz)	190	12	9	2
Breaded Breast Tenders	5 pieces (3 oz)	220	15	8	0
Breaded Chicken Chunks	6 pieces (3 oz)	220	14	11	1
Chick'n Quick Chick'n Cheddar	1 patty (2.6 oz)	220	14	12	1
Chicken Bits Southern Fried	6 pieces (2.9 oz)	260	19	11	0
Chicken Strips	1 serv (3 oz)	90	1	0	0
Chicken Strips Southwestern	1 serv (3 oz)	110	3	2	1

FOOD	PORTION	CAL	FAT	CARB	SUG
Country Fried Chicken Fritter	5 pieces (2.9 oz)	260	18	13	0
Drumsticks Hot BBQ Style	2 (3.5 oz)	160	7	3	2
Glazed Grilled Breast Pattie	1 (2.7 oz)	120	7	1	0
Grilled Chicken Pattie	1 (2.9 oz)	170	12	1	0
Nuggets Breaded White Meat	6 pieces (2.9 oz)	250	18	12	0
Patties Southern Fried	1 (2.9 oz)	260	19	11	0
Roasted Drumsticks	3 (5.6 oz)	320	15	2	2
Roasted Drumsticks w/o Skin	2 (3.3 oz)	140	5	1	1
Roasted Half Chicken	1 serv (3 oz)	160	11	1	1
Roasted Whole Chicken	1 serv (3 oz)	160	11	1	1
Roasted Breast Boneless w/o Skin	1 (3.7 oz)	130	3	1	1
Roasted Breast Half w/o Skin	1 (4.3 oz)	150	3	1	1
Roasted Half Breast w/ Skin	1 (5.1 oz)	260	13	1	1
Roasted Half Chicken w/o Skin	1 serv (3 oz)	120	6	1	1
Roasted Tabasco Wings	3 (3 oz)	190	13	1	1
Roasted Thigh w/ Skin	1 (3.6 oz)	270	21	1	1
Roasted Thighs w/o Skin	1 (2.9 oz)	150	8	1	1
Roll White Meat	2 oz	90	6	0	0
Southern Fried Breaded Breast Pattie	1 (2.6 oz)	180	12	8	0
Southern Fried Breast Fillets	2 pieces (3.4 oz)	210	11	14	0

FOOD	PORTION	CAL	FAT	CARB	SUG
Southern Fried Chunks	6 pieces (2.9 oz)	260	19	11	0
Tenders Breaded Honey Battered	5 pieces (2.9 oz)	230	15	12	3
Tenders Breaded Pattie	3 pieces (3.2 oz)	100	0	11	1
Thick'n Crispy Pattie	1 (2.6 oz)	200	14	10	1
Wings BBQ	3 pieces (3.2 oz)	200	13	2	2
Wings Hot N'Spicy	4 (3.2 oz)	210	14	1	0
Wings Teriyaki	4 pieces (3.4 oz)	190	12	2	1
Wings Of Fire	4 pieces (3.4 oz)	220	15	1	0
take-out					
oven roasted breast of chicken	2 oz	60	1	0	0

CHICKEN DISHES
canned
Bumble Bee

Chicken Salad	1 pkg (3.5 oz)	230	10	25	8
mix					
Chicken Skillet Helper					
Stir-Fried Chicken as prep	1 cup	270	9	30	1
Tyson					
Mandarin Wrap Kit	1½ wraps (14.6 oz)	630	15	92	8
shelf-stable					
Lunch Bucket					
Chicken Fiesta	1 pkg (7.5 oz)	160	2	30	6
Dumplings'n Chicken	1 pkg (7.5 oz)	140	5	21	2
take-out					
boneless breaded & fried w/ barbecue sauce	6 pieces (4.6 oz)	330	18	25	—
boneless breaded & fried w/ honey	6 pieces (4 oz)	339	18	27	—

FOOD	PORTION	CAL	FAT	CARB	SUG
boneless breaded & fried w/ mustard sauce	6 pieces (4.6 oz)	323	17	21	—
boneless breaded & fried w/ sweet & sour sauce	6 pieces (4.6 oz)	346	18	29	—
breast & wing breaded & fried	2 pieces (5.7 oz)	494	30	20	—
chicken & dumplings	¾ cup	256	12	12	—
chicken & noodles	1 cup	365	18	26	—
chicken a la king	1 cup	470	34	12	—
chicken cacciatore	¾ cup	394	24	9	—
chicken pie w/ top crust	1 slice (5.6 oz)	472	31	32	—
drumstick breaded & fried	2 pieces (5.2 oz)	430	27	16	—
groundnut stew hkatenkwan	1 serv (15.7 oz)	576	40	18	3
jamaican jerk wings	4 wings (9.9 oz)	709	51	3	tr
thigh breaded & fried	2 pieces (5.2 oz)	430	27	16	—

CHICKEN SUBSTITUTES

Health Is Wealth

Buffalo Wings	3 pieces (2.2 oz)	100	2	11	0
Chicken-Free Nuggets	3 pieces (2.25 oz)	90	1	11	0
Chicken-Free Patties	1 (3 oz)	120	2	15	0

Loma Linda

Chicken Supreme Mix not prep	⅓ cup (0.9 oz)	90	1	6	0
Chik Nuggets	5 pieces (3 oz)	240	16	13	tr
Fried Chik'n w/ Gravy	2 pieces (2.8 oz)	160	10	4	tr

Morningstar Farms

Chik Nuggets	4 pieces (3 oz)	160	4	17	2

FOOD	PORTION	CAL	FAT	CARB	SUG
Chik Patties	1 (2.5 oz)	150	6	15	1
Meatless Buffalo Wings	5 pieces (3 oz)	200	9	16	1
Quorn					
Cutlets	1 (3.5 oz)	200	8	20	2
Nuggets	3–4 pieces (3 oz)	180	8	18	2
Patties	1 patty (2.6 oz)	160	7	12	2
Tenders	1 cup (3 oz)	90	2	8	1
Worthington					
Chic-Ketts	2 slices (1.9 oz)	120	7	2	0
Chicken Sliced or Roll	2 slices (2 oz)	80	5	1	0
ChikStiks	1 (1.6 oz)	110	7	3	tr
CrispyChik Patties	1 (2.5 oz)	150	6	15	1
Cutlets	1 slice (2.1 oz)	70	1	3	0
Diced Chik	¼ cup (1.9 oz)	40	0	1	0
FriChik	2 pieces (3.2 oz)	120	8	1	0
FriChik Low Fat	2 pieces (3 oz)	80	3	2	0
Golden Croquettes	4 pieces (3 oz)	210	10	14	1
Yves					
Veggie Chicken Burgers	1 (3 oz)	120	3	6	1
CHICKPEAS					
canned					
Progresso					
Chick Peas	½ cup (4.6 oz)	120	3	20	3
Garbanzo	½ cup (4.4 oz)	110	2	18	tr
dried					
cooked	1 cup	269	4	45	—
CHILI					
chile pepper paste	1 tbsp	6	1	1	—
dried ancho	1 tsp	3	tr	1	—
dried casabel	1 tsp	3	tr	1	—
dried guajillo	1 tsp	3	tr	1	—

FOOD	PORTION	CAL	FAT	CARB	SUG
dried mulato	1 tsp	3	tr	1	—
dried pasilla	1 tsp	3	tr	1	—
dried smoked chipotle	1 tsp	3	tr	1	—
powder	1 tsp	8	tr	1	—
Carroll Shelby's					
Original Texas Chili Kit	2 tbsp	60	1	12	0
Chef Boyardee					
Chili Mac	½ can (7 oz)	260	11	30	5
Gebhardt					
Chili Powder	¼ tsp (0.3 g)	1	tr	tr	tr
Chili Quik Seasoning	1 tbsp (0.3 oz)	43	1	8	1
Plain	1 cup (9.4 oz)	232	19	11	0
With Beans	1 cup (9.4 oz)	322	15	32	tr
Health Valley					
Vegetarian w/ Black Beans Spicy	1 cup	160	1	28	7
Healthy Choice					
Bowls Chili & Cornbread	1 meal (9.5 oz)	350	8	49	18
Hunt's					
Chili Beans	½ cup (4.5 oz)	87	1	17	8
Chili Sauce	2 tbsp (1.2 oz)	35	tr	8	8
Just Rite					
With Beans	1 cup (9 oz)	379	27	31	0
Lean Cuisine					
Everyday Favorites Three Bean Chili w/ Rice	1 pkg (10 oz)	250	6	37	7
Manwich					
Homestyle Fixins	½ cup (4.6 oz)	84	1	19	7
Marie Callender's					
Chili & Cornbread	1 meal (16 oz)	560	21	67	25

FOOD	PORTION	CAL	FAT	CARB	SUG
McCormick					
Original Chili Seasoning	1⅓ tbsp (9 g)	30	1	5	tr
Natural Touch					
Vegetarian	1 cup (8.1 oz)	170	1	21	2
Nature's Entree					
Texas Chili	1 pkg (12 oz)	320	7	43	5
Open Range					
Plain	1 cup (8.8 oz)	353	26	19	6
With Beans	1 cup (9 oz)	281	16	25	7
Van Camp					
Beanee Weenee Chilee	1 cup (7.7 oz)	240	12	27	1
Chili With Beans	1 cup (8.9 oz)	350	21	28	1
Mexican Style Chili Beans	½ cup (4.6 oz)	110	2	21	1
Wick Fowler's					
2 Alarm Chili Kit	3 tbsp	60	2	10	0
False Alarm Chili Kit	2 tbsp	50	2	9	0
Worthington					
Chili	1 cup (8.1 oz)	290	15	21	2
Low Fat	1 cup (8.1 oz)	170	1	21	2
Yves					
Veggie Chili	1 pkg (10.5 oz)	230	1	37	7

CHILI PEPPERS

(*see* PEPPERS)

CHINESE CABBAGE

(*see* CABBAGE)

CHINESE FOOD

(*see* ASIAN FOOD)

CHINESE PRESERVING MELON

cooked	½ cup	11	tr	3	—

FOOD	PORTION	CAL	FAT	CARB	SUG
CHIPS					
Barbara's Bakery					
Potato	1¼ cup (1 oz)	150	10	15	0
Potato No Salt Added	1¼ cups (1 oz)	150	10	15	0
Potato Ripple	1¼ cup (1 oz)	150	10	15	0
Potato Yogurt & Green Onion	1¼ cup (1 oz)	150	9	15	tr
Tortilla Blue Corn	15 chips (1 oz)	140	7	16	tr
Tortilla Blue Corn No Salt	15 chips (1 oz)	140	7	16	tr
Tortilla Pinta Salsa	15 chips (1 oz)	130	6	19	0
Cape Cod					
Potato Golden Russet	1 pkg (0.5 oz)	70	4	8	0
Durangos					
Tortilla	15 (1 oz)	150	7	20	0
Fritos					
Chili Cheese	31 (1 oz)	160	10	16	tr
Corn Chips King Size	12 (1 oz)	150	10	16	0
Original	32 (1 oz)	160	10	15	tr
Lance					
Ripple	15 (1 oz)	160	11	14	0
Lay's					
Baked Original	11 (1 oz)	110	2	23	2
Baked Sour Cream & Onion	12 (1 oz)	120	2	21	3
Classic	20 (1 oz)	150	10	15	0
Wavy Original	11 pieces (1 oz)	160	10	15	0
Wow Original	20 (1 oz)	75	0	18	0
Old Dutch Foods					
Potato	12–15 chips (1 oz)	150	8	16	1
Potato BBQ	12–15 chips (1 oz)	150	9	15	1
Potato BBQ Ripple	12–15 chips (1 oz)	150	9	16	1

FOOD	PORTION	CAL	FAT	CARB	SUG
Potato Cajun Ripple	12–15 chips (1 oz)	150	10	15	tr
Potato Cheddar & Sour Cream Ripple	12–15 chips (1 oz)	160	9	16	tr
Potato Cheddar & Sour Cream Ripples	12–15 chips (1 oz)	150	9	15	1
Potato Dill	12–15 chips (1 oz)	140	8	16	2
Potato Dutch Crunch	15–20 chips (1 oz)	130	6	18	0
Potato French Onion Ripple	12–15 chips (1 oz)	150	10	15	2
Potato Jalapeno & Cheddar Dutch Crunch	15–20 chips (1 oz)	130	6	17	0
Potato Jalapeno Cheese	12–15 chips (1 oz)	150	9	16	tr
Potato Mesquite BBQ Dutch Crunch	15–20 chips (1 oz)	130	6	19	1
Potato Onion & Garlic	12–15 chips (1 oz)	140	8	16	1
Potato Outback Spicy BBQ	12–15 chips (1 oz)	150	10	15	1
Potato Ripples	12–15 chips (1 oz)	150	9	15	0
Potato Salt & Vinegar Dutch Crunch	15–20 chips (1 oz)	130	6	18	1
Potato Sour Cream & Onion	12–15 chips (1 oz)	150	9	15	2
Tortilla Bite Size White Corn	20 chips (1 oz)	150	8	18	0
Tortilla Nacho Cheese	15 chips (1 oz)	150	7	19	0
Tortilla Restaurant Style White	9 chips (1 oz)	140	7	20	0
Tostados White Corn	11 chips (1 oz)	140	7	20	0
Tostados Yellow	11 chips (1 oz)	140	6	21	0
Pita-Snax					
Cheddar Cheese	34 (1 oz)	110	2	21	1
Chili & Lime	34 (1 oz)	120	2	20	1

FOOD	PORTION	CAL	FAT	CARB	SUG
Cinnamon	34 (1 oz)	120	2	22	2
Dill Ranch	34 (1 oz)	120	2	21	0
Garlic	34 (1 oz)	120	2	22	0
Lightly Salted	34 (1 oz)	110	1	22	0
Pringles					
BBQ	14 chips (1 oz)	150	10	15	1
Cheese & Onion	14 chips (1 oz)	160	11	15	1
Cheez-ums	14 chips (1 oz)	150	10	14	1
Pizzalicious	14 chips (1 oz)	160	11	14	1
Ranch	14 chips (1 oz)	150	10	15	1
Salt & Vinegar	14 chips (1 oz)	160	11	15	1
Sour Cream & Onion	14 chips (1 oz)	160	10	15	1
Robert's American Gourmet					
Spirulina Spirals	1 oz	120	2	22	4
Ruffles					
Baked	10 (1 oz)	110	2	23	2
Baked Cheddar & Sour Cream	9 (1 oz)	120	3	21	2
Buffalo Style	11 chips (1 oz)	160	10	16	0
Cheddar & Sour Cream	11 chips (1 oz)	160	10	14	2
French Onion	11 (1 oz)	150	10	15	tr
MC Masterpiece Mesquite BBQ	11 (1 oz)	150	10	15	tr
Original	12 chips (1 oz)	150	10	14	0
Ranch	13 (1 oz)	150	9	15	1
Reduced Fat	16 (1 oz)	130	7	18	0
The Works	12 (1 oz)	160	11	14	2
Wow Cheddar & Sour Cream	15 (1 oz)	75	0	16	tr
Wow Original	17 (1 oz)	75	0	17	0

FOOD	PORTION	CAL	FAT	CARB	SUG
Snyder's Of Hanover					
BBQ Rib	1 oz	140	7	17	tr
Barbeque Corn	1.5 oz	230	14	22	0
Cheddar Bacon	1 oz	150	6	20	tr
Corn Chips	1.5 oz	230	15	22	0
Grilled Steak & Onion	1 oz	140	6	20	0
Hot Buffalo	1 oz	150	7	20	0
Kosher Dill	1 oz	140	6	20	1
No Salt	1 oz	140	6	19	0
Potato	1 oz	140	6	19	0
Ripple	1 oz	140	6	18	0
Salt & Vinegar	1 oz	140	6	19	tr
Sausage Pizza	1 oz	150	6	20	tr
Sour Cream & Onion	1 oz	150	7	19	tr
Tasty Veggie Potato Chips	1 oz	150	6	20	1
Tortilla Nacho	1 oz	140	7	19	tr
Tortilla No Salt Yellow Corn	1 oz	140	6	19	tr
Tortilla White Corn	1 oz	140	6	20	tr
Tortilla Yellow Corn	1 oz	140	6	19	tr
Tortilla Yellow Corn Mini	1 oz	160	8	20	tr
Sunchips					
Original	14 (1 oz)	140	6	19	2
Torengos					
Chips	13 chips (1 oz)	140	9	15	0
Tostitos					
Baked Original	13 (1 oz)	110	1	21	0
Wow Original	6 (1 oz)	90	1	20	0
Utz					
Potato	20 (1 oz)	150	9	14	0
Tortilla Restaurant Style	6 (1 oz)	140	7	18	0

FOOD	PORTION	CAL	FAT	CARB	SUG
CHITTERLINGS					
pork cooked	3 oz	258	24	0	0
CHIVES					
freeze-dried	1 tbsp	1	tr	tr	—
fresh chopped	1 tbsp	1	tr	tr	—
CHOCOLATE					
baking					
Baker's					
Bittersweet	½ square (0.5 oz)	70	6	7	5
German's Sweet	2 squares (0.5 oz)	60	4	8	8
Semi-Sweet	½ square (0.5 oz)	70	5	8	7
Unsweetened	½ square (0.5 oz)	70	7	4	0
White	½ square (0.5 oz)	80	5	8	8
Nestle					
Choco Bake	½ oz	80	8	5	0
Premier White Bar	½ oz	80	5	8	8
Premier White Morsels	1 tbsp	80	4	9	9
Semi-Sweet Bar	½ oz	70	4	9	8
Unsweetened Bar	½ oz	80	7	4	0
chips					
Nestle					
Crunch Baking Pieces	1½ tbsp	80	4	10	8
Milk Chocolate Morsels	1 tbsp	70	4	9	8
Mint Chocolate Morsels	1 tbsp	70	4	9	8
Morsels Semi-Sweet	1 tbsp	70	4	9	8
Semi-Sweet Mega Morsels	1 tbsp	70	4	9	8
Semi-Sweet Mini Morsels	1 tbsp	70	4	9	8
mix					
Quik					
Chocolate Powder	2 tbsp (0.8 oz)	90	1	19	18

FOOD	PORTION	CAL	FAT	CARB	SUG
Chocolate Powder No Sugar	2 tbsp (0.4 oz)	40	1	7	1

CHOCOLATE MILK

(*see* CHOCOLATE, COCOA, MILK DRINKS, MILK SUBSTITUTES)

CHOCOLATE SYRUP

Estee

Chocolate	2 tbsp	15	0	5	—

Quik

Chocolate	2 tbsp (1.3 oz)	100	1	23	17

Smucker's

Plate Scapers Chocolate	2 tbsp	100	5	23	11

Toll House

Mint Chocolate	2 tbsp (1.5 oz)	130	3	25	22
Semi-Sweet	2 tbsp (1.5 oz)	130	4	24	22

CHUTNEY

apple	1.2 oz	68	0	18	—
apple cranberry	1 tbsp	16	0	4	—
coconut	¼ cup	74	7	4	—
mango	1 tbsp	54	2	10	—
tomato	1 tbsp	32	tr	8	—

Sonoma

Dried Tomato	1 tbsp (0.7 g)	35	0	9	8

CILANTRO

fresh	1 tsp (2 g)	tr	tr	tr	—
fresh	1 cup (1.6 oz)	11	tr	2	—

CINNAMON

ground	1 tsp	6	tr	2	—
sticks	0.5 oz	39	tr	8	0

CISCO

smoked	1 oz	50	3	0	0

FOOD	PORTION	CAL	FAT	CARB	SUG
CLAMS					
canned					
Bumble Bee					
Baby	2 oz	50	1	2	0
Progresso					
Creamy Clam Sauce	½ cup (4.2 oz)	110	6	8	0
Minced	¼ cup (2.1 oz)	25	0	2	0
Red Clam Sauce	½ cup (4.4 oz)	60	1	8	4
White Clam Sauce	½ cup (4.4 oz)	150	10	5	tr
fresh					
cooked	20 sm	133	2	5	—
raw	20 sm (6.3 oz)	133	2	5	—
take-out					
breaded & fried	20 sm	379	21	19	—
CLOVES					
ground	1 tsp	7	tr	1	—
COCOA					
Carnation					
Hot Cocoa 70 Calorie	1 pkg (0.7 oz)	70	0	15	15
Hot Cocoa Double Chocolate Meltdown	1 pkg (1.2 oz)	150	4	27	24
Hot Cocoa Fat Free Raspberry	1 pkg (0.3 oz)	30	0	4	3
Hot Cocoa Fat Free w/ Marshmallows	1 pkg (0.4 oz)	45	0	10	7
Hot Cocoa Lactose Free	1 pkg (1 oz)	120	2	25	19
Hot Cocoa Marshmallow Blizzard	1 pkg (1.5 oz)	180	2	39	33
Hot Cocoa Milk Chocolate	3 tbsp (1 oz)	110	1	24	20

FOOD	PORTION	CAL	FAT	CARB	SUG
Hot Cocoa Rich Chocolate	3 tbsp (1 oz)	110	1	24	21
Hot Cocoa Rich Chocolate Fat Free	1 pkg (0.3 oz)	25	0	4	3
Hot Cocoa Rich Chocolate No Sugar Added	3 tbsp (0.5 oz)	50	0	8	7
Hot Cocoa Rich Chocolate w/ Marshmallows	3 tbsp (1 oz)	110	1	24	21
Nestle					
Cocoa	1 tbsp	15	1	3	0
Hot Cocoa Rich Chocolate	1 pkg (1 oz)	110	1	24	19
Hot Cocoa Rich w/ Marshmallows	1 pkg (1 oz)	110	1	24	19
Swiss Miss					
Hot Cocoa And Cream	1 serv	153	5	25	21
Hot Cocoa Chocolate Sensation	1 serv	148	4	27	23
Hot Cocoa Diet	1 serv	22	tr	4	2
Hot Cocoa Fat Free	1 serv	52	tr	9	7
Hot Cocoa Fat Free Marshmallow Lovers	1 serv	65	tr	13	10
Hot Cocoa Lite	1 serv	76	1	18	15
Hot Cocoa Marshmallow Lovers	1 serv	142	3	27	22
Hot Cocoa Milk Chocolate	1 serv	118	3	22	16
Hot Cocoa Milk Chocolate No Sugar Added	1 serv	55	1	10	6

FOOD	PORTION	CAL	FAT	CARB	SUG
Hot Cocoa Milk Chocolate w/ Marshmallows	1 serv	118	3	22	17
Hot Cocoa Rich Chocolate	1 serv	110	2	23	21
Hot Cocoa White Chocolate	1 serv	109	1	21	21
Hot Cocoa w/ Marshmallows No Sugar Added	1 serv	56	1	10	6
Premiere Hot Cocoa Almond Mocha	1 serv	144	3	28	26
Premiere Hot Cocoa English Toffee	1 serv	142	2	29	26
Premiere Hot Cocoa Raspberry Truffle	1 serv	144	3	28	26
Premiere Hot Cocoa Suisse Truffle	1 serv	142	2	28	26
Rich Hot Cocoa No Sugar Added	1 serv	54	1	10	6
Sidewalk Cafe Cappuccino	1 serv	119	4	18	17
Sidewalk Cafe Cinnamon	1 serv	126	4	21	20
Sidewalk Cafe French Vanilla	1 serv	121	4	19	15
Sidewalk Cafe Mocha	1 serv	120	4	20	19
Weight Watchers					
Hot Cocoa Mix as prep	1 pkg	70	0	7	6

COCONUT

FOOD	PORTION	CAL	FAT	CARB	SUG
fresh	1 piece (1.5 oz)	159	15	7	—
fresh shredded	1 cup	283	27	12	—

FOOD	PORTION	CAL	FAT	CARB	SUG
Baker's					
Angel Flake	1 tbsp (0.5 oz)	70	5	6	5
Angel Flake (canned)	2 tbsp (0.5 oz)	70	6	6	5
Premium Shred	2 tbsp (0.5 oz)	70	5	6	5
COD					
atlantic canned	3 oz	89	1	0	0
atlantic dried	3 oz	246	2	0	0
atlantic fresh cooked	3 oz	89	1	0	0
pacific fresh baked	3 oz	95	1	0	0
roe canned	1 oz	34	1	tr	—
roe baked w/ butter & lemon juice	1 oz	36	1	tr	—
roe tarama	3.5 oz	547	55	6	tr
COFFEE					
instant					
Nescafe					
Decafe	1 tsp (2 g)	0	0	tr	0
Decafe w/ Chicory	1 tsp (2 g)	0	0	tr	0
French Vanilla	1 tsp (2 g)	5	0	1	0
French Vanilla Decaf	1 tsp (2 g)	5	0	1	0
Hazelnut	1 tsp (2 g)	5	0	1	0
Irish Creme	1 tsp (2 g)	5	0	1	0
Regular	1 tsp (2 g)	0	0	tr	0
With Chicory	1 tsp (2 g)	5	0	1	0
regular					
brewed	6 oz	4	0	1	—
roasted beans	1 oz	64	4	18	—
Folgers					
Colombian Supreme	1 tbsp	16	tr	3	—
Custom Roast	1 tbsp	16	tr	3	—
Decaffeinated	1 tbsp	17	tr	3	—

FOOD	PORTION	CAL	FAT	CARB	SUG
French Roast	1 tbsp	16	tr	3	—
Instant	1 tsp	8	tr	1	—
Instant Decaffeinated	1 tsp	8	tr	2	—
Maryland Club					
Ground	1 tbsp	16	tr	3	—
Nescafe					
Cafe Mocha	1 can (10 oz)	140	3	27	24
Caffe Latte	1 can (10 oz)	130	3	22	20
Caffe Latte Decaffeinated	1 can (10 oz)	130	3	22	20
Espresso	1 tsp (2 g)	0	0	tr	0
Espresso Cafe Latte	1 pkg (0.6 oz)	70	2	10	6
Espresso Cafe Mocha	1 pkg (1 oz)	110	3	20	15
Espresso Cappuccino	1 pkg (0.6 oz)	80	3	11	6
Espresso Roast	1 can (10 oz)	90	1	21	14
French Vanilla	1 can (10 oz)	150	4	25	21
Hazelnut	1 can (10 oz)	130	3	22	20
Roasted Ground Decaffeinated as prep	1 cup (6 oz)	0	0	tr	0
Roasted Ground as prep	1 cup (6 oz)	0	0	tr	0
take-out					
cafe au lait	1 cup (8 fl oz)	77	4	6	7
cafe brulot	1 cup (4.8 fl oz)	48	0	3	3
cappuccino	1 cup (8 fl oz)	77	4	6	7
coffee con leche	1 cup (8 fl oz)	77	4	6	7
espresso	1 cup (3 fl oz)	2	0	tr	0
irish coffee	1 serv (9 fl oz)	107	3	3	0
latte w/ skim milk	13 oz	88	tr	12	11
latte w/ whole milk	13 oz	152	8	12	11
mocha	1 mug (9.6 fl oz)	202	15	17	12

FOOD	PORTION	CAL	FAT	CARB	SUG
COFFEE BEVERAGES					
Chock full o'Nuts					
New York Cappuccino French Vanilla	1 pkg (0.9 oz)	90	2	19	14
New York Cappuccino Hazelnut	1 pkg. (0.9 oz)	90	2	19	14
Coffee House USA					
All Flavors	1 bottle (9.5 oz)	100	4	29	28
General Foods					
International Coffees Italian Cappuccino as prep	1 serv (8 oz)	10	2	10	8
International Coffees Sugar Free Fat Free French Vanilla Cafe as prep	1 serv (8 oz)	15	0	5	0
Maxwell House					
Cafe Cappuccino Decaffeinated Vanilla as prep	1 serv (8 oz)	10	1	19	18
Cafe Cappuccino Mocha as prep	1 serv (8 oz)	100	3	17	16
Cafe Cappuccino Sugar Free Mocha as prep	1 serv (8 oz)	10	3	7	0
Cafe Cappuccino Sugar Free Vanilla as prep	1 serv (8 oz)	10	3	7	0
COFFEE SUBSTITUTES					
Natural Touch					
Kaffree Roma	1 tsp (2 g)	10	0	2	0
Roma Cappuccino	3 tbsp (0.4 oz)	50	3	5	4

FOOD	PORTION	CAL	FAT	CARB	SUG
Postum					
Instant Coffee Flavor as prep	1 serv (8 oz)	10	0	3	0
Instant as prep	1 serv (8 oz)	10	0	3	0

COFFEE WHITENERS
N-Rich

Coffee Creamer	1 tsp (2 g)	10	1	1	0

COLESLAW
take-out

coleslaw w/ dressing	½ cup	42	2	7	—
vinegar & oil coleslaw	3.5 oz	150	9	16	—

COLLARDS

fresh cooked	½ cup	17	tr	4	—
Birds Eye					
Chopped Greens frzn	1 cup (3.1 oz)	30	0	2	1

COOKIES
mix

Betty Crocker

Chocolate Peanut Butter as prep	1 bar	180	9	25	18
Date Bar as prep	1 bar	150	6	23	14
Oatmeal as prep	2	150	6	22	12
ready-to-eat					
hermits	1 (1 oz)	117	5	18	10
jumbles coconut	1 (1 oz)	121	7	13	7
ladyfingers	1 (0.38 oz)	40	1	7	—
macaroons	1 (0.8 oz)	97	3	17	—
madeleines	1 (0.8 oz)	86	5	10	5
merinque	1 (0.3 oz)	20	0	5	5
molasses	1 (0.5 oz)	65	2	11	—
neapolitan tri-color cookie	1 (0.6 oz)	79	5	8	5

FOOD	PORTION	CAL	FAT	CARB	SUG
pinenut cookies	1 (1.1 oz)	134	9	11	8
spritz	1 (0.4 oz)	42	2	6	3
zeppole	1 (0.8 oz)	78	6	6	4
Bahlsen					
Deloba	4 (0.9 oz)	130	5	19	8
Girl Scout					
Samoas	2 (1 oz)	160	9	17	12
Tagalongs	2 (0.9 oz)	150	10	13	8
Thin Mints	4 (1 oz)	140	8	18	10
Trefoils	5 (1.1 oz)	160	8	20	7
Godiva					
Biscotti Dipped In Milk Chocolate	1 (0.9 oz)	120	6	15	6
Keebler					
Droxies	3 (1.1 oz)	140	6	21	12
E.L. Fudge Fudge w/ Fudge Filling	2 (0.9 oz)	120	6	17	7
Fudge Shoppe Deluxe Grahams	3 (1 oz)	140	7	19	10
Fudge Shoppe Fudge Sticks	3 (1 oz)	150	8	20	15
Golden Fruit Raisin	1 (0.7 oz)	80	2	15	9
Graham Original	8 (1 oz)	130	3	23	7
Sandies Simply Shortbread	1 (0.5 oz)	80	5	9	3
Vienna Fingers	2 (1 oz)	140	6	21	8
LU					
Le Chocolatiers	3 (1 oz)	150	8	17	11
Le Petit Beurre	4 (1.2 oz)	150	4	25	7
La Choy					
Fortune	4 (1 oz)	112	tr	26	11

FOOD	PORTION	CAL	FAT	CARB	SUG
Lance					
Choc-O-Lunch	1 pkg (1.5 oz)	200	8	31	17
Lem-O-Lunch	1 pkg (3.4 oz)	240	11	32	11
Peanut Butter	1 (2 oz)	140	8	14	10
Van-O-Lunch	1 pkg (1.5 oz)	210	8	31	13
Little Debbie					
Caramel Bars	1 (1.2 oz)	160	8	22	16
Coconut Rounds	1 (1.2 oz)	150	7	23	13
Fudge Delights	1 (1.1 oz)	110	2	24	14
Jelly Creme Pies	1 (1.2 oz)	160	7	23	15
Marshmallow Crispy Bar	1 (1.3 oz)	140	4	26	13
Nutty Bar	1 (2 oz)	310	18	32	20
Peanut Butter Bars	1 (1.9 oz)	270	15	32	19
Yo-Yo's	1 (1.2 oz)	130	6	21	12
MoonPie					
Chocolate	1 (2.75 oz)	330	10	56	24
Murray's					
Sugar Free Double Fudge	3 (1.2 oz)	140	6	23	0
Sugar Free Ginger Snap	6 (1 oz)	110	4	21	0
Sugar Free Peanut Butter	6 (1 oz)	130	7	17	0
Sugar Free Vanilla Sandwich Creme	3 (1 oz)	120	5	21	0
Sugar Free Vanilla Wafers	9 (1.1 oz)	120	4	23	0
Nabisco					
Biscos Sugar Wafers	8 (1 oz)	140	6	21	13
Cameo	2 (1 oz)	130	5	21	10

FOOD	PORTION	CAL	FAT	CARB	SUG
Chips Ahoy!	3 (1.1 oz)	160	8	21	10
Famous Chocolate Wafers	5 (1.1 oz)	140	4	24	11
Grahams	4 (1 oz)	120	3	22	6
Lorna Doone	4 (1 oz)	140	7	19	6
Mallomars	2 (0.9 oz)	120	5	17	12
Mystic Mint	1 (0.5 oz)	90	5	11	8
National Arrowroot	1 (5 g)	20	1	4	1
Newtons Fig	2 (1.1 oz)	110	3	22	14
Nilla Wafers	8 (1.1 oz)	140	5	24	12
Oreo	3 (1.2 oz)	160	7	23	13
Social Tea	6 (1 oz)	120	4	20	7
Teddy Grahams Honey	24 (1 oz)	130	4	23	8
Newman's Own					
Fig Newman's Organic	2 (1.3 oz)	120	0	28	15
Nonni's					
Biscotti Original	1 (1 oz)	100	4	15	8
Olde World					
Pizzelle Chocolate	3 (1 oz)	100	5	11	5
Pizzelle Vanilla	3 (1 oz)	90	4	12	4
Otis Spunkmeyer					
Butter Sugar	1 (2 oz)	250	12	35	21
Chocolate Chip	1 (2 oz)	250	11	36	21
Chocolate Chip Walnut	1 (2 oz)	270	14	34	21
Otis Express Chocolate Chunk	1 (2 oz)	280	13	37	22
Otis Express Oatmeal Raisin	1 (2 oz)	240	10	35	17
Otis Express Peanut Butter	1 (2 oz)	270	15	31	17

FOOD	PORTION	CAL	FAT	CARB	SUG
Pally					
Butter	5 (1 oz)	140	3	23	6
Tea Biscuits	5 (1 oz)	150	4	23	6
Peek Freans					
Petit Beurre	4 (1 oz)	130	4	22	5
Pepperidge Farm					
Brussels	3	150	7	20	11
Chessman	3	120	8	18	5
Chocolate Chip	3	140	7	18	9
Geneva	3	160	9	19	8
Ginger Man	4 (1 oz)	130	4	21	11
Lemon Nut Crunch	3	170	9	18	7
Lido	1	90	5	10	5
Milano	3	180	10	21	11
Real Torino					
Lady Fingers	3 (1 oz)	110	1	23	11
Royal					
Devilfood	1 (1 oz)	110	5	17	10
Salerno					
Scotter Pie	1 (1.2 oz)	140	5	23	14
Season					
Hamantashen Poppy	1 (1 oz)	150	7	20	4
Hamantasken Apricot	1 (1 oz)	150	7	20	4
SnackWell's					
Caramel Delights	1 (0.6 oz)	70	2	13	8
Chocolate Sandwich	2 (0.8 oz)	110	3	20	11
Creme Sandwich	2 (0.9 oz)	110	3	20	10
Golden Devil's Food	1 (0.5 oz)	50	1	11	7
Mint Creme	2 (0.9 oz)	110	4	19	14
Stella D'Oro					
Angel Wings	2 (0.9 oz)	140	9	13	3

FOOD	PORTION	CAL	FAT	CARB	SUG
Angelica	1 (0.8 oz)	100	4	15	6
Anisette Toast	3 (1.2 oz)	130	1	27	17
Breakfast Treats	1 (0.8 oz)	100	3	16	7
Egg Jumbo	2 (0.8 oz)	90	1	18	9
Fruit Slices Fat Free	1 (0.6 oz)	50	0	12	6
Sesame Regina	3 (1.1 oz)	150	6	21	8
Streit's					
Wafers	3 (1 oz)	160	9	19	12
Sunshine					
Hydrox	3 (1.1 oz)	150	7	21	11
Vanilla Wafers	7 (1.1 oz)	150	7	21	9
Vienna Fingers	2 (1 oz)	140	6	21	8
Tastykake					
Fudge Bar	1 (2 oz)	250	10	37	21
Lemon Bar	1 (2 oz)	260	10	41	23
Voortman					
Sugar	1 (0.6 oz)	80	4	11	5
Walkers					
Shortbread Triangles	2 (0.7 oz)	100	6	12	4
White Eagle Bakery					
Chruscik	2 (1 oz)	140	8	16	5
refrigerated					
Pillsbury					
Sugar	2	130	3	19	10
Toll House					
Brownie Dough	½ pkg (1.5 oz)	180	7	26	18
take-out					
black & white	1 lg (3 oz)	302	9	52	31
finikia	1 (1.2 oz)	171	5	16	5
koulourakia butter cookie twist	1 (0.9 oz)	113	6	14	5

FOOD	PORTION	CAL	FAT	CARB	SUG
CORIANDER					
leaf dried	1 tsp	2	tr	tr	—
leaf fresh	¼ cup	1	tr	tr	—
seed	1 tsp	5	tr	1	—
CORN					
canned					
Green Giant					
Cream Style	½ cup (4.5 oz)	100	1	22	11
Mexicorn	⅓ cup (2.7 oz)	60	0	14	4
Niblets	⅓ cup (2.7 oz)	70	0	15	4
Niblets 50% Less Sodium	⅓ cup (2.7 oz)	60	0	14	3
Niblets Extra Sweet	⅓ cup (2.6 oz)	50	1	10	4
White Shoepeg	⅓ cup	80	1	16	3
fresh					
on-the-cob w/ butter cooked	1 ear	155	3	32	—
frozen					
Birds Eye					
Gold & White Blend	½ cup (3.5 oz)	60	1	11	4
Green Giant					
Butter Sauce Niblets	⅔ cup (4.3 oz)	130	3	23	5
Extra Sweet Niblets	⅔ cup (3.1 oz)	70	1	13	6
Harvest Fresh Niblets	⅔ cup (3.4 oz)	80	1	17	3
Niblets	⅔ cup (2.9 oz)	80	1	17	3
On The Cob Extra Sweet	1 ear (4.4 oz)	120	2	22	13
Stouffer's					
Souffle	½ cup (6 oz)	170	7	21	7
take-out					
fritters	1 (1 oz)	62	2	9	—
scalloped	½ cup	258	7	43	—

FOOD	PORTION	CAL	FAT	CARB	SUG
CORN CHIPS					
(see CHIPS)					
CORNISH HENS					
(see CHICKENS)					
CORNMEAL					
Albers					
White	3 tbsp	110	0	24	0
Yellow	3 tbsp	110	0	24	0
mix					
Hodgson Mill					
Cornbread Mix Jalapeno Mexican	¼ cup (1 oz)	100	1	21	1
Yellow Organic	¼ cup (1 oz)	100	1	22	0
Yellow Self Rising	¼ cup (1 oz)	90	1	21	0
Kentucky Kernal					
Sweet Cornbread Mix	¼ cup (1 oz)	120	2	24	6
take-out					
hush puppies	1 (0.75 oz)	74	3	10	—
CORNSTARCH					
Armour					
Cream Cornstarch	1 tbsp (0.4 oz)	40	0	9	0
COTTAGE CHEESE					
Breakstone's					
2% Fat Large Curd	½ cup (4.2 oz)	90	3	4	3
2% Fat Small Curd	½ cup (4.2 oz)	90	3	4	3
4% Fat Large Curd	½ cup (4.2 oz)	120	5	5	4
4% Fat Small Curd	½ cup (4.2 oz)	120	5	5	4
Cottage Doubles Peach	1 pkg (5.5 oz)	140	3	16	13
Dry Curd	¼ cup (1.9 oz)	45	0	3	3
Free	½ cup (4.4 oz)	80	0	6	5

FOOD	PORTION	CAL	FAT	CARB	SUG
Horizon Organic					
Cottage Cheese	½ cup (3.9 oz)	110	5	4	3
Light N'Lively					
1% Fat	½ cup (4 oz)	80	1	5	4
Fat Free	½ cup (4.4 oz)	80	0	6	4
COTTONSEED					
kernels roasted	1 tbsp	51	4	2	—
COUSCOUS					
cooked	1 cup (5.5 oz)	176	tr	36	—
COWPEAS					
catjang dried cooked	1 cup (2.9 oz)	200	1	35	—
common canned	1 cup	184	1	33	—
frozen cooked	½ cup	112	tr	20	—
leafy tips chopped cooked	1 cup	12	tr	1	—
CRAB					
canned					
Bumble Bee					
Fancy Lump Meat	½ can (1.9 oz)	40	1	0	0
Fancy White Meat	½ can (1.9 oz)	28	0	1	0
fresh					
alaska king cooked	1 leg (4.7 oz)	129	2	0	0
alaska king cooked	3 oz	82	1	0	0
blue cooked	3 oz	87	2	0	0
blue cooked	1 cup	138	2	0	0
queen steamed	3 oz	98	1	0	0
take-out					
baked	1 (3.8 oz)	160	2	4	—
cake	1 (2 oz)	160	10	5	—
kenagi korean crab cooked	1 serv (3 oz)	71	tr	0	0
soft-shell fried	1 (4.4 oz)	334	18	31	—

FOOD	PORTION	CAL	FAT	CARB	SUG
CRACKER CRUMBS					
Baker's Harvest					
Graham	⅓ cup (1 oz)	130	4	23	7
Kellogg's					
Corn Flake Crumbs	2 tbsp (0.4 oz)	40	0	9	1
CRACKERS					
Ak-mak					
100% Whole Wheat	5 (1 oz)	116	2	19	2
Armenian Cracker Bread	1 sheet (1 oz)	100	2	19	2
Armenian Cracker Bread Whole Wheat	1 sheet (1 oz)	116	2	19	2
Round Cracker Bread No Seeds	1 (1 oz)	100	1	20	2
Round Cracker Bread Seeded	1 (1 oz)	100	2	19	2
Round Cracker Bread Whole Wheat	1 (1 oz)	116	2	19	2
Austin					
Cracker Sandwich Cheese On Cheese	6 (1.3 oz)	170	7	25	4
Cracker Sandwich Cheese Peanut Butter	6 (1.3 oz)	170	7	24	3
Cracker Sandwich Toasty Peanut Butter	6 (1.3 oz)	170	7	24	4
Cracker Sandwich Whole Wheat Cheese	6 (1.3 oz)	170	7	25	4
Baker's Harvest					
Cheese	23 (1 oz)	150	6	18	0
Cheese Reduced Fat	29 (1 oz)	130	4	21	0
Oyster	35 (0.5 oz)	70	2	11	0

FOOD	PORTION	CAL	FAT	CARB	SUG
Snackers	9 (1.1 oz)	160	8	19	2
Snackers Reduced Fat	10 (1.1 oz)	140	4	23	2
Barbara's Bakery					
Cheese Bites	26 (1 oz)	120	2	24	0
Right Lite Rounds Original	5 (0.5 oz)	55	5	12	1
Rite Lite Rounds Savory Poppy	5 (0.5 oz)	70	2	11	tr
Rite Lite Rounds Tamari Sesame	5 (0.5 oz)	70	2	12	tr
Wheatines All Flavors	1 lg sq (0.5 oz)	50	2	10	tr
Blue Diamond					
Nut Thins Almond	16 (1 oz)	130	5	19	0
Nut Thins Hazelnut	16 (1 oz)	120	4	20	0
Nut Thins Pecan	16 (1 oz)	130	5	20	0
Cheez It					
Big	13 (1 oz)	150	8	16	tr
Original	27 (1 oz)	160	8	16	tr
Courtney's					
Sun-Dried Tomato Organic	4 (0.5 oz)	60	1	10	0
Estee					
Sugar Free Cracked Pepper	18	120	2	24	0
Sugar Free Golden	10	130	2	28	0
Sugar Free Wheat	17	100	2	18	0
Keebler					
Club 33% Reduced Fat	5 (0.6 oz)	70	2	12	2
Club Orignal	4 (0.5 oz)	70	3	9	1
Elfin	23 (1 oz)	130	2	24	8
Export Soda	3 (0.5 oz)	60	2	10	0

FOOD	PORTION	CAL	FAT	CARB	SUG
Harvest Bakery Multigrain	2 (0.6 oz)	70	3	10	2
Munch'ems Cheddar	30 (1 oz)	130	4	21	2
Toasteds Buttercrisp	5 (0.6 oz)	80	4	10	1
Toasteds Sesame	5 (0.6 oz)	80	4	10	1
Toasteds Wheat	5 (0.6 oz)	80	4	10	2
Town House	5 (0.6 oz)	80	5	9	1
Town House Reduced Fat	6 (0.6 oz)	70	2	11	2
Wheatables Original	12 (1 oz)	140	6	10	4
Zesta Saltine Fat Free	5 (0.5 oz)	50	0	11	0
Zesta Saltine Original	5 (0.5 oz)	60	2	10	0
Zesta Soup & Oyster	42 (0.5 oz)	80	3	10	0
Lance					
Bonnie	6 (1⅛ oz)	160	7	23	7
Cheese-On-Wheat	1 pkg (1.3 oz)	190	10	21	4
Lanchee	1 pkg (1¼ oz)	190	11	18	3
Nekot	1 pkg (1.5 oz)	210	10	25	12
Nip-Chee	1 pkg (1.3 oz)	190	10	21	3
Toastchee	1 pkg (1.4 oz)	200	12	19	0
Little Debbie					
Cheese Crackers With Peanut Butter	1 (0.9 oz)	140	8	16	2
Wheat Crackers With Cheddar Cheese	1 (0.9 oz)	140	8	15	2
Nabisco					
Royal Lunch	1 (0.4 oz)	60	2	8	1
Zwieback	1 (8 g)	35	1	6	1
Pepperidge Farm					
Butter Thins	4 (0.5 oz)	70	3	10	1
Goldfish Cheddar	55	140	6	19	0
Goldfish Original	55	140	6	19	0

FOOD	PORTION	CAL	FAT	CARB	SUG
Goldfish Pizza Flavored	55 (1 oz)	140	6	19	0
Goldfish Pretzel	43 (1 oz)	120	3	22	tr
Hearty Wheat	3 (0.6 oz)	80	4	10	2
Premium					
Saltine Multigrain	5 (0.5 oz)	60	2	10	0
Ralston					
Oyster	35 (0.5 oz)	70	2	11	0
RedOval Farms					
Stoned Wheat Thins Cracked Pepper	4 (0.6 oz)	70	3	10	0
Smucker's					
Snackers Grape	1 pkg (3.3 oz)	410	20	47	23
Snackers Strawberry	1 pkg (3.3 oz)	410	20	47	23
Sunshine					
Hi Ho	4 (0.5 oz)	70	4	8	1
Hi Ho Reduced Fat	5 (0.5 oz)	70	3	10	1
Krispy	5 (0.5 oz)	60	2	10	tr
Krispy Fat Free	5 (0.5 oz)	50	0	11	0
Venus					
Fat Free Garlic & Herb	11 (0.5 oz)	10	0	12	1
Wisecrackers					
Low Fat Poblano Chili & Sweet Onion	4 (0.5 oz)	45	1	8	1
Wortz					
Oyster	35 (0.5 oz)	70	2	11	0
CRANBERRIES					
fresh chopped	1 cup	54	tr	14	—
Ocean Spray					
Craisins	⅓ cup (1.4 oz)	130	0	33	31
Cranberry Sauce Jellied	¼ cup	110	0	27	26

FOOD	PORTION	CAL	FAT	CARB	SUG
Fresh	2 oz	25	0	6	0
Whole Berry Sauce	¼ cup	110	0	28	27

CRANBERRY BEANS

canned	1 cup	216	1	39	—
dried cooked	1 cup	240	1	43	—

CRANBERRY JUICE

Ocean Spray

Cocktail	8 oz	140	0	34	34
Cocktail Reduced Calorie	8 oz	50	0	13	13
White Cranberry	1 cup (8 oz)	120	0	29	29
White Cranberry Peach	1 cup (8 oz)	120	0	30	30
White Cranberry Strawberry	1 cup (8 oz)	120	0	31	31

Veryfine

Cocktail	1 bottle (10 oz)	180	0	45	44

Wellfleet Farms

Cranberry	8 oz	130	0	33	33

CRAYFISH

cooked	3 oz	97	1	0	0

CREAM

clotted cream	2 tbsp (1 oz)	164	18	1	—
creme fraiche	2 tbsp (1 oz)	100	11	1	—
heavy whipping whipped	1 cup (4.1 oz)	411	44	7	—
light coffee	1 cup (8.4 oz)	196	46	9	—
light whipping cream whipped	1 cup (4.2 oz)	345	37	7	—

Land O Lakes

Fat Free Half & Half	2 tbsp (1 oz)	20	0	3	2
Half & Half	2 tbsp (1 oz)	40	4	1	1
Heavy Whipping	1 tbsp (0.5 oz)	50	6	0	0

FOOD	PORTION	CAL	FAT	CARB	SUG
Organic Valley					
Half & Half	2 tbsp (1 oz)	40	3	1	1

CREAM CHEESE
Alpine Lace

Reduced Fat Roasted Garlic & Herbs	1 tsp (1 oz)	60	4	2	1
Reduced Fat Sundried Tomato & Basil	2 tsp (1 oz)	70	5	2	1
Boar's Head					
Cream Cheese	2 tbsp (1 oz)	100	10	2	2
Horizon Organic					
Spreadable	2 tbsp	100	10	1	0
Organic Valley					
Cream Cheese	1 oz	100	9	1	tr
Philadelphia					
Free	1 oz	30	0	2	1
Regular	1 oz	100	10	tr	tr
Soft	2 tbsp (1 oz)	100	10	1	1
Soft Garden Vegetable	2 tbsp (1.1 oz)	110	11	1	tr
Soft Free Strawberries	2 tbsp (1.2 oz)	15	0	6	5
Soft Light Jalapeno	2 tbsp (1.1 oz)	10	5	2	2
Whipped	2 tbsp (0.7 oz)	70	7	tr	tr

CREAM OF TARTAR

cream of tartar	1 tsp	8	0	2	—

CREPES
Frieda's

Ready-To-Use	2 (0.8 oz)	50	1	9	4

CRESS

garden cooked	½ cup	16	tr	3	—
garden raw	½ cup	8	tr	1	—

FOOD	PORTION	CAL	FAT	CARB	SUG
CROAKER					
atlantic breaded & fried	3 oz	188	11	6	—
CROCODILE					
cooked	3 oz	78	1	0	0
CROISSANT					
Sara Lee					
Broccoli & Cheese	1 (3.7 oz)	280	13	30	0
French Style	1 (1.5 oz)	170	8	20	0
Ham & Swiss	1 (3.7 oz)	300	16	27	1
Petite	2 (2 oz)	230	11	26	0
take-out					
w/ egg & cheese	1 (4.5 oz)	368	25	24	—
w/ egg cheese & bacon	1 (4.5 oz)	413	28	24	—
w/ egg cheese & ham	1 (5.3 oz)	474	34	24	—
w/ egg cheese & sausage	1 (5.6 oz)	523	38	25	—
CROUTONS					
Pepperidge Farm					
Garlic	6 (0.2 oz)	30	1	5	0
Homestyle	6 (0.2 oz)	30	1	5	0
Sourdough	6 (0.2 oz)	35	2	4	0
CUCUMBER					
fresh					
Chiquita					
Cucumber	⅛ med (3.5 oz)	15	0	3	2
take-out					
cucumber salad	3.5 oz	50	tr	11	—
kimchee	½ cup (1.8 oz)	36	2	4	3
tzatziki	½ cup (3.4 oz)	72	6	4	3

FOOD	PORTION	CAL	FAT	CARB	SUG
CUMIN					
seed	1 tsp	8	tr	1	—
CURRANT JUICE					
black currant nectar	7 oz	110	0	26	—
red currant nectar	7 oz	108	tr	26	—
CURRANTS					
black fresh	½ cup	36	tr	9	—
zante dried	½ cup	204	tr	53	—
CUSK					
fillet baked	3 oz	106	1	0	0
CUSTARD					
mix					
Betty Crocker					
Flan w/ Caramel Sauce as prep	1 serv	330	7	60	23
Jell-O					
Flan as prep w/ 2% milk	½ cup (5.1 oz)	140	3	26	25
ready-to-eat					
Swiss Miss					
Egg Custard	1 pkg (4 oz)	153	5	22	21
take-out					
flan	½ cup (5.4 oz)	220	6	35	—
zabaione	½ cup (57.2 g)	135	5	13	—
CUTTLEFISH					
steamed	3 oz	134	1	1	—
DANDELION GREENS					
fresh cooked	½ cup	17	tr	3	—
raw chopped	½ cup	13	tr	3	—

FOOD	PORTION	CAL	FAT	CARB	SUG
DANISH PASTRY					
frozen					
Morton					
Honey Buns	1 (2.28 oz)	270	13	35	16
Honey Buns Mini	1 (1.3 oz)	160	8	19	6
ready-to-eat					
Dolly Madison					
Danish Rollers	3 (2.8 oz)	290	10	46	21
Tastykake					
Cheese	1 (3 oz)	290	14	44	22
Lemon	1 (3 oz)	290	14	44	22
Raspberry	1 (3 oz)	290	14	44	22
take-out					
almond	1 (4¼ in) (2.3 oz)	280	16	30	—
apple	1 (4¼ in) (2.5 oz)	264	13	34	—
cheese	1 (3.2 oz)	353	25	29	—
cheese	1 (4¼ in) (2.5 oz)	266	16	26	—
cinnamon	1 (3.1 oz)	349	17	47	—
cinnamon	1 (4¼ in) (2.3 oz)	262	15	29	—
cinnamon nut	1 (4¼ in) (2.3 oz)	280	16	30	—
fruit	1 (3.3 oz)	335	16	45	—
lemon	1 (4¼ in) (2.5 oz)	264	13	34	—
raisin	1 (4¼ in) (2.5 oz)	264	13	34	—
raspberry	1 (4¼ in) (2.5 oz)	264	13	34	—
strawberry	1 (4¼ in) (2.5 oz)	264	13	34	—
DATES					
jujube dried	1 oz	75	tr	19	—
jujube preserved in sugar	1 oz	91	tr	22	—
Calavo					
Dried Pitted	5–6 (1.4 oz)	120	0	31	20

FOOD	PORTION	CAL	FAT	CARB	SUG
California Redi-Date					
Deglet Noor Dried	5–6 (1.4 oz)	120	0	31	29
Sonoma					
Dried	5–6 (1.4 oz)	110	0	30	21

DEER

(*see* VENISON)

DELI MEATS/COLD CUTS

(*see also* BEEF, CHICKEN, HAM, MEAT SUBSTITUTES, TURKEY)

blood sausage	1 oz	95	9	tr	—
braunschweiger pork	1 oz	102	9	1	—
headcheese pork	1 oz	60	5	tr	—
liverwurst pork	1 oz	92	8	1	—
olive loaf pork	1 oz	67	5	3	—
Boar's Head					
Bologna Beef	2 oz	150	13	0	0
Bologna Garlic	2 oz	150	13	1	1
Bologna Lowered Sodium	2 oz	150	13	0	0
Bologna Pork & Beef	2 oz	150	13	tr	tr
Braunschweiger Lite	2 oz	120	8	1	0
Head Cheese	2 oz	90	5	tr	0
Liverwurst Strassburger	2 oz	170	15	1	1
Olive Loaf	2 oz	130	12	tr	tr
Pastrami	2 oz	90	4	2	0
Prosciutto	1 oz	60	3	0	0
Red Pastrami	2 oz	90	4	2	0
Salami Beef	2 oz	120	9	0	0
Salami Cooked	2 oz	130	11	0	0
Salami Genoa	2 oz	180	14	1	0

FOOD	PORTION	CAL	FAT	CARB	SUG
Salami Hard	1 oz	110	9	tr	0
Spiced Ham	2 oz	120	10	1	0
Hormel					
Pepperoni Sliced	15 slices (1 oz)	140	13	0	0
Pillow Pack Genoa Salami	2 oz	160	18	0	0
Oscar Mayer					
Bologna	1 slice (1 oz)	90	8	1	tr
Braunschweiger Spread	2 oz	190	17	2	tr
Light Bologna	1 slice (1 oz)	60	4	2	tr
Liver Cheese	1 slice (1.3 oz)	120	10	1	0
Luncheon Loaf Spiced	1 slice (1 oz)	70	5	2	1
Old Fashioned Loaf	1 slice (1 oz)	70	5	2	1
Olive Loaf	1 slice (1 oz)	70	6	2	tr
Pepperoni	15 slices (1 oz)	140	13	0	0
Salami Cotto	1 slice (1 oz)	70	5	1	0
Salami Hard	3 slices (1 oz)	100	9	0	0
Spam					
Less Salt	2 oz	170	16	0	0
Lite	2 oz	110	8	0	0
Original	2 oz	170	16	0	0
Smoked	2 oz	170	16	0	0

DIETING AIDS

(*see* NUTRITION SUPPLEMENTS)

DILL

seed	1 tsp	6	tr	1	—
sprigs fresh	5	0	tr	tr	—
weed dry	1 tsp	3	tr	1	—

FOOD	PORTION	CAL	FAT	CARB	SUG
DINNER					
Banquet					
Beef Patty w/ Country Style Vegetables	1 meal (9.5 oz)	310	20	22	6
Boneless Pork Rib	1 meal (10 oz)	400	19	40	22
Boneless White Fried Chicken	1 meal (8.25 oz)	540	34	41	10
Chicken Parmigiana	1 meal (9.5 oz)	320	18	29	7
Chicken Fingers Meal	1 meal (7.1 oz)	740	43	67	24
Chicken Fried Beef Steak	1 pkg (10 oz)	420	23	39	9
Chicken Nuggets Meal	1 meal (6.75 oz)	430	23	42	11
Extra Helping Boneless Pork Riblet	1 meal (15.25 oz)	720	40	62	18
Extra Helping Fried Beef Steak	1 meal (16 oz)	820	50	63	13
Extra Helping Fried Chicken	1 meal (14.7 oz)	910	55	70	8
Extra Helping Meatloaf	1 meal (16 oz)	610	40	34	12
Extra Helping Salisbury Steak	1 meal (16.5 oz)	740	54	37	7
Extra Helping Turkey & Gravy w/ Dressing	1 meal (17 oz)	620	32	54	11
Extra Helping White Fried Chicken	1 meal (13 oz)	690	48	40	3
Extra Helping Yankee Pot Roast	1 meal (14.5 oz)	410	20	33	25
Family Size Brown Gravy & Salisbury Steak	1 serv	240	20	7	2
Family Size Brown Gravy & Sliced Beef	1 serv	140	8	5	2

FOOD	PORTION	CAL	FAT	CARB	SUG
Family Size Chicken & Broccoli Alfredo	1 serv	270	12	28	3
Family Size Country Style Chicken & Dumplings	1 serv	290	14	30	6
Family Size Creamy Broccoli Chicken Cheese & Rice	1 serv	280	14	25	6
Family Size Hearty Beef Stew	1 cup	170	7	18	4
Family Size Homestyle Gravy & Sliced Turkey	2 slices	140	10	5	1
Family Size Mushroom Gravy & Charbroiled Beef Patties	1 patty	250	20	6	2
Family Size Potato Ham & Broccoli Au Gratin	⅔ cup	210	13	16	6
Family Size Savory Gravy & Meatloaf	1 slice	120	13	7	2
Fish Sticks	1 meal (6.6 oz)	290	13	33	14
Grilled Chicken	1 meal (9.9 oz)	330	13	37	18
Honey Roast Turkey Breast	1 meal (9 oz)	270	12	29	8
Meatloaf	1 meal (9.5 oz)	280	16	23	9
Our Original Fried Chicken	1 meal (9 oz)	470	27	35	4
Pork Cutlet Meal	1 meal (10.25 oz)	420	25	36	21
Salisbury Steak	1 meal (9.5 oz)	380	24	28	4
Sliced Beef	1 meal (9 oz)	270	10	19	12
Turkey	1 meal (9.25 oz)	270	11	30	7
Veal Parmagiana	1 meal (8.75 oz)	330	14	37	7
Western Style Beef Patty	1 meal (9.5 oz)	360	21	28	4

FOOD	PORTION	CAL	FAT	CARB	SUG
White Meat Fried Chicken	1 meal (8.75 oz)	460	28	40	4
Yankee Pot Roast	1 meal (9.4 oz)	230	10	20	8
Birds Eye					
Chicken Voila! Alfredo	1 cup (6.1 oz)	230	8	26	5
Chicken Voila! Garden Herb	1 cup	310	15	28	8
Chicken Voila! Grilled Salsa	1 cup	240	5	35	5
Chicken Voila! Teriyaki	2 cups (6.4 oz)	240	9	26	7
Chicken Voila! Zesty Garlic Chicken	2 cups (6.2 oz)	260	11	28	6
Easy Recipe Creations Sweet & Sour w/ Pineapple Tidbits as prep	1⅜ cups (8.7 oz)	200	1	45	41
Steak Voila! Beef Sirloin Steak And Garlic Potatoes	1 cup	240	9	26	5
Turkey Voila! Homestyle w/ Roasted Potatoes	1 cup	200	6	24	4
Healthy Choice					
Beef Pepper Steak Oriental	1 meal (9.5 oz)	260	5	34	5
Beef Pot Roast	1 meal (11 oz)	300	6	41	24
Beef Stoganoff	1 meal (11 oz)	320	8	40	14
Beef Tips Francais	1 meal (9.5 oz)	300	7	40	6
Beef Tips Portabello	1 meal (11.25 oz)	270	5	34	14
Bowls Chicken Teriyaki w/ Rice	1 meal (9.5 oz)	270	4	41	7
Bowls Country Chicken Bake	1 meal (9.5 oz)	230	8	22	9
Bowls Fiesta Chicken	1 meal (9.5 oz)	220	2	34	6

FOOD	PORTION	CAL	FAT	CARB	SUG
Bowls Garlic Lemon Chicken w/ Rice	1 meal (9.5 oz)	300	4	48	6
Bowls Roasted Potatoes w/ Ham	1 meal (8.5 oz)	210	4	26	10
Bowls Turkey Divan	1 meal (9.5 oz)	250	6	31	7
Charbroiled Beef Patty	1 meal (11 oz)	310	9	40	8
Chicken Cantonese	1 meal (10.75 oz)	280	6	34	15
Chicken Parmigiana	1 meal (11.5 oz)	330	8	46	23
Chicken & Vegetables Marsala	1 meal (11.5 oz)	240	4	32	4
Chicken Broccoli Alfredo	1 meal (11.5 oz)	300	7	34	5
Chicken Dijon	1 meal (11 oz)	270	5	33	6
Chicken Teriyaki	1 meal (11 oz)	270	6	37	11
Country Breaded Chicken	1 meal (10.25 oz)	350	9	51	20
Country Glazed Chicken Breast	1 meal (8.5 oz)	250	5	31	6
Country Herb Chicken	1 meal (12.15 oz)	320	8	44	23
Country Inn Roast Turkey	1 meal (10 oz)	250	6	28	16
Garlic Chicken Milano	1 meal (9.5 oz)	260	6	34	4
Grilled Chicken Sonoma	1 meal (9 oz)	200	4	30	9
Grilled Chicken w/ Mashed Potatoes	1 meal (8 oz)	180	4	18	3
Herb Baked Fish	1 meal (10.9 oz)	340	7	54	11
Herb Breaded Pork Patty	1 meal (8 oz)	280	6	38	4
Homestyle Chicken & Pasta	1 meal (9 oz)	270	6	32	6
Honey Glazed Chicken	1 meal (10 oz)	270	7	32	11
Honey Mustard Chicken	1 meal (9.5 oz)	290	6	38	7
Lemon Pepper Fish	1 meal (10.7 oz)	320	7	50	20

FOOD	PORTION	CAL	FAT	CARB	SUG
Mandarin Chicken	1 meal (10 oz)	280	3	44	9
Mesquite Beef w/ Barbecue Sauce	1 meal (11 oz)	320	9	36	16
Mesquite Chicken Barbecue	1 meal (10.5 oz)	310	5	48	15
Oriental Style Chicken & Vegetable Stir Fry	1 meal (11.9 oz)	360	6	57	16
Oven Roasted Beef	1 meal (10.15 oz)	280	8	35	10
Roast Turkey Breast	1 meal (8.5 oz)	220	5	28	0
Roasted Chicken	1 meal (11 oz)	230	5	23	9
Sesame Chicken	1 meal (10.8 oz)	360	7	54	17
Shrimp & Vegetables	1 meal (11.8 oz)	270	6	39	6
Sweet & Sour Chicken	1 meal (11 oz)	360	7	53	25
Traditional Meatloaf	1 meal (12 oz)	330	7	52	17
Tradtional Breast Of Turkey	1 meal (10.5 oz)	290	5	40	20
Tradtional Salisbury Steak	1 meal (11.5 oz)	330	7	48	24
Tuna Casserole	1 meal (8 oz)	240	5	33	7
Kid Cuisine					
Circus Show Corn Dog	1 meal (8.8 oz)	490	20	70	46
Cosmic Chicken Nuggets	1 meal (9.1 oz)	500	25	50	19
Futuristic Fish Sticks	1 meal (8.25 oz)	410	16	57	30
Game Time Taco Roll Up	1 meal (7.35 oz)	420	18	55	25
High Flying Fried Chicken	1 meal (10.1 oz)	440	20	48	20
Parachuting Pork Ribettes	1 meal (7.55 oz)	390	19	39	16
Lean Cuisine					
Cafe Classics Baked Chicken	1 pkg (8.6 oz)	240	5	33	4

FOOD	PORTION	CAL	FAT	CARB	SUG
Cafe Classics Baked Fish	1 pkg (9 oz)	290	6	40	6
Cafe Classics Beef Peppercorn	1 pkg (8.75 oz)	260	7	32	5
Cafe Classics Beef Portobello	1 pkg (9 oz)	220	7	24	6
Cafe Classics Beef Pot Roast	1 pkg (9 oz)	210	6	25	4
Cafe Classics Chicken Carbonara	1 pkg (9 oz)	280	7	36	5
Cafe Classics Chicken Medallions w/ Creamy Cheese Sauce	1 pkg (9.37 oz)	300	7	40	5
Cafe Classics Chicken Mediterranean	1 pkg (10.5 oz)	260	4	38	6
Cafe Classics Chicken & Vegetables	1 pkg (10.5 oz)	240	5	30	5
Cafe Classics Chicken In Peanut Sauce	1 pkg (9 oz)	260	6	32	7
Cafe Classics Chicken In Wine Sauce	1 pkg (8.1 oz)	220	5	23	7
Cafe Classics Chicken L'Orange	1 pkg (9 oz)	230	2	33	9
Cafe Classics Chicken Parmesan	1 pkg (10.9 oz)	300	6	41	8
Cafe Classics Chicken Piccata	1 pkg (9 oz)	300	9	41	9
Cafe Classics Chicken w/ Basil Cream Sauce	1 pkg (8.5 oz)	260	7	33	4
Cafe Classics Country Vegetables & Beef	1 pkg (9 oz)	210	4	33	9
Cafe Classics Fiesta Chicken	1 pkg (9.25 oz)	270	5	40	3

FOOD	PORTION	CAL	FAT	CARB	SUG
Cafe Classics Glazed Chicken	1 pkg (8.5 oz)	240	6	25	7
Cafe Classics Glazed Turkey Tenderloins	1 pkg (9 oz)	260	5	41	20
Cafe Classics Grilled Chicken	1 pkg (9.4 oz)	250	5	29	6
Cafe Classics Herb Roasted Chicken	1 pkg (8 oz)	190	4	22	6
Cafe Classics Honey Mustard Chicken	1 pkg (8 oz)	270	4	40	8
Cafe Classics Honey Roasted Chicken	1 pkg (8.5 oz)	270	6	41	13
Cafe Classics Honey Roasted Pork	1 serv (9.5 oz)	250	6	32	11
Cafe Classics Meatloaf w/ Whipped Potatoes	1 pkg (9.4 oz)	260	7	28	5
Cafe Classics Oriental Beef	1 pkg (9.25 oz)	210	4	30	8
Cafe Classics Oven Roasted Beef	1 pkg (9.25 oz)	260	8	28	7
Cafe Classics Roasted Turkey Breast	1 pkg (9.75 oz)	270	2	49	27
Cafe Classics Salisbury Steak	1 pkg (9.5 oz)	280	8	29	2
Cafe Classics Southern Beef Tips	1 pkg (8.75 oz)	270	6	37	10
Everyday Favorites Chicken Chow Mein	1 pkg (9 oz)	240	4	37	3
Everyday Favorites Chicken Florentine	1 pkg (8 oz)	220	5	32	3
Everyday Favorites Homestyle Turkey	1 pkg (9.4 oz)	240	5	27	6
Everyday Favorites Hunan Beef & Broccoli	1 pkg (8.5 oz)	240	4	40	9

FOOD	PORTION	CAL	FAT	CARB	SUG
Everyday Favorites Mandarin Chicken	1 pkg (9 oz)	260	5	38	9
Everyday Favorites Roasted Chicken	1 pkg (8.1 oz)	260	7	34	3
Everyday Favorites Stuffed Cabbage	1 pkg (9.5 oz)	210	8	25	4
Everyday Favorites Vegetable Lasagna	1 pkg (10.5 oz)	260	7	36	9
Hearty Portions Cheese & Spinach Manicotti	1 serv	370	8	50	14
Hearty Portions Chicken & Barbecue Sauce	1 serv	370	6	60	31
Hearty Portions Homestyle Beef Stroganoff	1 serv	350	9	44	12
Hearty Portions Jumbo Rigatoni w/ Meatballs	1 serv	440	9	64	12
Hearty Portions Oriental Glazed Chicken	1 serv	370	2	66	12
Hearty Portions Roasted Chicken w/ Mushrooms	1 serv	330	4	49	5
Skillet Sensations Beef Teriyaki & Rice	1 serv	280	3	48	11
Skillet Sensations Chicken Primavera	1 serv	320	5	50	7
Skillet Sensations Chicken Oriental	1 serv	280	3	46	10
Skillet Sensations Fiesta Beef & Rice	1 serv	300	4	48	6

FOOD	PORTION	CAL	FAT	CARB	SUG
Skillet Sensations Garlic Chicken	1 serv	340	5	56	6
Skillet Sensations Herb Chicken & Roasted Potatoes	1 serv	270	5	39	10
Skillet Sensations Roasted Turkey	1 serv	220	2	37	10
Skillet Sensations Savory Beef & Vegetables	1 serv	290	7	38	9
Skillet Sensations Three Cheese Chicken	1 serv	370	10	45	9
Luzianne					
Cajun Creole Dirty Rice	1 serv	160	1	35	0
Cajun Creole Etouffee	1 serv	200	1	42	2
Cajun Creole Gumbo	1 serv	160	1	33	3
Cajun Creole Jambalaya	1 serv	200	1	43	0
Marie Callender's					
Beef Stroganoff w/ Noodles	1 meal (13 oz)	600	27	59	9
Beef Tips In Mushroom Sauce	1 meal (13 oz)	430	19	39	11
Breaded Chicken Parmigiana	1 meal (16 oz)	860	32	63	18
Cheesy Rice w/ Chicken & Broccoli	1 meal (12 oz)	390	13	44	8
Chicken & Dumplings	1 meal (14 oz)	390	20	34	14
Chicken & Noodles	1 meal (13 oz)	520	30	42	7
Chicken Cordon Bleu	1 meal (13 oz)	610	28	58	9
Chicken Fried Beef Steak & Gravy	1 meal (15 oz)	650	37	50	9

FOOD	PORTION	CAL	FAT	CARB	SUG
Chicken Teriyaki	1 meal (13 oz)	510	12	71	22
Country Fried Chicken & Gravy	1 meal (16 oz)	620	30	63	16
Country Fried Pork Chop	1 meal (15 oz)	540	28	50	23
Escalloped Noodles & Chicken	1 meal (13 oz)	740	46	60	10
Glazed Chicken	1 meal (13 oz)	490	25	40	2
Grilled Southwestern Style Chicken	1 meal (14 oz)	410	11	43	9
Grilled Chicken & Mashed Potatoes	1 meal (10 oz)	340	16	20	2
Grilled Chicken Breast & Rice Pilaf	1 meal (11.75 oz)	360	14	36	14
Grilled Chicken In Mushroom Sauce	1 meal (14 oz)	480	15	54	0
Grilled Turkey Breast & Rice Pilaf	1 meal (11.75 oz)	310	10	34	8
Herb Roasted Chicken & Mashed Potatoes	1 meal (14 oz)	580	34	26	16
Homestyle Turkey & Noodles	1 meal (12 oz)	600	35	52	12
Honey Roasted Chicken	1 meal (14 oz)	440	17	27	7
Honey Smoked Ham Steak w/ Macroni & Cheese	1 meal (14 oz)	490	13	63	32
Meatloaf & Gravy w/ Mashed Potatoes	1 meal (14 oz)	540	30	42	30
Old Fashioned Beef Pot Roast & Gravy	1 meal (15 oz)	500	17	55	13
Roast Beef	1 meal (14.5 oz)	390	19	30	7
Sirloin Salisbury Steak & Gravy	1 meal (14 oz)	550	25	51	14

FOOD	PORTION	CAL	FAT	CARB	SUG
Skillet Meal Au Gratin Potatoes	⅔ cup (5 oz)	190	10	19	4
Skillet Meal Beef Pot Roast	½ pkg	290	9	33	5
Skillet Meal Beef Stroganoff	½ pkg	310	11	31	7
Skillet Meal Chicken & Rice w/ Broccoli & Cheese	½ pkg	440	14	47	5
Skillet Meal Chicken Teriyaki	½ pkg	340	1	61	14
Skillet Meal Herb Chicken	½ pkg	290	4	42	1
Skillet Meal Roasted Chicken & Vegetables	½ pkg	260	6	30	1
Skillet Meal White & Wild Rice In Cheese Sauce	1 cup	300	13	35	7
Swedish Meatballs	1 meal (12.5 oz)	520	26	44	3
Sweet & Sour Chicken	1 meal (14 oz)	570	15	66	55
Turkey w/ Gravy & Dressing	1 meal (14 oz)	500	19	52	11
Morton					
Breaded Chicken Pattie	1 meal (6.75 oz)	290	17	24	12
Chicken Nuggets	1 meal (7 oz)	340	19	31	12
Chili Gravy w/ Beef Enchilada & Tamale	1 meal (10 oz)	270	9	40	3
Fried Chicken	1 meal (9 oz)	470	30	30	4
Gravy & Charbroiled Beef Patty	1 meal (9 oz)	310	18	26	3
Gravy & Salisbury Steak	1 meal (9 oz)	310	20	24	7
Gravy & Turkey w/ Stuffing	1 meal (9 oz)	240	10	27	5

FOOD	PORTION	CAL	FAT	CARB	SUG
Tomato Sauce w/ Meat Loaf	1 meal (9 oz)	250	13	24	17
Veal Parmagiana w/ Tomato Sauce	1 meal (8.75 oz)	290	15	30	8
Nature's Choice					
Broccoli Parmesan Alfredo	1 pkg (12 oz)	270	9	29	4
Nature's Entree					
Hearty Stew	1 pkg (12 oz)	290	9	34	6
Tuscany White Bean	1 pkg (12 oz)	330	8	42	4
Patio					
Ranchera	1 pkg (13 oz)	470	22	55	4
Swanson					
Beef Pot Roast	1 pkg (14 oz)	320	8	44	15
Chicken Parmigiana w/ Spaghetti	1 pkg (11 oz)	380	17	41	18
Turkey Breast	1 pkg (11.7 oz)	330	6	50	18
Weight Watchers					
Smart Ones Swedish Meatballs	1 pkg (9 oz)	280	70	34	2
Yves					
Voggie Country Stew	1 pkg (10.5 oz)	170	0	24	2

DIP

FOOD	PORTION	CAL	FAT	CARB	SUG
Snyder's Of Hanover					
Microwavable Hot Nacho Cheese	2 tbsp	48	3	5	2
Microwavable Mild Cheese	2 tbsp	45	3	2	1
Mustard Pretzel	2 tbsp	60	2	12	11
Sour Cream & Onion	2 tbsp	60	5	2	1

FOOD	PORTION	CAL	FAT	CARB	SUG
DOCK					
fresh cooked	3½ oz	20	1	3	—
DOLPHINFISH					
fresh baked	3 oz	93	1	0	0
DOUGHNUTS					
Dolly Madison					
Chocolate Frosted	1 (1.1 oz)	140	8	15	9
Donut Gems Chocolate	4 (2 oz)	260	15	28	17
Donut Gems Powdered	4 (2 oz)	230	11	30	14
Glazed Whirl	1 (1.6 oz)	210	11	25	9
Glazed Yeast	1 (1.5 oz)	190	9	23	6
Old Fashioned	1 (2.1 oz)	280	16	28	23
Plain	1 (1.2 oz)	140	7	15	3
Powdered	1 (1 oz)	120	6	14	7
Dutch Mill					
Cinnamon	1 (1.8 oz)	210	11	26	12
Double-Dipped Chocolate	1 (2.1 oz)	280	17	31	9
Glazed	1 (2.1 oz)	250	12	34	23
Plain	1 (1.8 oz)	210	12	25	9
Sugared	1 (1.8 oz)	220	11	27	12
Hostess					
Donettes Crumb	3 (1.5 oz)	170	8	23	16
Donettes Frosted	3 (1.5 oz)	200	12	21	13
Donettes Powdered	3 (1.5 oz)	180	9	23	10
Old Fashioned Glazed	1 (2.1 oz)	260	13	33	14
Plain	1 (1.1 oz)	140	7	15	3
Powdered	1 (1.3 oz)	150	8	19	9
Little Debbie					
Donut Sticks	1 (1.6 oz)	210	12	24	15
Mini Powdered	1 pkg (2.5 oz)	290	14	38	19

FOOD	PORTION	CAL	FAT	CARB	SUG
Tastykake					
Mini Plain Glaze	1 pkg (2.5 oz)	260	11	40	23
Mini Rich Frosted	1 pkg (3 oz)	370	22	43	23
Tom's					
Chocolate Gem	1 pkg (2.5 oz)	320	18	37	19
Dunkin' Sticks	1 pkg (2.5 oz)	370	22	43	20
Powdered Gems	1 pkg (2.5 oz)	320	18	41	23

DRESSING

(*see* STUFFING/DRESSING)

DRINK MIXERS

FOOD	PORTION	CAL	FAT	CARB	SUG
Daily's					
Bloody Mary Original	1 serv (6 oz)	50	0	14	14
Margarita Daiquiri Strawberry	1 serv (4 oz)	180	0	47	45
Margarita Green Demon	1 serv (3 oz)	80	0	19	19
Pina Colada	1 serv (3 oz)	160	2	37	36
Tabasco					
Bloody Mary Mix	1 serv (8.4 oz)	56	tr	11	8
Bloody Mary Mix Extra Spicy	1 serv (8.4 oz)	58	tr	11	10

DRUM

FOOD	PORTION	CAL	FAT	CARB	SUG
freshwater baked	3 oz	130	5	0	0

DUCK

FOOD	PORTION	CAL	FAT	CARB	SUG
w/ skin roasted	1 cup (4.9 oz)	472	40	0	0
w/ skin w/ bone leg roasted	3 oz	184	10	0	0
w/ skin w/o bone breast roasted	3 oz	172	9	0	0
w/o skin roasted	1 cup (4.9 oz)	281	16	0	0
w/o skin w/o bone breast broiled	1 cup (6.1 oz)	244	4	0	0

FOOD	PORTION	CAL	FAT	CARB	SUG
Grimaud Farms					
Muscovy Duck Confit	1 serv (3 oz)	170	10	tr	—
DUMPLING					
Health Is Wealth					
Potstickers Chicken Free	2 (1.6 oz)	80	4	11	1
Potstickers Pork Free	2 (1.6 oz)	80	4	11	1
Potstickers Vegetable	2 (1.6 oz)	90	3	11	0
Steamed Dumpling	2 (1.6 oz)	50	2	12	0
Pepperidge Farm					
Apple	1 (3 oz)	230	11	30	11
Peach	1 (3 oz)	320	11	50	15
DURIAN					
fresh	3.5 oz	141	2	29	—
EDAMAME					
(*see* SOYBEANS)					
EEL					
fresh cooked	3 oz	200	13	0	0
smoked	3.5 oz	330	28	0	0
EGG					
chicken					
fresh	1	75	5	1	—
hard cooked	1	77	5	1	—
hard cooked chopped	1 cup	210	14	2	—
poached	1	74	5	1	—
white only	1	17	0	tr	—
Horizon Organic					
Medium	1 (1.5 oz)	70	4	1	—

FOOD	PORTION	CAL	FAT	CARB	SUG
Organic Valley					
Brown Extra Large	1 (2.2 oz)	90	6	tr	—
Brown Large	1 (2 oz)	80	6	tr	—
Brown Medium	1 (1.8 oz)	70	5	tr	—
other poultry					
duck	1 (2.5 oz)	130	10	1	—
duck 100 year old	1 (1 oz)	49	3	1	—
duck salted	1 (1 oz)	54	4	2	—
goose	1 (5 oz)	267	19	2	—
quail	1 (9 g)	14	1	tr	—
turkey	1 (2.7 oz)	135	9	1	—

EGG DISHES

take-out

FOOD	PORTION	CAL	FAT	CARB	SUG
deviled	2 halves	145	13	1	—
omelette plain	1 serv (3.5 oz)	172	13	tr	tr
salad	½ cup	307	28	2	—
scotch egg	1 (4.2 oz)	301	21	16	—
scrambled plain	2 (3.3 oz)	199	15	2	—
scrambled w/ whole milk & margarine	1 serv	365	27	5	—
sunny side up	1	91	7	1	—

EGG ROLLS

Chun King

FOOD	PORTION	CAL	FAT	CARB	SUG
Chicken Mini	6	210	9	25	3
Chicken Restaurant Style	1 (3 oz)	190	9	22	4
Pork & Shrimp Mini	6	210	9	27	4
Shrimp Mini	6	190	6	28	3
Shrimp Restaurant Style	1 (3 oz)	180	7	25	6

FOOD	PORTION	CAL	FAT	CARB	SUG
Health Is Wealth					
Broccoli	1 (3 oz)	150	5	23	0
Oriental Vegetable	1 (3 oz)	160	4	23	0
Oriental Chicken Free	1 (3 oz)	120	4	21	0
Pizza	1 (3 oz)	200	9	23	0
Spinach	1 (3 oz)	180	8	20	0
Spring Rolls	1 (1.6 oz)	70	2	10	0
Veggie	1 (3 oz)	130	4	21	0
La Choy					
Chicken Mini	6	210	9	25	3
Chicken Restaurant Style	1 (3 oz)	210	9	25	4
Pork Restaurant Style	1 (3 oz)	220	11	24	6
Pork & Shrimp Bite Size	12	210	10	25	3
Pork & Shrimp Mini	6	210	9	27	4
Shrimp Mini	6	190	6	28	3
Shrimp Restaurant Style	1 (3 oz)	180	7	25	6
Sweet & Sour Chicken Restaurant Style	1 (3 oz)	220	9	29	10
Vegetable w/ Lobster Mini	6	190	7	27	3
take-out					
lobster	1 (4.8 oz)	270	7	43	4
lumpia vegetable & shrimp	2 (3 oz)	120	0	26	1
meat & shrimp	1 (4.8 oz)	320	12	41	3
pork & shrimp	1 (5 oz)	300	10	41	6
shrimp	1 (3 oz)	170	5	24	5
spicy pork	1 (3 oz)	200	9	23	3
vegetable	1 (3 oz)	170	4	28	4

FOOD	PORTION	CAL	FAT	CARB	SUG
EGG SUBSTITUTES					
Better'n Eggs					
Fat Free Cholesterol Free	¼ cup (2 oz)	30	0	1	1
Morningstar Farms					
Breakfast Sandwich Bagel Scramblers Pattie Cheese	1 (5.9 oz)	320	5	40	6
Scramblers	¼ cup (2 oz)	35	0	2	2
EGGNOG					
eggnog	1 qt	1368	76	138	—
Oberweis					
Egg Nog	½ cup	240	15	25	21
EGGPLANT					
cubed cooked	½ cup	13	tr	3	—
slices grilled	4 (7 oz)	38	0	0	0
Progresso					
Caponata	2 tbsp (1 oz)	25	2	2	2
take-out					
baba ghannouj	¼ cup	55	4	5	—
caponata	2 tbsp (1 oz)	30	2	3	2
iman bayildi eggplant w/ onion & tomato	1 serv (15.6 oz)	345	28	25	6
indian eggplant runi	1 serv	180	14	13	1
papoutsakis little shoes	1 serv (15.5 oz)	245	16	15	1
ELDERBERRIES					
fresh	1 cup	105	1	27	—
ELDERBERRY JUICE					
elderberry	7 oz	76	0	16	—

FOOD	PORTION	CAL	FAT	CARB	SUG
ELK					
roasted	3 oz	124	2	0	0
ENDIVE					
raw chopped	½ cup	4	tr	1	—
ENERGY BARS					
AllGoode Organics					
Amazin' Peanut Raisin	1 bar	210	11	25	15
Banana Nut Nirvana	1 bar	190	8	30	21
Cashew Almond Passion	1 bar	210	9	25	16
Chocolate Peanut Pleasure	1 bar	200	9	29	22
Honey Nut Harvest	1 bar	210	9	29	17
Nutty Chocolate Apricot	1 bar	200	10	26	19
Balance					
Oasis Strawberry Cheesecake	1 bar (1.69 oz)	180	3	28	16
Better Bar					
Chocolate Coated Peanut	1 bar (1.8 oz)	180	4	15	10
Yogurt Coated Raspberry	1 bar (1.8 oz)	180	3	15	11
Carbolite					
Chocolate Peanut Butter Sugar Free	1 bar (1 oz)	144	12	2	0
Clif Bar					
Apricot	1 bar (2.4 oz)	220	3	43	21
Carrot Cake	1 bar (2.4 oz)	240	4	43	21
Chocolate Brownie	1 bar (2.4 oz)	240	4	41	20
Chocolate Almond Fudge	1 bar (2.4 oz)	230	5	36	20

FOOD	PORTION	CAL	FAT	CARB	SUG
Chocolate Chip	1 bar (2.4 oz)	240	4	41	21
Chocolate Chip Peanut Crunch	1 bar (2.4 oz)	240	5	39	20
Cookies'N Cream	1 bar (2.4 oz)	230	4	39	21
Cranberry Apple Cherry	1 bar (2.4 oz)	220	2	44	22
Crunchy Peanut Butter	1 bar (2.4 oz)	240	5	39	18
GingerSnap	1 bar (2.4 oz)	230	4	42	20
Ensure					
All Flavors	1 bar (2.1 oz)	230	6	35	23
Glucerna					
All Flavors	1 bar (1.3 oz)	140	4	24	7
Jenny Craig					
Meal Bar Chocolate Peanut	1 bar (2 oz)	220	5	33	20
Meal Bar Lemon Meringue	1 bar (2 oz)	210	5	31	23
Meal Bar Milk Chocolate	1 bar (2 oz)	210	5	33	20
Meal Bar Oatmeal Raisin	1 bar (1.97 oz)	210	3	35	22
Meal Bar Yogurt Peanut	1 bar (2 oz)	220	5	33	20
Kashi					
GoLean Chocolate Peanut Butter	1 (2.7 oz)	280	6	50	26
GoLean Honey Vanilla Yogurt	1 (2.7 oz)	280	4	53	26
GoLean Strawberry Vanilla Yogurt	1 (2.7 oz)	280	4	53	28
Luna					
Chai Tea	1 bar (1.7 oz)	180	4	27	12
Chocolate Pecan Pie	1 bar (1.7 oz)	180	5	24	12
LemonZest	1 bar (1.7 oz)	180	4	24	12

FOOD	PORTION	CAL	FAT	CARB	SUG
Nutz Over Chocolate	1 bar (1.7 oz)	180	5	24	12
S'Mores	1 bar (1.7 oz)	180	4	26	12
Sesame Raisin Crunch	1 bar (1.7 oz)	170	3	26	13
Toasted Nuts 'n Cranberry	1 bar (1.7 oz)	170	3	26	12
Tropical Crisp	1 bar (1.7 oz)	180	5	24	11
Met-Rx					
Big 100 Gram Bar Peanut Butter	1 bar (3.5 oz)	340	4	52	38
Source/One Chocolate Cheesecake	1 bar (2.1 oz)	160	5	21	4
Nutiva					
Flaxseed & Raisin Organic	1 bar (1.4 oz)	280	19	12	5
Hempseed Bar Organic	1 bar (1.4 oz)	210	14	11	5
Odwalla Bar!					
Peanut Crunch	1 bar (2.2 oz)	260	7	40	17
PermaLean					
Protein Crunch Chocoholic Chocolate	1 bar (1.8 oz)	170	3	10	1
Protein Crunch Chocolate Raspberry	1 bar (1.8 oz)	180	2	9	1
Protein Crunch Stark Raving Peanutz	1 bar (1.8 oz)	180	4	9	2
PowerBar					
Essentials Chocolate	1 bar (1.9 oz)	180	4	28	20
Harvest Blueberry	1 bar (2.3 oz)	240	4	45	18
Vanilla Crisp	1 bar (2.3 oz)	230	3	45	20
Revival					
Marshmallow Krunch	1 bar (2.1 oz)	220	3	30	21
Protein Bars Chocolate Temptation	1 bar (2.1 oz)	220	4	31	22

FOOD	PORTION	CAL	FAT	CARB	SUG
Protein Bars Peanut Butter Chocolate Pal	1 bar (2.1 oz)	240	6	30	18
Protein Bars Peanut Butter Pal	1 bar (2.1 oz)	240	5	29	19
Slim-Fast					
Crispy Peanut Caramel	1 bar	120	4	21	13
Dutch Chocolate	1 bar	140	5	20	13
Meal On-The-Go Apple Cobbler	1 bar	220	5	33	23
Meal On-The-Go Chocolate Cookie Dough	1 bar	220	5	35	22
Meal On-The-Go Honey Peanut	1 bar	220	5	34	23
Meal On-The-Go Milk Chocolate Peanut	1 bar	220	5	36	24
Meal On-The-Go Oatmeal Raisin	1 bar	220	5	36	19
Meal On-The-Go Rich Chocolate Brownie	1 bar	220	5	34	23
Meal On-The-Go Toasted Oat & Spice	1 bar	220	5	35	20
Peanut Butter	1 bar	150	5	19	10
Peanut Butter Crunch	1 bar	130	4	21	20
Rich Chewy Caramel	1 bar	120	4	22	11
Sweet Success					
Chewy Chocolate Brownie	1 bar (1.2 oz)	120	4	23	12
ZonePerfect					
Honey Peanut	1 bar (1.8 oz)	200	7	22	20

FOOD	PORTION	CAL	FAT	CARB	SUG
ENERGY DRINKS					
Hansen's					
D-Stress	1 can (8.2 oz)	110	0	31	29
Energy	1 can (8.3 oz)	120	0	32	32
Kashi					
GoLean Shake Man	1 pkg (2.5 oz)	260	1	34	23
GoLean Shake Woman	1 pkg (2.5 oz)	250	2	32	21
Red Bull					
Energy Drink	1 can (8.3 oz)	113	0	28	28
Slim-Fast					
Chocolate as prep w/ fat free milk	1 serv	190	1	32	29
Chocolate Malt as prep w/ fat free milk	1 serv	190	1	32	29
JumpStart Chocolate as prep w/ fat free milk	1 serv	240	2	39	33
JumpStart Vanilla as prep w/ fat free milk	1 serv	240	2	39	32
Strawberry as prep w/ fat free milk	1 serv	190	1	32	30
Vanilla as prep w/ fat free milk	1 serv	190	1	32	30
SoBe					
Adrenaline Rush	1 can (8.3 oz)	140	0	36	34
Edge	8 fl oz	110	0	30	29
Elixir 3C Strawberry Carrot	8 fl oz	90	0	25	24
Lean Sugar Free Metabolic Enhancer Diet Green Tea	8 fl oz	5	0	1	0

FOOD	PORTION	CAL	FAT	CARB	SUG
Lean Sugar Free Metabolic Enhancer Diet Orange Carrot	8 fl oz	10	0	2	2
Tsunami Orange Cream	8 fl oz	110	0	29	27
Sweet Success					
Creamy Milk Chocolate	1 can	200	3	36	30
Creamy Milk Chocolate as prep w/ skim milk	1 serv	180	1	36	8
TwinLab					
Ultra Fuel	1 bottle (16 oz)	400	0	100	30
Ultra Slim-Fast					
Cafe Mocha as prep w/ fat free milk	1 serv	200	2	36	30
Chocolate Fudge as prep w/ fat free milk	1 serv	200	3	36	28
Chocolate Malt as prep w/ fat free milk	1 serv	200	2	36	30
Chocolate Royale as prep w/ fat free milk	1 serv	200	2	36	29
Fruit Juice Mixable as prep w/ juice	1 serv	200	1	44	34
Milk Chocolate as prep w/ fat free milk	1 serv	210	2	34	25
Ready-To-Drink Cappuccino Delight	1 serv	220	2	42	36
Ready-To-Drink Apple Cranberry Raspberry	1 serv	220	2	46	41
Ready-To-Drink Chocolate Royale	1 serv	220	3	38	33

FOOD	PORTION	CAL	FAT	CARB	SUG
Ready-To-Drink Creamy Milk Chocolate	1 serv	220	3	42	35
Ready-To-Drink Dark Chocolate Fudge	1 serv	220	3	42	34
Ready-To-Drink Orange Strawberry Banana	1 serv	220	2	46	41
Ready-To-Drink Orange Pineapple	1 serv	220	2	46	40
Ready-To-Drink Strawberries N' Cream	1 serv	220	3	40	35
Strawberry as prep w/ fat free milk	1 serv	200	1	37	32
Vanilla as prep w/ fat free milk	1 serv	200	1	37	31

ENGLISH MUFFIN
ready-to-eat

crumpets	1 (1.5 oz)	80	0	16	1

Wonder

Original	1 (2 oz)	130	1	25	4

take-out

w/ butter	1 (2.2 oz)	189	6	30	—
w/ cheese & sausage	1 (4 oz)	393	24	29	—
w/ egg cheese & canadian bacon	1 (4.8 oz)	289	13	28	—
w/ egg cheese & sausage	1 (5.8 oz)	487	31	31	—

EPAZOTE

fresh	1 tbsp (1 g)	tr	0	tr	—
fresh sprig	1 (2 g)	1	tr	tr	—

FOOD	PORTION	CAL	FAT	CARB	SUG
EPPAW					
raw	½ cup	75	1	16	—
FALAFEL					
take-out					
falafel	1 (1.2 oz)	57	3	5	—
FAST FOODS					
(*see individual names in Part 2*)					
FAT					
beef cooked	1 oz	193	20	0	0
chicken	1 tbsp	115	13	0	0
duck	1 tbsp (13 g)	115	13	0	0
goose	1 tbsp	115	13	0	0
lard	1 tbsp (13 g)	115	13	0	0
pork backfat	1 oz	230	25	0	0
salt pork	1 oz	212	23	0	0
shortening	1 tbsp	113	13	0	0
turkey	1 tbsp	115	13	0	0
Crisco					
Butter Flavor	1 tbsp	110	12	0	0
Shortening	1 tbsp (0.4 oz)	110	12	0	0
FAT SUBSTITUTES					
Smucker's					
Baking Healthy 100% Fat Free	1 tbsp	30	0	7	4
FAVA BEANS					
Progresso					
Fava Beans	½ cup (4.6 oz)	110	1	20	0
FEIJOA					
fresh	1 (1.75 oz)	25	tr	5	—
puree	1 cup	119	2	26	—

FOOD	PORTION	CAL	FAT	CARB	SUG
FENNEL					
fresh bulb	1 (8.2 oz)	72	tr	17	—
fresh sliced	1 cup	27	tr	6	—
seed	1 tsp	7	tr	1	—
FENUGREEK					
seed	1 tsp	12	tr	2	—
FIBER					
Apple Fiber					
Pure	2 tbsp (7 g)	16	0	7	—
Benefiber					
Supplement	1 pkg (4 g)	20	0	4	—
Metamucil					
Fiber Wafers Apple Crisp	2	120	5	17	—
ND Labs					
Pure Apple Fiber	1 tbsp (7 g)	16	0	7	—
FIDDLEHEAD FERNS					
fresh	3.5 oz	34	tr	6	—
FIGS					
canned in heavy syrup	3	75	tr	19	—
canned in light syrup	3	58	tr	15	—
fresh	1 med	50	tr	10	—
Sonoma					
Dried White Misson	3–4 (1.4 oz)	110	0	26	20
FIREWEED					
leaves chopped	1 cup (0.8 oz)	24	1	4	—
FISH					

(*see also individual names and* SUSHI)

FOOD	PORTION	CAL	FAT	CARB	SUG
frozen					
Gorton's					
Baked Au Gratin	1 piece (4.6 oz)	130	5	7	1
Baked Broccoli Cheddar	1 piece (4.6 oz)	130	5	7	1
Baked Primavera	1 piece (4.6 oz)	120	5	4	2
Batter Dipped Portions	1 piece (2.5 oz)	170	11	12	2
Crunchy Golden Fillets Breaded	2 (3.8 oz)	250	14	21	3
Crunchy Golden Sticks	6 (3.8 oz)	250	13	21	3
Garlic & Herb	2 pieces (3.6 oz)	220	11	21	6
Garlic Butter Crumb	1 piece (4.6 oz)	170	9	5	1
Grilled Cajun Blackened	1 piece (3.8 oz)	120	6	1	1
Grilled Garlic Butter	1 piece (3.8 oz)	120	6	1	1
Grilled Italian Herb	1 piece (3.8 oz)	130	6	2	2
Grilled Lemon Butter	1 piece (3.8 oz)	120	6	1	1
Grilled Lemon Pepper	1 piece (3.8 oz)	120	6	1	1
Parmesan	2 pieces (3.6 oz)	260	15	20	4
Ranch	1 piece (3.6 oz)	240	13	22	3
Southern Fried Country Style	2 pieces (3.6 oz)	230	14	10	3
Tenders	3.5 pieces (4 oz)	250	14	20	2
take-out					
fish cake	1 (4.7 oz)	166	7	6	—
jamaican brown fish stew	1 serv	426	22	9	—
kedgeree	5.6 oz	242	11	15	—
mousse	1 serv (3.5 oz)	185	14	3	tr
stew	1 cup (7.9 oz)	157	4	10	—
taramasalata	2 tbsp	124	14	1	—

FOOD	PORTION	CAL	FAT	CARB	SUG
FISH OIL					
cod liver	1 tbsp	123	14	0	0
herring	1 tbsp	123	14	0	0
menhaden	1 tbsp	123	14	0	0
salmon	1 tbsp	123	14	0	0
sardine	1 tbsp	123	14	0	0
shark	1 oz	270	29	0	0
whale	1 oz	270	29	0	0
FISH PASTE					
fish paste	2 tsp	15	1	tr	—
FISH SUBSTITUTES					
Loma Linda					
Ocean Platter not prep	⅓ cup (0.9 oz)	90	1	8	0
Worthington					
Fillets	2 (3 oz)	180	10	8	tr
FLAXSEED					
Bite Me					
Flax Bar	1 bar (1.8 oz)	242	11	30	5
FLOUNDER					
fresh					
cooked	3 oz	99	1	0	0
take-out					
battered & fried	3.2 oz	211	11	15	—
breaded & fried	3.2 oz	211	11	15	—
FLOUR					
buckwheat whole groat	1 cup (4.2 oz)	402	4	85	—
corn masa	1 cup (4 oz)	416	4	87	—
potato	1 cup (6.3 oz)	628	1	143	—
rye light	1 cup (3.6 oz)	374	1	82	—

FOOD	PORTION	CAL	FAT	CARB	SUG
All Trump					
Flour	¼ cup (1 oz)	100	0	22	tr
Betty Crocker					
Softasilk Velvet Cake Flour	¼ cup (1 oz)	100	0	23	tr
Gold Medal					
All Purpose	¼ cup (1 oz)	100	0	22	tr
Better For Bread	¼ cup (1 oz)	100	0	22	0
Organic All Purpose	¼ cup (1 oz)	100	0	22	—
Self Rising	¼ cup (1 oz)	100	0	22	—
Unbleached	¼ cup (1 oz)	100	0	22	tr
Wondra	¼ cup	100	0	23	—
Hodgson Mill					
White Unbleached Organic	¼ cup (1 oz)	100	0	23	0
Whole Wheat Graham Organic	¼ cup (1 oz)	100	1	22	0
La Pina					
Flour	¼ cup (1 oz)	100	0	23	tr
Red Band					
All Purpose	¼ cup (1 oz)	100	0	23	—
Self-Rising	¼ cup (1 oz)	100	0	22	—
Robin Hood					
All Purpose	¼ cup (1 oz)	100	0	22	tr
Self-Rising	¼ cup (1 oz)	100	0	22	tr
Unbleached	¼ cup (1 oz)	100	0	22	tr
Whole Wheat	¼ cup (1 oz)	90	1	21	—

FRANKFURTER

(*see* HOT DOG)

FRENCH BEANS

dried cooked	1 cup	228	1	43	—

FOOD	PORTION	CAL	FAT	CARB	SUG
FRENCH FRIES					
(*see* POTATOES)					
FRENCH TOAST					
take-out					
w/ butter	2 slices (4.7 oz)	356	19	36	—
FROG'S LEGS					
take-out					
as prep w/ seasoned flour & fried	1 (0.8 oz)	70	5	15	—
FROSTING					
(*see* CAKE ICING)					
FRUCTOSE					
Estee					
Fructose	1 tsp	15	0	4	4
Packet	1 pkg	10	0	3	3
FRUIT DRINKS					
mix					
Crystal Light					
Fruit Punch as prep	1 serv (8 oz)	5	0	0	0
Lemon-Lime Drink as prep	1 serv (8 oz)	5	0	0	0
Kool-Aid					
Cherry as prep	1 serv (8 oz)	60	0	16	16
Strawberry Raspberry Drink as prep	1 serv (8 oz)	60	0	16	16
Strawberry Raspberry Drink as prep w/ sugar	1 serv (8 oz)	100	0	25	25
Sugar Free Tropical Punch as prep	1 serv (8 oz)	5	0	0	0
Tropical Punch as prep	1 serv (8 oz)	60	0	16	16

FOOD	PORTION	CAL	FAT	CARB	SUG
Tropical Punch as prep w/ sugar	1 serv (8 oz)	100	0	25	25
ready-to-drink					
Apple & Eve					
Apple Cranberry	8 oz	120	0	30	26
Crystal Light					
Fruit Punch	1 serv (8 oz)	5	0	0	0
Guzzler					
Citrus Punch	8 fl oz	140	0	25	25
Island Punch	8 fl oz	140	0	29	22
Juicy Juice					
Apple Grape	1 box (8.45 oz)	140	0	34	32
Berry	1 box (8.45 oz)	130	0	37	31
Punch	1 box (4.23 oz)	70	0	17	15
Punch	1 box (8.45 oz)	140	0	34	32
Tropical	1 box (8.45 oz)	140	0	34	31
Mott's					
Berry	1 box (8 oz)	100	0	26	—
Fruit Punch	1 box (8 oz)	110	0	27	—
Fruit Punch	8 fl oz	130	0	32	—
Nantucket Nectars					
Fruit Punch	8 oz	130	0	32	30
Oberweis					
Fruit Punch	8 oz	120	0	30	29
Ocean Spray					
Cranapple	8 oz	160	0	41	40
Cranapple Reduced Calorie	8 oz	50	0	13	13
Snapple					
Cranberry Raspberry	8 fl oz	120	0	29	27
Diet Cranberry Raspberry	8 fl oz	10	0	2	2

FOOD	PORTION	CAL	FAT	CARB	SUG
Fruit Punch	8 fl oz	110	0	29	27
Kiwi Strawberry	8 fl oz	110	0	28	26
Tropicana					
Citrus Punch	8 fl oz	140	0	36	33
Tangerine Orange Juice	8 fl oz	110	0	25	—
Tropics Orange Pineapple	8 fl oz	110	0	27	24
Veryfine					
Apple Cranberry	1 bottle (10 oz)	190	0	48	48
Fruit Punch	1 bottle (10 oz)	170	0	42	41

FRUIT MIXED
canned

FOOD	PORTION	CAL	FAT	CARB	SUG
fruit cocktail in heavy syrup	½ cup	93	tr	24	—
fruit cocktail juice pack	½ cup	56	tr	15	—
fruit cocktail water pack	½ cup	40	tr	10	—
fruit salad in heavy syrup	½ cup	94	tr	24	—
fruit salad in light syrup	½ cup	73	tr	19	—
fruit salad juice pack	½ cup	62	tr	16	—
fruit salad water pack	½ cup	37	tr	10	—
mixed fruit in heavy syrup	½ cup	92	tr	24	—
tropical fruit salad in heavy syrup	½ cup	110	tr	29	—
Del Monte					
Orchard Select Premium Mixed	½ cup (4.4 oz)	80	0	20	18
SunFresh Ambrosia Salad	½ cup	70	0	16	13
Tropical Fruit Salad	½ cup (4.4 oz)	80	0	21	20

FOOD	PORTION	CAL	FAT	CARB	SUG
Dole					
FruitBowls Tropical Fruit	1 pkg (4 oz)	60	0	16	14
Tropical Fruit Salad	½ cup (4.3 oz)	80	0	20	18
Mott's					
Fruitsations Mixed Berry	1 pkg (4 oz)	90	0	22	20
Healthy Harvest Peach Medley	1 pkg (3.9 oz)	50	0	13	11
Ocean Spray					
Cran*Fruit Cranberry Raspberry	¼ cup	120	0	29	27
Sunfresh					
Tropical Salad	½ cup	80	0	20	16
dried					
Sonoma					
Diced	⅓ cup (1.4 oz)	120	0	31	8
Mixed Fruit	5–8 pieces (1.4 oz)	120	0	30	9
Sun-Maid					
Tropical Medley	¼ cup (1.4 oz)	130	0	32	29
frozen					
Birds Eye					
Mixed Fruit	½ cup (4.4 oz)	90	0	23	21
FRUIT SNACKS					
Health Valley					
Fruit Bars Apricot	1	140	0	35	12
Weight Watchers					
Apple & Cinnamon	1 pkg (0.5 oz)	50	0	13	9
Apple Chips	1 pkg (0.75 oz)	70	0	18	13
Peach & Strawberry	1 pkg (0.5 oz)	50	0	13	11

GARBANZO

(*see* CHICKPEAS)

FOOD	PORTION	CAL	FAT	CARB	SUG
GARLIC					
clove	1	4	tr	1	—
powder	1 tsp	9	tr	2	—
Dorot					
Frozen Crushed Cubes	1 cube (4 g)	5	0	1	0
GEFILTE FISH					
sweet	1 piece (1.5 oz)	35	1	3	—
GELATIN					
mix					
mix artificially sweetened as prep	1 pkg 4 serv (16.5 oz)	33	0	3	tr
mix as prep	½ cup (4.7 oz)	80	0	19	11
mix as prep	1 pkg 4 serv (19 oz)	319	0	76	43
Jell-O					
Cherry as prep	½ cup (5 oz)	80	0	19	19
Grape as prep	½ cup (5 oz)	80	0	19	19
Lemon as prep	½ cup (5 oz)	80	0	19	19
Lime as prep	½ cup (5 oz)	80	0	19	19
Mixed Fruit as prep	½ cup (5 oz)	80	0	19	19
Orange as prep	½ cup (5 oz)	80	0	19	19
Raspberry as prep	½ cup (5 oz)	80	0	19	19
Sparkling White Grape as prep	½ cup (5 oz)	80	0	19	19
Strawberry as prep	½ cup (5 oz)	80	0	19	19
Sugar Free Cherry as prep	½ cup (4.2 oz)	10	0	0	0
Sugar Free Mixed Fruit as prep	½ cup (4.2 oz)	10	0	0	0

FOOD	PORTION	CAL	FAT	CARB	SUG
Sugar Free Orange as prep	½ cup (4.2 oz)	10	0	0	0
Sugar Free Raspberry as prep	½ cup (4.2 oz)	10	0	0	0
Sugar Free Strawberry as prep	½ cup (4.2 oz)	10	0	0	0
ready-to-eat					
Handi-Snacks					
Gels Cherry	1 serv (4 oz)	80	0	20	20
Gels Orange	1 serv (3.5 oz)	80	0	20	20
Gels Strawberry	1 serv (3.5 oz)	80	0	20	20
Hunt's					
Snack Pack Gels Cherry	1 serv (3.5 oz)	100	0	25	24
Snack Pack Gels Raspberry Berry	1 serv (3.5 oz)	100	0	25	24
Snack Pack Gels Strawberry	1 serv (3.5 oz)	100	0	25	24
Snack Pack Gels Strawberry Orange	1 serv (3.5 oz)	100	0	25	24
Jell-O					
Cherry	1 serv (3.5 oz)	70	0	17	17
Orange	1 serv (3.5 oz)	70	0	17	17
Raspberry	1 serv (3.5 oz)	70	0	17	17
Strawberry	1 serv (3.5 oz)	70	0	17	17
Sugar Free Orange	1 serv (3.2 oz)	10	0	0	0
Sugar Free Strawberry	1 serv (3.2 oz)	10	0	0	0
Swiss Miss					
Gels Berry Strawberry	1 pkg (3.5 oz)	79	0	18	18
Gels Berry Lemon	1 pkg (3.5 oz)	79	0	18	18
Gels Raspberry Orange	1 pkg (3.5 oz)	79	0	18	18
Gels Strawberry Raspberry	1 pkg (3.5 oz)	79	0	18	18

FOOD	PORTION	CAL	FAT	CARB	SUG
GIBLETS					
capon simmered	1 cup (5 oz)	238	8	0	0
chicken floured & fried	1 cup (5 oz)	402	19	6	—
chicken simmered	1 cup (5 oz)	228	7	1	—
turkey simmered	1 cup (5 oz)	243	7	3	—
GINGER					
ground	1 tsp (1.8 g)	6	tr	1	—
pickled	0.5 oz	5	0	1	—
root fresh	¼ cup	17	tr	4	—
root fresh sliced	¼ cup	17	tr	4	—
GINKGO NUTS					
canned	1 oz	32	tr	6	—
dried	1 oz	99	tr	21	—
GINSENG					
dried	1 oz	90	tr	20	—
fresh	1 oz	28	tr	6	—
GIZZARDS					
chicken simmered	1 cup (5 oz)	222	5	2	—
turkey simmered	1 cup (5 oz)	236	6	1	—
GOAT					
roasted	3 oz	122	3	0	0
GOOSE					
w/ skin roasted	6.6 oz	574	41	0	0
w/o skin roasted	5 oz	340	18	0	0
GOOSEBERRIES					
canned in light syrup	½ cup	93	tr	24	—
fresh	1 cup	67	1	15	—
GRANOLA					

(see CEREAL, CEREAL BARS)

FOOD	PORTION	CAL	FAT	CARB	SUG
GRAPE JUICE					
Juicy Juice					
Drink	1 box (8.45 oz)	140	0	34	32
Drink	1 box (4.23 oz)	70	0	17	16
Kool-Aid					
Drink as prep w/ sugar	1 serv (8 oz)	100	0	25	25
Sugar Free Drink Mix as prep	1 serv (8 oz)	5	0	0	0
Veryfine					
100% Juice	1 bottle (10 oz)	200	0	47	43
Welch's					
100% White	8 oz	160	0	39	37
GRAPE LEAVES					
canned	1 (4 g)	3	tr	tr	—
fresh raw	1 (3 g)	3	tr	1	—
GRAPEFRUIT **fresh**					
pink	½	37	tr	9	—
pink sections	1 cup	69	tr	18	—
red	½	37	tr	9	—
red sections	1 cup	69	tr	18	—
white	½	39	tr	10	—
white sections	1 cup	76	tr	19	—
Ocean Spray					
Fresh	2 oz	50	0	14	31
GRAPEFRUIT JUICE					
Everfresh					
Juice	1 can (8 oz)	90	0	22	22
Nantucket Nectars					
100% Ruby Red	8 oz	100	0	25	20

FOOD	PORTION	CAL	FAT	CARB	SUG
Ocean Spray					
100% Juice	8 oz	100	0	24	23
Veryfine					
Pink	1 bottle (10 oz)	150	0	38	34
GRAPES					
Chiquita					
Grapes	1½ cups (4.8 oz)	90	1	24	23
GRAVY					
canned					
Campbell					
Beef	¼ cup	29	1	4	1
Brown	¼ cup	46	3	4	1
Chicken	¼ cup	42	2	4	tr
Turkey	¼ cup	29	1	3	tr
mix					
Bournvita					
Extract	2 heaping tsp	34	1	7	—
Bovril					
Extract	1 heaping tsp	9	0	tr	—
Durkee					
Au Jus as prep	¼ cup	5	0	1	0
Brown as prep	¼ cup	10	1	3	0
Chicken as prep	¼ cup	20	1	4	0
Pork as prep	¼ cup	10	0	3	0
Turkey as prep	¼ cup	20	0	4	1
French's					
Au Jus as prep	¼ cup	5	0	1	0
Brown as prep	¼ cup	10	1	3	0
Chicken as prep	¼ cup	25	1	4	0
Herb Brown as prep	¼ cup	15	1	3	0
Mushroom as prep	¼ cup	10	1	3	0

FOOD	PORTION	CAL	FAT	CARB	SUG
Onion	¼ cup	15	1	4	0
Turkey as prep	¼ cup	20	0	4	1
Loma Linda					
Gravy Quik Brown	1 tbsp (5 g)	20	0	4	0
Gravy Quik Chicken	1 tbsp (5 g)	20	0	3	0
Quik Gravy Country	1 tbsp (5 g)	25	1	4	0
Quik Gravy Mushroom	1 tbsp (5 g)	15	0	3	0
Quik Gravy Onion	1 tbsp (5 g)	20	0	3	0
Marmite					
Extract	1 heaping tsp	9	0	tr	—
McCormick					
Beef & Herb as prep	¼ cup	30	1	3	1
Chicken as prep	¼ cup	20	0	4	1
Turkey as prep	¼ cup	20	0	3	1

GREAT NORTHERN BEANS
canned
Green Giant

FOOD	PORTION	CAL	FAT	CARB	SUG
Great Northern	½ cup (4.4 oz)	100	1	18	0
dried					
cooked	1 cup	210	1	37	—

GREEN BEANS
canned
Green Giant

FOOD	PORTION	CAL	FAT	CARB	SUG
Cut	½ cup (4.2 oz)	20	0	4	2
French Style	½ cup (4.1 oz)	20	0	4	2
fresh					
cooked	½ cup	22	tr	5	—
raw	½ cup	17	tr	4	—
frozen					
Green Giant					
Cut	¾ cup (2.8 oz)	25	0	5	2

FOOD	PORTION	CAL	FAT	CARB	SUG
GROUNDCHERRIES					
fresh	½ cup	37	tr	8	—
GROUPER					
cooked	3 oz	100	1	0	0
GUAVA					
fresh	1	45	1	11	—
guava sauce	½ cup	43	tr	11	—
GUINEA HEN					
w/ skin raw	½ hen (12.1 oz)	545	22	0	0
w/o skin raw	½ hen (9.3 oz)	292	7	0	0
HADDOCK					
fresh cooked	3 oz	95	1	0	0
roe raw	1 oz	37	tr	tr	—
smoked	1 oz	33	tr	0	0
take-out					
breaded & fried	1 piece (3.5 oz)	187	9	3	0
HALIBUT					
atlantic & pacific cooked	3 oz	119	2	0	0
greenland baked	3 oz	203	15	0	0
HAM					
prosciutto	1 oz	55	2	tr	—
steak boneless extra lean	1 (2 oz)	69	2	0	0
westphalian smoked	1 oz	105	10	0	0
Alpine Lace					
Boneless Cooked 98% Fat Free	2 slices (2 oz)	60	1	2	1
Honey Ham 98% Fat Free	2 slices (2 oz)	60	1	2	1

FOOD	PORTION	CAL	FAT	CARB	SUG
Smoked Virginia 98% Fat Free	2 slices (2 oz)	60	1	2	1
Armour					
Deviled Ham Spread	1 pkg (3 oz)	210	18	0	0
Boar's Head					
Black Forest Smoked	2 oz	60	1	2	2
Cappy	2 oz	60	2	3	2
Deluxe	2 oz	60	1	2	2
Deluxe Lowered Sodium	2 oz	50	1	tr	0
Maple Glazed Honey	2 oz	60	1	3	3
Pepper	2 oz	60	1	2	1
Rosemary & Sundried Tomato	2 oz	70	3	2	0
Sweet Slice Smoked	3 oz	100	3	1	0
Virgina	2 oz	60	1	3	3
Virginia Smoked	2 oz	60	1	2	2
Hormel					
Ham & Cheese Patties	1 patty (2 oz)	190	17	0	0
Ham Patties	1 (2 oz)	180	17	1	1
Oscar Mayer					
Boiled	3 slices (2.2 oz)	60	3	0	0
Dinner Steaks	1 (2 oz)	60	2	0	0
Smoked	3 slices (2.2 oz)	60	3	0	0
Spam					
Spread	4 tbsp (2 oz)	140	12	1	1
HAM DISHES take-out					
croquettes	1 (3.1 oz)	217	14	11	—
salad	½ cup	287	23	5	—

FOOD	PORTION	CAL	FAT	CARB	SUG
HAM SUBSTITUTES					
Yves					
Veggie Ham Deli Slices	1 serv (2.2 oz)	80	0	6	2
HAMBURGER					
Kid Cuisine					
Buckaroo Beef Patty Sandwich w/ Cheese	1 meal (8.5 oz)	410	15	58	27
White Castle					
Cheeseburger	2 (3.6 oz)	310	17	23	0
Hamburger	2 (3.2 oz)	270	14	23	0
take-out					
double patty w/ bun	1 reg	544	28	43	—
double patty w/ cheese & bun	1 reg	457	28	22	—
double patty w/ cheese & double bun	1 reg	461	22	44	—
double patty w/ cheese ketchup mayonnaise onion pickle tomato & bun	1 reg	416	21	35	—
double patty w/ ketchup mayonnaise onion pickle tomato & bun	1 reg	649	35	53	—
double patty w/ ketchup cheese mayonnaise mustard pickle tomato & bun	1 lg	706	44	40	—

FOOD	PORTION	CAL	FAT	CARB	SUG
double patty w/ ketchup mustard mayonnaise onion pickle tomato & bun	1 lg	540	27	40	—
double patty w/ ketchup mustard onion pickle & bun	1 reg	576	32	39	—
single patty w/ bacon ketchup cheese mustard onion pickle & bun	1 lg	609	37	37	—
single patty w/ bun	1 reg	275	12	31	—
single patty w/ bun	1 lg	400	23	25	—
single patty w/ cheese & bun	1 reg	320	15	32	—
single patty w/ cheese & bun	1 lg	608	33	47	—
single patty w/ ketchup cheese ham mayonnaise pickle tomato & bun	1 lg	745	48	38	—
single patty w/ ketchup mustard mayonnaise onion pickle tomato & bun	1 reg	279	13	27	—
triple patty w/ cheese & bun	1 lg	769	51	27	—
triple patty w/ ketchup mustard pickle & bun	1 lg	693	41	29	—

FOOD	PORTION	CAL	FAT	CARB	SUG

HAMBURGER SUBSTITUTES

Boca Burgers

FOOD	PORTION	CAL	FAT	CARB	SUG
Vegan Original	1 patty (2.5 oz)	84	0	9	0
Gardenburger					
Fire Roasted Vegetable	1 (2.5 oz)	120	3	17	2
Hamburger Style	1 (2.5 oz)	90	0	7	0
Lightlife					
Barbecue Grilles	1 patty (2.7 oz)	120	4	11	3
Lemon Grilles	1 patty (2.7 oz)	140	6	11	2
Light Burgers	1 (3 oz)	130	1	12	2
Tamari Grilles	1 patty (2.7 oz)	120	5	9	2
Loma Linda					
Patty Mix not prep	⅓ cup (0.9 oz)	90	1	7	0
Redi-Burger	⅝ in slice (3 oz)	120	3	7	1
Vege-Burger	¼ cup (1.9 oz)	70	2	2	0
Morningstar Farms					
Better'n Burger	1 (2.7 oz)	80	0	8	tr
Garden Grille	1 patty (2.5 oz)	120	3	18	1
Garden Veggie Patties	1 patty (2.4 oz)	100	3	9	1
Hard Rock Cafe Veggie Burger	1 (3 oz)	170	8	18	3
Harvest Burger Italian Style	1 patty (3.2 oz)	140	5	8	tr
Harvest Burger Original	1 (3.2 oz)	140	4	8	tr
Harvest Burger Southwestern	1 (3.2 oz)	140	4	9	1
Spicy Black Bean Burger	1 (2.7 oz)	110	1	16	2
Natural Touch					
Garden Veggie Pattie	1 (2.4 oz)	110	3	8	0
Okara Pattie	1 (2.2 oz)	110	5	4	0

FOOD	PORTION	CAL	FAT	CARB	SUG
Original Veggie Burger Kit not prep	¼ pkg (0.8 oz)	80	0	6	0
Southwestern Veggie Burger Kit not prep	¼ pkg (0.9 oz)	90	0	9	tr
Spicy Black Bean Burger	1 (2.7 oz)	100	1	15	2
Vegan Burger	1 (2.7 oz)	70	0	6	0
Superburgers					
Vegan Organic Original	1 (3 oz)	98	2	14	0
Vegan Organic Smoked	1 (3 oz)	98	2	14	0
Vegan Organic Tex Mex	1 (3 oz)	110	1	14	0
V'dora					
Vegetable BurgerLites	1 (3.3 oz)	58	0	4	1
Worthington					
Granburger not prep	3 tbsp (0.6 oz)	60	1	3	0
Prosage Patties	1 (1.3 oz)	80	3	3	0
Yves					
Black Bean & Mushroom Burgers	1 (3 oz)	100	0	13	1
Garden Vegetable Pattioo	1 (3 oz)	90	0	11	1
Veggie Burger	1 (3 oz)	119	2	9	2
HAZELNUTS					
oil roasted	1 oz	187	18	5	—
HEART					
beef simmered	3 oz	148	5	tr	—
chicken simmered	1 cup (5 oz)	268	11	tr	—
lamb braised	3 oz	158	7	2	—
pork braised	1 cup	215	7	1	—
turkey simmered	1 cup (5 oz)	257	9	3	—
veal braised	3 oz	158	6	tr	—

FOOD	PORTION	CAL	FAT	CARB	SUG
HEARTS OF PALM					
canned	1 cup (5.1 oz)	41	1	7	—
canned	1 (1.2 oz)	9	tr	2	—
HEMP					
HempNut					
Shelled Hempseed	1 oz	162	13	3	1
Nutiva					
Hempseed	1½ tbsp (0.5 oz)	70	5	3	0
HERBAL TEA					
(*see* TEA/HERBAL TEA)					
HERBS/SPICES					
(*see also individual names*)					
chinese five spice	1 tsp	7	tr	2	—
curry powder	1 tsp	6	tr	1	—
garam masala	1 tsp	8	tr	1	—
poultry seasoning	1 tsp	5	tr	1	—
pumpkin pie spice	1 tsp	6	tr	1	—
McCormick					
Big'n Season Buffalo Wings	1 tbsp (8 g)	30	0	5	3
Meat Loaf Seasoning	1 tsp (4 g)	15	0	2	2
HERRING					
atlantic cooked	3 oz	172	10	0	0
pacific baked	3 oz	213	15	0	0
roe canned	1 oz	34	1	tr	—
smoked	3.5 oz	210	14	0	0
take-out					
atlantic kippered	1 fillet (1.4 oz)	87	5	0	0
atlantic pickled	½ oz	39	3	1	—
fried	1 serv (3.5 oz)	233	15	2	—

FOOD	PORTION	CAL	FAT	CARB	SUG
HICKORY NUTS					
dried	1 oz	187	18	5	—
HOMINY					
canned					
Van Camp					
Golden	½ cup (4.3 oz)	80	1	17	0
White	½ cup (4.3 oz)	80	1	16	0
HONEY					
honey	1 tbsp (0.7 oz)	64	0	17	17
wild honey	1 tbsp	60	0	17	16
HONEYDEW					
fresh					
Chiquita					
Wedge	⅒ melon (4.7 oz)	50	0	13	12
HORSE					
roasted	3 oz	149	5	0	0
HORSERADISH					
Boar's Head					
Horseradish	1 tsp (5 g)	5	0	0	0
Kraft					
Cream Style	1 tsp (5 g)	0	0	0	0
HOT CAKES					
(*see* PANCAKES)					
HOT COCOA					
(*see* COCOA)					
HOT DOG					
Boar's Head					
Beef	1 (2 oz)	160	14	1	0
Beef Lite	1 (1.6 oz)	90	6	0	0
Pork & Beef	1 (2 oz)	150	14	0	0

FOOD	PORTION	CAL	FAT	CARB	SUG
Healthy Choice					
Beef Low Fat	1 (1.8 oz)	70	3	7	2
Low Fat Turkey Pork Beef	1 (1.4 oz)	60	2	5	1
Kid Cuisine					
Mystical Mini Corn Dogs	4 pieces	230	14	18	7
Louis Rich					
Bun Length	1 (2 oz)	110	8	3	1
Cheese	1 (1.6 oz)	90	6	2	tr
Oscar Mayer					
Beef	1 (1.6 oz)	140	13	1	tr
Bun-Length Beef	1 (2 oz)	180	17	2	1
Cheese	1 (1.6 oz)	140	13	1	tr
Wieners Little	6 (2 oz)	180	17	2	1
take-out					
corndog	1	460	19	56	—
w/ bun chili	1	297	13	31	—
w/ bun plain	1	242	15	18	—

HOT DOG SUBSTITUTES

FOOD	PORTION	CAL	FAT	CARB	SUG
Lightlife					
Smart Deli Jumbo's	1 link (2.7 oz)	80	0	4	1
Smart Dogs	1 (1.5 oz)	45	0	2	0
Tofu Pups	1 (1.4 oz)	60	3	2	0
Wonder Dogs	1 (1.5 oz)	60	2	2	0
Loma Linda					
Big Franks	1 (1.8 oz)	110	7	2	0
Big Franks Low Fat	1 (1.8 oz)	80	3	3	0
Corn Dogs	1 (2.5 oz)	150	4	22	4
Morningstar Farms					
America's Original Veggie Dog	1 (2 oz)	80	1	6	2

FOOD	PORTION	CAL	FAT	CARB	SUG
Meatfree Corn Dog	1 (2.5 oz)	150	4	22	4
Meatfree Mini Corn Dog	4 (2.7 oz)	170	5	21	6
Natural Touch					
Vege Frank	1 (1.6 oz)	100	6	2	0
Yves					
Good Dog	1 (1.8 oz)	70	2	2	1
Tofu Dogs	1 (1.3 oz)	45	1	2	0
Veggie Dogs	1 (1.6 oz)	60	0	1	0
Veggie Dogs Chili	1 (1.6 oz)	50	0	3	1
Veggie Dogs Jumbo	1 (2.7 oz)	100	2	7	1
Veggie Dogs Jumbo Hot N' Spicy	1 (2.7 oz)	106	2	4	2

HUMMUS
take-out

FOOD	PORTION	CAL	FAT	CARB	SUG
hummus	⅓ cup	140	7	17	—

HYACINTH BEANS

FOOD	PORTION	CAL	FAT	CARB	SUG
dried cooked	1 cup	228	1	40	—

ICE CREAM AND FROZEN DESSERTS

FOOD	PORTION	CAL	FAT	CARB	SUG
dixie cup chocolate	1 (3.5 fl oz)	125	6	16	11
dixie cup strawberry	1 (3.5 fl oz)	112	5	16	9
dixie cup vanilla	1 (3.5 fl oz)	116	6	14	9
strawberry	½ cup (4 fl oz)	127	6	18	10
vanilla	½ cup (4 fl oz)	132	7	16	10
Better Than Ice Creme					
Soy Vanilla as prep	½ cup	110	3	21	8
Bon Bons					
Dark Chocolate	5 pieces	190	13	16	12
Milk Chocolate	5 pieces	200	14	17	13
Butterfinger					
Bar	1 (2.5 oz)	190	13	16	14

FOOD	PORTION	CAL	FAT	CARB	SUG
Carnation					
Cup Chocolate	1 (3 oz)	140	8	16	14
Cup Chocolate Malt	1 (12 oz)	270	6	48	36
Cup Strawberry	1 (3 oz)	100	5	12	10
Cup Vanilla	1 (5 oz)	170	10	19	16
Cup Vanilla	1 (3 oz)	100	6	11	9
Cup Vanilla Malt	1 (12 oz)	260	6	48	37
Sundae Cup Strawberry	1 (5 oz)	200	8	29	23
Sunday Cup Chocolate	1 (5 oz)	210	9	30	22
Cool Creations					
Cookies & Cream Sandwich	1 (3.5 oz)	240	11	34	18
Mickey Mouse Bar	1 (2.5 oz)	120	8	10	9
Mini Sandwich	1 (2.3 oz)	110	5	16	8
Dippin' Dots					
Dipping Dots Chocolate	⅝ cup (3 oz)	190	9	22	22
Drumstick					
Cone Chocolate	1 (4.6 oz)	320	17	36	20
Cone Chocolate Dipped	1 (4.6 oz)	320	16	40	20
Cone Vanilla	1 (4.6 oz)	340	19	35	20
Cone Vanilla Caramel	1 (4.6 oz)	360	20	38	24
Cone Vanilla Fudge	1 (4.6 oz)	360	20	39	25
Flintstones					
Cool Cream	1 (2.75 oz)	90	2	18	14
Push-Up Pebbles Treats	1 (2.75 oz)	120	6	15	14
Healthy Choice					
Butter Pecan Crunch	½ cup	120	2	22	21
Cappuccino Chocolate Chunk	½ cup	120	2	22	19
Cappuccino Mocha Crunch	½ cup	120	2	22	19

FOOD	PORTION	CAL	FAT	CARB	SUG
Cherry Chocolate Chunk	½ cup	110	2	19	19
Chocolate Chocolate Chunk	½ cup	120	2	21	18
Coconut Cream Pie	½ cup	120	2	23	17
Cookies 'N Cream	½ cup	120	2	21	19
Cookies Creme De Mint	½ cup	130	2	24	20
Fudge Brownie	½ cup	120	2	22	20
Mint Chocolate Chip	½ cup	120	2	21	20
Old Fashioned Blueberry Hill	½ cup	120	2	23	17
Old Fashioned Butterscotch Blonde	½ cup	140	2	26	22
Old Fashioned Cherry Vanilla	½ cup	120	2	22	17
Old Fashioned Strawberry	½ cup	110	2	20	17
Peanut Butter Cup	⅛ cup	110	2	19	18
Praline & Caramel	½ cup	130	2	25	24
Praline Caramel Cluster	½ cup	130	2	25	24
Rocky Road	½ cup	140	2	28	19
Turtle Fudge Cake	½ cup	130	2	25	23
Vanilla	½ cup	100	2	18	17
Vanilla Bean	½ cup	110	2	19	18
Wild Raspberry Truffle	½ cup	120	2	22	15
Klondike					
Choco Taco Fudge Grande	1 bar (3.2 oz)	310	17	36	24
Oreo Ice Cream Cookie Sandwich	1 (2.6 oz)	240	10	35	19
Original	1 (3.3 oz)	290	19	25	22

FOOD	PORTION	CAL	FAT	CARB	SUG
Nestle Crunch					
Chocolate	1 bar (3 oz)	200	14	17	14
Crunch King	1 (4 oz)	270	19	21	16
Nuggets	8 pieces	310	21	25	19
Reduced Fat	1 (2.5 oz)	130	7	14	6
Vanilla	1 bar (3 oz)	200	14	16	13
Rice Dream					
Cappuccino	½ cup (3.2 oz)	150	6	23	17
Carob	½ cup (3.2 oz)	150	6	24	17
Carob Almond	½ cup (3.2 oz)	170	8	24	17
Cherry Vanilla	½ cup (3.2 oz)	150	6	24	18
Cocoa Marble Fudge	½ cup (3.2 oz)	150	6	25	15
Cookies N' Dream	½ cup (3.2 oz)	170	7	26	17
Mint Chocolate Chip	½ cup (3.2 oz)	170	8	26	19
Neapolitan	½ cup (3.2 oz)	150	6	24	18
Orange Vanilla Swirl	½ cup (3.2 oz)	250	6	23	17
Strawberry	½ cup (3.2 oz)	140	5	24	19
Vanilla Swiss Almond	½ cup (3.2 oz)	180	8	25	18
Rice Dream Supreme					
Cappuccino Almond Fudge	½ cup (3.2 oz)	170	8	24	15
Cherry Chocolate Chunk	½ cup (3.2 oz)	170	7	27	19
Chocolate Almond Chunk	½ cup (3.2 oz)	170	8	25	18
Chocolate Fudge Brownie	½ cup (3.2 oz)	170	7	28	16
Double Espresso Bean	½ cup (3.2 oz)	160	7	24	17
Mint Chocolate Cookie	½ cup (3.2 oz)	170	8	26	18
Peanut Butter Cup	½ cup (3.2 oz)	180	8	25	18
Pralines N' Dream	½ cup (3.2 oz)	180	9	25	16

FOOD	PORTION	CAL	FAT	CARB	SUG
Turkey Hill					
Black Cherry	½ cup	140	7	18	16
Butter Pecan	½ cup	170	11	16	15
Cookies 'N Cream	½ cup	160	9	19	17
Light Butter Pecan	½ cup	130	6	17	16
Light Choco Mint Chip	½ cup	140	5	19	18
Light Vanilla & Chocolate	½ cup	110	3	18	18
Light Vanilla Bean	½ cup	110	3	18	17
Neapolitan	½ cup	150	8	18	17
Rocky Road	½ cup	170	8	23	19
Tin Roof Sundae	½ cup	160	9	19	18
Vanilla & Chocolate	½ cup	150	8	17	16
Vanilla Bean	½ cup	140	8	16	16
Weight Watchers					
Chocolate Mousse	1 bar	40	1	9	3
Chocolate Treat	1 bar	100	1	20	17
Orange Vanilla Treat	1 bar	40	1	10	3
Vanilla Sandwich	1 bar	150	3	28	14
take-out					
gelato chocolate hazelnut	½ cup (5.3 oz)	370	29	26	21
gelato vanilla	½ cup (3 oz)	211	15	18	18

ICE CREAM CONES AND CUPS

FOOD	PORTION	CAL	FAT	CARB	SUG
Dutch Mill					
Chocolate Covered Wafer Cups	1 (0.5 oz)	80	5	8	6
Keebler					
Chocolatey Cone	1 (0.4 oz)	50	1	10	4
Fudge Dipped Cup	1 (0.3 oz)	35	2	6	2
Ice Creme Cup	1 (0.2 oz)	15	0	4	0

FOOD	PORTION	CAL	FAT	CARB	SUG
Sugar Cone	1 (0.4 oz)	50	1	10	4
Waffle Bowl	1 (0.4 oz)	50	1	10	4
Waffle Cone	1 (0.4 oz)	50	1	10	4

ICED TEA
mix

Crystal Light

Iced Tea as prep	1 serv (8 oz)	5	0	0	0

Lipton

100% Tea Decaffeinated as prep	1 serv	0	0	0	0
100% Tea Unsweetened as prep	1 serv	0	0	0	0
100% Tea as prep	1 serv	0	0	0	0
Calorie Free as prep	1 serv	0	0	0	0
Decaffeinated Lemon as prep	1 serv	90	0	22	22
Diet Decaffeinated Lemon as prep	1 serv	5	0	1	0
Diet Lemon as prep	1 serv	5	0	1	0
Herbal Iced Collection	1 tea bag	0	0	tr	0
Ice Tea Brew as prep	1 serv (8 oz)	0	0	0	0

Nestea

100% Tea	2 tsp (1 g)	0	0	tr	0
100% Tea Decafe	2 tsp (1 g)	0	0	tr	0
Ice Teasers Lemon	1 serv (0.5 oz)	5	0	1	0
Ice Teasers Orange	1 serv (0.5 oz)	5	0	1	0
Ice Teasers Wild Cherry	1 serv (0.5 oz)	5	0	1	0
Lemon	2 tsp (1 g)	5	0	1	0

FOOD	PORTION	CAL	FAT	CARB	SUG
Lemon & Sugar	2 tbsp (0.7 oz)	80	0	19	19
Lemonade Tea	2 tbsp (0.7 oz)	80	0	19	17
Sugar Free	2 tbsp (0.7 oz)	5	0	1	0
Sugar Free Decafe	1 tbsp (0.7 oz)	5	0	1	0
Sun Tea	1 tsp (1 g)	0	0	tr	0
ready-to-drink					
Lipton					
Sweetened Lemon	8 oz	10	0	20	20
Mad River					
Red Tea w/ Guarana	8 oz	90	0	24	23
Nantucket Nectars					
Diet	8 oz	5	0	1	0
Diet Green Tea	8 oz	5	0	1	0
Snapple					
Diet Lemon	8 fl oz	0	0	1	0
Diet Peach	8 fl oz	0	0	1	0
Diet Raspberry	8 fl oz	0	0	1	0
Ginseng Tea	8 fl oz	80	0	20	18
Green Tea w/ Lemon	8 fl oz	100	0	25	24
Lemon	8 fl oz	100	0	25	23
Lemonade Ice Tea	8 fl oz	110	0	28	28
Peach	8 fl oz	100	0	26	24
Raspberry	8 fl oz	100	0	26	25
Turkey Hill					
Blueberry Oolong w/ Vitamins C & E	1 cup	100	0	24	24
Decaffeinated	1 cup	80	0	20	20
Decaffeinated Orange	1 cup	10	0	2	2
Diet	1 cup	0	0	0	0
Diet Decaffeinated	1 cup	0	0	0	0
Diet Green Tea w/ Ginseng & Honey	1 cup	5	0	tr	tr

FOOD	PORTION	CAL	FAT	CARB	SUG
Lemon	1 cup	100	0	24	24
Mint Tea w/ Chamomile	1 cup	90	0	21	21
Oolong w/ Ginkgo Biloba & Ginseng	1 cup	100	0	25	25
Orange	1 cup	100	0	25	25
Peach	1 cup	110	0	28	28
Raspberry Tea	1 cup	110	0	28	28
Regular	1 cup	90	0	22	22

ICES AND ICE POPS

FOOD	PORTION	CAL	FAT	CARB	SUG
fruit & juice bar	1 (3 fl oz)	75	tr	19	17
gelatin pop	1 (1.5 oz)	31	0	7	7
Carnation					
Cup Orange Sherbet	1 (5 oz)	150	2	32	28
Cup Orange Sherbet	1 (3 oz)	90	1	19	17
Cold Fusion					
Protein Juice Bar All Flavors	1 bar (3.8 oz)	130	0	23	23
Cool Creations					
Ice Pop	1 pop (2 oz)	50	0	13	13
Mickey Mouse Bar	1 (4 oz)	170	11	17	10
Surprise Pops	1 (2 oz)	60	0	14	13
Dole					
Fruit'n Juice Coconut	1 bar (4 oz)	210	7	33	30
Fruit'n Juice Lemonade	1 bar (4 oz)	120	0	28	24
Fruit'n Juice Lime	1 bar (4 oz)	110	0	28	24
Fruit'n Juice Peach Passion	1 bar (2.5 oz)	70	0	17	15
Fruit'n Juice Pineapple Coconut	1 bar (4 oz)	150	4	27	24
Fruit'n Juice Pineapple Orange Banana	1 bar (2.5 oz)	70	0	16	15

FOOD	PORTION	CAL	FAT	CARB	SUG
Fruit'n Juice Pineapple Orange Banana	1 bar (4 oz)	110	0	26	24
Fruit'n Juice Raspberry	1 bar (2.5 oz)	70	0	16	13
Fruit'n Juice Strawberry	1 bar (4 oz)	110	0	26	24
Fruit'n Juice Strawberry	1 bar (2.5 oz)	70	0	17	15
Grape No Sugar Added	1 bar (1.75 oz)	25	0	6	3
Raspberry	1 bar (1.75 oz)	45	0	11	10
Raspberry No Sugar Added	1 bar (1.75 oz)	25	0	6	3
Strawberry	1 bar (1.75 oz)	45	0	11	10
Strawberry No Sugar Added	1 bar (1.75 oz)	25	0	6	3
Flinstones					
Push-Up Sherbet Treats	1 (2.75 oz)	100	2	20	14
Frozfruit					
Cherry	1 bar (4 oz)	70	0	18	17
Lemon	1 bar (4 oz)	90	0	22	20
Lime	1 bar (4 oz)	90	0	21	19
Orange	1 bar (4 oz)	90	0	21	19
Pineapple	1 bar (4 oz)	80	0	19	18
Raspberry	1 bar (4 oz)	80	0	20	18
Strawberry	1 bar (4 oz)	80	0	20	18
Tropical	1 bar (4 oz)	90	0	23	22
Watermelon	1 bar (4 oz)	50	0	13	12
Mr. Freeze					
Assorted	2 bars (3 oz)	45	0	11	11
Tropical	2 bars (3 oz)	45	0	11	11

ICING

(*see* CAKE ICING)

INSTANT BREAKFAST

(*see* BREAKFAST DRINKS)

FOOD	PORTION	CAL	FAT	CARB	SUG
JACKFRUIT					
fresh	3.5 oz	70	tr	4	—
JALAPENO					
(*see* PEPPERS)					
JAM/JELLY/PRESERVES					
all flavors jam	1 tbsp (0.7 oz)	48	0	13	10
all flavors jam	1 pkg (0.5 oz)	34	0	9	7
all flavors jelly	1 tbsp (0.7 oz)	52	0	14	12
all flavors jelly	1 pkg (0.5 oz)	38	0	10	9
all flavors preserve	1 pkg (0.5 oz)	34	0	9	7
all flavors preserve	1 tbsp (0.7 oz)	48	0	13	10
apple jelly	1 tbsp (0.7 oz)	52	0	14	12
linganberry jam	0.5 oz	23	tr	6	4
strawberry jam	1 pkg (0.5 oz)	34	0	9	7
strawberry jam	1 tbsp (0.7 oz)	48	0	13	10
strawberry preserve	1 pkg (0.5 oz)	34	0	9	7
strawberry preserve	1 tbsp (0.7 oz)	48	0	13	10
Estee					
Fruit Spread Apple Spice	1 tbsp	16	0	4	4
Fruit Spread Apricot	1 tbsp	16	0	4	4
Fruit Spread Grape	1 tbsp	16	0	4	4
Fruit Spread Peach	1 tbsp	16	0	4	4
Fruit Spread Red Raspberry	1 tbsp	16	0	4	4
Fruit Spread Strawberry	1 tbsp	16	0	4	4
Smucker's					
Concord Grape Jelly	1 tbsp	50	0	13	12
Peach Preserves	1 tbsp	50	0	13	12
Simply Fruit Red Raspberry	1 tbsp	40	0	10	8

FOOD	PORTION	CAL	FAT	CARB	SUG
Tabasco					
Spicy Pepper Jelly	1 tbsp (0.6 oz)	50	0	12	11
White House					
Apple Butter	1 tbsp (0.6 oz)	35	0	9	7
JAPANESE FOOD					
(*see* ASIAN FOOD, SUSHI)					
JAVA PLUM					
fresh	1 cup	82	tr	21	—
fresh	3	5	tr	1	—
KALE					
fresh					
chopped cooked	½ cup	21	tr	4	—
scotch chopped cooked	½ cup	18	tr	4	—
KEFIR					
kefir	7 oz	132	8	10	—
KETCHUP					
Estee					
Ketchup	1 tbsp	15	0	5	1
Healthy Choice					
Ketchup	1 tbsp (0.5 oz)	9	tr	2	2
Heinz					
Ketchup	1 tbsp (0.6 oz)	15	0	4	4
Hunt's					
Ketchup	1 tbsp (0.6 oz)	16	tr	3	4
No Salt Added	1 tbsp (0.6 oz)	16	tr	3	4
McIlhenny					
Spicy	1 tbsp (0.6 oz)	20	0	5	2
Muir Glen					
Organic	1 tbsp (0.6 oz)	15	0	3	3
Smucker's					
Tomato	1 tbsp	25	0	7	6

FOOD	PORTION	CAL	FAT	CARB	SUG
KIDNEY					
beef simmered	3 oz	122	3	0	0
lamb braised	3 oz	117	3	1	—
pork cooked	3 oz	128	4	0	0
veal braised	3 oz	139	5	0	0
KIDNEY BEANS					
canned					
Green Giant					
Dark Red	½ cup (4.5 oz)	110	0	18	tr
Light Red	½ cup (4.5 oz)	110	0	20	2
Hunt's					
Kidney	½ cup (4.5 oz)	94	1	20	6
Progresso					
Dark Red	½ cup (4.5 oz)	110	0	20	2
Red	½ cup (4.6 oz)	110	1	20	0
S&W					
Dark Red Premium	½ cup (4.6 oz)	100	1	23	7
Van Camp					
Dark Red	½ cup (4.6 oz)	90	0	20	2
Light Red	½ cup (4.6 oz)	90	0	20	3
dried					
cooked	1 cup	225	1	40	—
KIWIS					
Sonoma					
Dried	7-8 pieces (1 oz)	90	1	19	—
Chiquita					
Fresh	2 med (5.2 oz)	100	1	24	16
KNISH					
take-out					
cheese & blueberry	1 (7 oz)	378	13	40	—

FOOD	PORTION	CAL	FAT	CARB	SUG
cheese & cherry	1 (7 oz)	378	13	40	—
everything	1 (7 oz)	221	8	34	—
kashe	1 (7 oz)	270	8	45	—
potato	1 med (3.5 oz)	166	6	25	2
potato	1 lg (7 oz)	332	12	49	5
potato w/ broccoli & cheese	1 (7 oz)	312	15	33	—
potato w/ spinach & mushroom	1 (7 oz)	214	8	32	—
KOHLRABI					
raw sliced	½ cup	19	tr	4	—
sliced cooked	½ cup	24	tr	5	—
KRILL					
fresh	1 oz	22	1	tr	—
KUMQUATS					
fresh	1	12	tr	3	—
LAMB					
cubed lean only braised	3 oz	190	7	0	0
cubed lean only broiled	3 oz	158	6	0	0
ground broiled	3 oz	240	17	0	0
leg lean & fat Choice roasted	3 oz	219	14	14	—
loin chop w/ bone lean & fat Choice broiled	1 chop (2.3 oz)	201	15	0	0
loin chop w/ bone lean only Choice broiled	1 chop (1.6 oz)	100	5	0	0
rib chop lean & fat Choice broiled	3 oz	307	25	0	0

FOOD	PORTION	CAL	FAT	CARB	SUG
rib chop lean only Choice broiled	3 oz	200	11	0	0
shank lean & fat Choice braised	3 oz	206	11	0	0
shank lean & fat Choice roasted	3 oz	191	11	0	0
shoulder chop w/ bone lean & fat Choice braised	1 chop (2.5 oz)	244	17	0	0
shoulder chop w/ bone lean only Choice braised	1 chop (1.9 oz)	152	8	0	0
sirloin lean & fat Choice roasted	3 oz	248	21	0	0

LAMB DISHES
take-out

curry	¾ cup	345	17	22	—
moussaka	5.6 oz	312	21	16	—
stew	¾ cup	124	5	11	—

LAMBSQUARTERS

chopped cooked	½ cup	29	1	5	—

LECITHIN

(*see* SOY)

LEEKS

cooked	1 (4.4 oz)	38	tr	9	—
freeze dried	1 tbsp	1	0	tr	—

LEMON

fresh	1 med	22	tr	12	—
peel	1 tbsp	0	tr	1	—
wedge	1	5	tr	3	—

FOOD	PORTION	CAL	FAT	CARB	SUG
LEMON CURD					
lemon curd made w/ egg	2 tsp	29	1	4	—
LEMON GRASS					
fresh	1 tbsp (5 g)	5	tr	1	—
LEMON JUICE					
fresh	1 tbsp	4	0	1	—
Canarino					
Italian Hot Lemon Beverage	1 cup oz)	0	0	0	0
LEMONADE					
mix					
Country Time					
Lem'n Berry Sippers Cranberry Raspberry Lemonade as prep	1 serv (8 oz)	90	0	21	21
Lem'n Berry Sippers Raspberry Lemonade as prep	1 serv (8 oz)	90	0	21	21
Lem'n Berry Sippers Strawberry Lemonade as prep	1 serv (8 oz)	90	0	21	21
Lem'n Berry Sippers Wildberry Lemonade as prep	1 serv (8 oz)	90	0	21	21
Lem'n Berry Sippers Sugar Free Strawberry Lemonade as prep	1 serv (8 oz)	5	0	0	0
Lemonade as prep	1 serv (8 oz)	70	0	17	17
Pink as prep	1 serv (8 oz)	70	0	17	17
Sugar Free Pink as prep	1 serv (8 oz)	5	0	0	0

FOOD	PORTION	CAL	FAT	CARB	SUG
Sugar Free as prep	1 serv (8 oz)	5	0	0	0
Crystal Light					
Lemonade as prep	1 serv (8 oz)	5	0	0	0
Pink as prep	1 serv (8 oz)	5	0	0	0
Kool-Aid					
Lemonade as prep	1 serv (8 oz)	70	0	17	17
Mix as prep w/ sugar	1 serv (8 oz)	100	0	25	25
Pink as prep w/ sugar	1 serv (8 oz)	100	0	25	25
Soarin' Strawberry Lemonade as prep	1 serv (8 oz)	70	0	17	17
Soarin' Strawberry Lemonade as prep w/ sugar	1 serv (8 oz)	100	0	25	25
Sugar Free Soarin' Strawberry Lemonade as prep	1 serv (8 oz)	5	0	0	0
Sugar Free Mix as prep	1 serv (8 oz)	5	0	0	0
ready-to-drink					
Crystal Light					
Lemonade	1 serv (8 oz)	5	0	0	0
Pink	1 serv (8 oz)	5	0	0	0
Everfresh					
Lemonade	1 can (8 oz)	120	0	29	29
Ruby Red	1 can (8 oz)	110	0	27	27
Nantucket Nectars					
Authentic	8 oz	120	0	30	28
Pink	8 oz	120	0	30	27
Newman's Own					
Lemonade	1 bottle (10 oz)	140	0	34	34

FOOD	PORTION	CAL	FAT	CARB	SUG
Roadside Virginia	8 fl oz	110	0	27	27
Shasta Plus					
Lemonade	1 can (11.5 oz)	160	0	40	40
Snapple					
Diet Pink	8 fl oz	20	0	4	4
Lemonade	8 fl oz	120	0	30	28
Pink	8 fl oz	120	0	29	28
Turkey Hill					
Lemonade	1 cup	120	0	29	29
Raspberry	1 cup	120	0	29	29
Strawberry Kiwi	1 cup	120	0	29	29
Veryfine					
Chillers	1 can (11.5 oz)	190	0	48	48
Chillers Cherry	8 fl oz	120	0	29	29
Chillers Peach	8 fl oz	120	0	31	31
Chillers Pink	1 can (11.5 oz)	180	0	45	45
Chillers Strawberry	1 can (11.5 oz)	170	0	43	42

LENTILS

Eden

Organic w/ Sweet Onion & Bay Leaf	¼ cup (4.6 oz)	90	0	13	0
Natural Touch					
Lentil Rice Loaf	1 in slice (3.2 oz)	170	9	14	tr
Shiloh Farms					
Organic Green not prep	¼ cup (1.6 oz)	150	0	27	2
take-out					
indian sambar	1 serv	236	5	37	—
yemiser selatta ethiopian lentil salad	1 serv (3 oz)	115	7	11	1

FOOD	PORTION	CAL	FAT	CARB	SUG
LETTUCE					
arugula	½ cup (0.4 oz)	3	tr	tr	—
bibb	1 head (6 oz)	21	tr	4	—
boston	2 leaves	2	tr	tr	—
cornsalad field salad	1 cup (1.9 oz)	7	tr	1	—
looseleaf shredded	½ cup	5	tr	1	—
Dole					
Iceberg	1½ cup (3 oz)	15	0	3	2
Romaine	1½ cups (3 oz)	15	0	2	2
Shredded	1½ cup (3 oz)	15	0	3	2
Earthbound Farm					
Romaine Salad Organic	1½ cups (2.9 oz)	15	0	3	2
LIMA BEANS					
canned					
lima beans	½ cup	93	tr	17	—
dried					
cooked	½ cup	104	tr	20	—
Hurst					
HamBeens Baby Limas w/ Ham	1 serv	120	1	22	1
HamBeens Large Limas w/ Ham	1 serv	120	1	22	1
frozen					
Birds Eye					
Baby	½ cup	130	0	24	2
Fordhook	½ cup	100	0	19	3
Green Giant					
Butter Sauce	⅔ cup (3.6 oz)	120	3	18	1
Harvest Fresh Baby	½ cup (2.7 oz)	80	0	15	tr

FOOD	PORTION	CAL	FAT	CARB	SUG
LIME					
fresh	1	20	tr	7	—
LIME JUICE					
Realime					
Juice	1 tsp (5 ml)	0	0	0	0
LING					
fresh baked	3 oz	95	1	0	0
LINGCOD					
baked	3 oz	93	1	0	0
LIQUOR/LIQUEUR					
anisette	⅔ oz	74	0	7	—
apricot brandy	⅔ oz	64	0	6	—
aquavit	1 oz	65	0	0	0
benedictine	⅔ oz	69	0	7	—
bloody mary	5 oz	116	tr	5	—
bourbon & soda	4 oz	105	0	0	0
coffee liqueur	1½ oz	174	tr	24	—
coffee w/ cream liqueur	1½ oz	154	7	10	—
cognac	1 oz	67	0	tr	0
cosmopolitan	1 (4 oz)	213	tr	17	4
creme de menthe	1½ oz	186	tr	21	—
curacao liqueur	⅔ oz	54	0	6	—
daiquiri	2 oz	111	0	4	—
gin	1½ oz	110	0	0	0
gin & tonic	7.5 oz	171	0	16	—
long island ice tea	1 serv (7.5 oz)	159	0	14	13
manhattan	2 oz	128	0	2	—
martini	2½ oz	156	0	tr	—
mint julep	10 oz	210	0	3	—
old-fashioned	2½ oz	127	0	3	—

FOOD	PORTION	CAL	FAT	CARB	SUG
pina colada	4½ oz	262	3	40	—
rum	1½ oz	97	0	0	0
screwdriver	7 oz	174	tr	18	—
sloe gin fizz	2½ oz	132	0	4	—
tequila sunrise	5½ oz	189	tr	15	—
tom collins	7½ oz	121	0	3	—
vodka	1½ oz	97	0	0	0
whiskey	1½ oz	105	0	tr	—
whiskey sour	3 oz	123	tr	5	—

LIVER

FOOD	PORTION	CAL	FAT	CARB	SUG
beef pan-fried	3 oz	184	7	7	—
chicken stewed	1 cup (5 oz)	219	8	1	—
lamb braised	3 oz	187	7	2	—
pork braised	3 oz	140	4	3	—
turkey simmered	1 cup (5 oz)	237	8	5	—
veal fried	3 oz	208	10	3	—

LOBSTER

FOOD	PORTION	CAL	FAT	CARB	SUG
northern cooked	1 cup	142	1	2	—
spiny steamed	1 (5.7 oz)	233	3	5	—
Progresso					
Lobster Sauce	½ cup (4.3 oz)	100	7	6	3
take-out					
newburg	1 cup	485	27	13	—

LOGANBERRIES

FOOD	PORTION	CAL	FAT	CARB	SUG
frozen	1 cup	80	tr	19	—

LONGANS

FOOD	PORTION	CAL	FAT	CARB	SUG
fresh	1	2	0	tr	—

LOQUATS

FOOD	PORTION	CAL	FAT	CARB	SUG
fresh	1	5	tr	1	—

FOOD	PORTION	CAL	FAT	CARB	SUG
LOTUS					
root sliced cooked	10 slices	59	tr	14	—
seeds dried	1 oz	94	1	18	—
LOX					
(*see* SALMON)					
LUPINES					
dried cooked	1 cup	197	5	16	—
LYCHEES					
fresh	1	6	tr	2	—
MACADAMIA NUTS					
Hawaiian Host					
Chocolate Covered	1 piece (0.5 oz)	53	6	8	7
MacFarms of Hawaii					
Chocolate Covered	¼ cup (1.3 oz)	210	16	18	15
Dry Roasted Salted	¼ cup (1.3 oz)	220	23	4	1
Kona Coffee Dark Chocolate Covered	¼ cup (1.3 oz)	210	16	18	15
MACARONI					
(*see* PASTA)					
MACE					
ground	1 tsp	8	1	1	—
MACKEREL					
canned					
jack	1 cup	296	12	0	0
fresh					
atlantic cooked	3 oz	223	15	0	0
jack baked	3 oz	171	9	0	0
king baked	3 oz	114	2	0	0
pacific baked	3 oz	171	9	0	0
spanish cooked	3 oz	134	5	0	0

FOOD	PORTION	CAL	FAT	CARB	SUG
smoked					
atlantic	3.5 oz	296	24	0	0
MALANGA					
fresh	½ cup	137	tr	32	—
MALT					
nonalcoholic	12 fl oz	32	0	5	—
MALTED MILK					
Carnation					
Chocolate	3 tbsp (0.7 oz)	90	1	18	14
Original	3 tbsp (0.7 oz)	90	2	15	10
MAMMY-APPLE					
fresh	1	431	4	106	—
MANGO					
fresh	1	135	1	35	—
Rainforest Farms					
Slices Dried	6 slices (1.3 oz)	140	1	33	30
Sonoma					
Pieces Dried	8 pieces (2 oz)	180	1	44	44
MANGO JUICE					
After The Fall					
Mango Ginger	1 can (12 oz)	150	0	35	30
Guzzler					
Mango Passion	8 fl oz	140	0	22	0
Ocean Spray					
Mango Mango	8 oz	130	0	33	33
Snapple					
Mango Madness	8 fl oz	110	0	29	27
Tang					
Drink Mix as prep	1 serv (8 oz)	100	0	25	25

FOOD	PORTION	CAL	FAT	CARB	SUG
MARGARINE					
tub unsalted	1 tsp	34	4	0	0
Take Control					
Spread	1 tbsp (0.5 oz)	50	6	0	0
Weight Watchers					
Light	1 tbsp	45	4	2	0
Light Sodium Free	1 tbsp	45	4	2	0
MARJORAM					
dried	1 tsp	2	tr	tr	—
MARLIN					
raw	3 oz	110	3	0	0
MARSHMALLOW					
marshmallow	1 reg (0.3 oz)	23	0	6	—
Just Born					
Peeps	5 (1.5 oz)	160	0	40	36
MATZO					
egg	1 (1 oz)	111	1	22	—
plain	1 (1 oz)	112	tr	24	—
whole wheat	1 (1 oz)	99	tr	22	—
Manischewitz					
Matzo Meal	¼ cup (1 oz)	130	0	23	1
MAYONNAISE					
Blue Plate					
Squeeze	1 tbsp	100	11	0	0
Hellman's					
Mayonnaise	1 tbsp	100	11	0	0
Kraft					
Fat Free	1 tbsp (0.6 oz)	10	0	2	1
Light	1 tbsp (0.5 oz)	50	5	2	tr
Real	1 tbsp (0.5 oz)	100	11	0	0

FOOD	PORTION	CAL	FAT	CARB	SUG
Weight Watchers					
Fat Free	1 tbsp	10	0	3	2
Light	1 tbsp	25	2	1	1
Light Low Sodium	1 tbsp	25	2	1	0

MAYONNAISE TYPE SALAD DRESSING

Miracle Whip					
Free	1 tbsp (0.5 oz)	15	0	2	2
Light	1 tbsp (0.5 oz)	35	3	2	2
Salad Dressing	1 tbsp (0.6 oz)	70	7	2	1
Weight Watchers					
Fat Free Whipped Dressing	1 tbsp	15	0	3	2

MEAT STICKS

Big Ones					
BBQ	1 (1 oz)	130	12	1	1
Hot n'Spicy	1 (1 oz)	130	12	1	1
Original	1 (1 oz)	130	12	1	1
Teriyaki	1 (1 oz)	130	12	2	2
Jack Link's					
Kippered Beefsteak Teriyaki	1 oz	80	1	5	4
Lance					
Beef & Cheese	1 pkg (1.5 oz)	150	11	3	0
Beef Jerky	1 piece (0.25 oz)	30	2	tr	0
Beef Snack	1 piece (0.63 oz)	100	8	1	0
Hot Sausage	1 piece (0.9 oz)	60	5	1	1
Lowrey's					
Smokehouse Tender Hickory Smoked	1 pkg (1 oz)	80	2	5	4
Smokehouse Tender Original	1 pkg (1 oz)	60	1	2	1

FOOD	PORTION	CAL	FAT	CARB	SUG
Smokehouse Tender Peppered	1 pkg (1 oz)	60	1	2	1
Oberto					
Beef Jerky	1 pkg (1.3 oz)	100	1	8	9
Pemmican					
Original Tender Kippered Beef Steak	1	110	5	3	0
Peppered Tender Kippered Beef Steak	1	110	5	3	0
Rough Cut					
Beef Steak Hot	1 pkg (1 oz)	70	1	2	2
Beef Steak Original	1 pkg (1 oz)	60	1	2	2
Beef Steak Peppered	1 pkg (1 oz)	60	1	2	1
Rustlers Roundup					
Beef Jerky	1 serv (5 g)	20	2	tr	0
Flamin' Hot	1 serv (8 g)	40	3	1	tr
Smoky Steak	1 serv (0.8 oz)	60	2	1	tr
Spicy	1 serv (0.5 oz)	70	6	1	0
Slim Jim					
Spicy	1 (4½ in) (0.3 oz)	50	4	0	0
Spicy Big	1 (.44 oz)	70	6	1	0
Spicy Giant	1 (0.97 oz)	150	14	2	0
Spicy Super	1 (0.64 oz)	100	9	1	0

MEAT SUBSTITUTES

FOOD	PORTION	CAL	FAT	CARB	SUG
Amy's Organic					
Whole Meals Veggie Loaf	1 pkg (10 oz)	260	5	47	9
Boca Burgers					
Chef Max's Original	1 patty (2.5 oz)	110	2	9	0

FOOD	PORTION	CAL	FAT	CARB	SUG
Frieda's					
SoyTaco	1 oz	50	3	3	0
Soyrizo	4 tbsp (1.9 oz)	120	9	5	2
Ken & Robert's					
Veggie Pockets	1 (4.5 oz)	250	8	40	3
Veggie Pockets Bar B Que	1 (4.5 oz)	290	8	45	2
Veggie Pockets Broccoli & Cheddar	1 (4.5 oz)	250	8	38	2
Veggie Pockets Greek	1 (4.5 oz)	250	8	37	2
Veggie Pockets Indian	1 (4.5 oz)	260	8	40	2
Veggie Pockets Pizza	1 (4.5 oz)	270	8	41	2
Veggie Pockets Pot Pie	1 (4.5 oz)	250	9	38	2
Veggie Pockets Potato & Cheddar	1 (4.5 oz)	260	8	42	2
Veggie Pockets Santa Fe	1 (4.5 oz)	250	8	39	2
Veggie Pockets Tex Mex	1 (4.5 oz)	260	8	46	2
Lightlife					
Foney Baloney	3 slices (1.5 oz)	60	3	2	0
Gimme Lean Beef	2 oz	70	0	8	1
Smart Deli Bologna	3 slices (1.5 oz)	50	0	2	0
Smart Deli Ham	3 slices (1.5 oz)	50	0	2	0
Smart Deli Peppercorn	3 slices (1.5 oz)	45	0	1	0
Smart Deli Sticks Pepperoni	1 oz	45	0	2	1
Smart Deli Sticks Soylami	1 oz	40	0	1	0
Smart Ground Original	⅓ cup (1.9 oz)	70	0	5	1
Smart Ground Taco	⅓ cup (2 oz)	60	0	6	0

FOOD	PORTION	CAL	FAT	CARB	SUG
Loma Linda					
Dinner Cuts	2 slices (3.2 oz)	90	2	3	0
Nuteena	⅜ in slice (1.9 oz)	160	13	6	tr
Sandwich Spread	¼ cup (1.9 oz)	80	5	7	tr
Savory Dinner Loaf Mix not prep	⅓ cup (0.9 oz)	90	2	7	0
Swiss Stake	1 piece (3.2 oz)	120	6	8	tr
Tender Bits	6 pieces (3 oz)	110	5	7	0
Tender Rounds	6 pieces (2.8 oz)	120	5	5	tr
Vita Burger Chunks not prep	¼ cup (0.7 oz)	70	1	6	1
Vita Burger Granules	3 tbsp (0.7 oz)	70	1	6	1
Morningstar Farms					
Burger Style Recipe Crumbles	⅔ cup (1.9 oz)	80	3	4	tr
Ground Meatless	½ cup (1.9 oz)	60	0	4	0
Harvest Burger Recipe Crumbles	½ cup (2 oz)	70	0	5	0
Quarter Prime	1 patty (3.4 oz)	140	2	6	1
Natural Touch					
Dinner Entree	1 patty (3 oz)	220	15	2	0
Loaf Mix not prep	4 tbsp (1 oz)	100	1	10	tr
Stroganoff Mix not prep	4 tbsp (0.8 oz)	90	4	10	1
Taco Mix not prep	3 tbsp (0.6 oz)	60	1	5	tr
Vegan Burger Crumbles	½ cup (1.9 oz)	60	0	4	0
Worthington					
Beef Style Meatless	⅜ in slice (1.9 oz)	110	7	4	tr
Bolono	3 slices (2 oz)	80	4	2	0
Choplets	2 slices (3.2 oz)	90	2	3	0
Corned Beef Meatless	4 slices (2 oz)	140	9	5	tr

FOOD	PORTION	CAL	FAT	CARB	SUG
Country Stew	1 cup (8.4 oz)	210	9	20	2
Dinner Roast	¾ in slice (3 oz)	180	12	5	1
FriPats	1 patty (2.2 oz)	130	6	4	0
Multigrain Cutlets	2 slices (3.2 oz)	100	2	5	0
Numete	⅝ in slice (1.9 oz)	130	10	5	tr
Prime Stakes	1 piece (3.2 oz)	120	7	4	0
Prosage Roll	⅝ in slice (1.9 oz)	140	10	2	0
Protose	⅝ in slice (1.9 oz)	130	7	5	tr
Salami Meatless	3 slices (2 oz)	130	8	2	0
Savory Slices	3 slices (2.9 oz)	150	9	6	0
Smoked Beef Meatless	6 slices (2 oz)	120	6	6	1
Stakelets	1 piece (2.5 oz)	140	8	6	0
Veelets	1 patty (2.5 oz)	180	9	10	tr
Vegetable Skallops	½ cup (3 oz)	90	2	3	0
Vegetable Steaks	2 pieces (2.5 oz)	80	2	3	0
Wham	2 slices (1.6 oz)	80	5	1	1
Yves					
Veggie Bologna	4 slices (2.2 oz)	70	0	2	1
Veggie Ground Italian	⅓ cup (2 oz)	60	0	4	0
Veggie Ground Round Italian	⅓ cup (1.9 oz)	60	0	4	0
Veggie Ground Round Original	2 oz	60	0	4	0
Veggie Pizza Pepperoni Slices	1 serv (1.7 oz)	70	0	4	0
Veggie Salami Deli Slices	1 serv (2.2 oz)	90	0	5	1

MELON JUICE

Ocean Spray

Mega Melon	8 oz	130	0	33	33

MEXICAN FOOD

(*see* SALSA, SAUCE, SPANISH FOODS, TORTILLA)

FOOD	PORTION	CAL	FAT	CARB	SUG
MILK					
canned					
Carnation					
Evaporated	½ cup	150	8	3	3
Evaporated Fat Free	½ cup (4 fl oz)	100	0	4	4
Evaporated Lowfat	½ cup	110	2	3	3
Sweetened Condensed	⅓ cup	330	8	22	22
dried					
Carnation					
Nonfat	⅓ cup	80	0	12	12
Saco					
Cultured Buttermilk	4 tbsp (0.8 oz)	80	tr	13	12
Sanalac					
Powder	¼ cup (0.8 oz)	85	tr	13	12
refrigerated					
1%	1 cup	102	3	12	—
2%	1 cup	121	5	12	—
buttermilk	1 cup	99	2	12	—
goat	1 cup	168	10	11	—
nonfat	1 cup	86	tr	12	—
whole	1 cup	150	8	11	—
Cool Cow					
Low Fat	1 cup (8 oz)	110	3	12	12
Farmland					
Skim Plus	1 cup (8 oz)	110	0	17	16
Horizon Organic					
Fat Free	1 cup (8 oz)	80	0	12	11
Land O Lakes					
1% Lowfat	1 carton (10 oz)	120	3	13	13
Fat Free	1 carton (10 oz)	100	5	13	13
Whole	1 carton (10 oz)	180	10	13	13

FOOD	PORTION	CAL	FAT	CARB	SUG
Organic Valley					
Low Fat	1 cup	100	3	12	12
Nonfat	1 cup	80	0	13	12
Reduced Fat	1 cup	130	5	12	11
Whole	1 cup	150	8	12	11
Stonyfield Farm					
Organic Whole Milk	1 cup (8 oz)	180	10	12	12
Organic Whole Milk Vanilla	1 cup (8 oz)	230	8	30	30
Turkey Hill					
Cool Moos 2% Reduced Fat	1 cup	130	5	12	11
Cool Moos Whole Milk	1 cup	160	8	12	11

MILK DRINKS

FOOD	PORTION	CAL	FAT	CARB	SUG
Horizon Organic					
Lowfat Chocolate Milk	1 cup (8 oz)	160	3	26	24
Land O Lakes					
Chocolate	1 cup (8.4 oz)	200	7	27	26
Organic Valley					
Chocolate Milk Reduced Fat	1 cup	180	5	26	25
Quik					
Banana Lowfat	1 cup (8.4 oz)	200	5	31	30
Banana Powder	2 tbsp (0.8 oz)	90	0	27	20
Chocolate	1 cup (8.4 oz)	230	8	33	30
Chocolate Lowfat	1 carton (8.4 oz)	200	5	30	29
Cookies n Cream Powder	2 tbsp (0.8 oz)	100	1	21	14
Strawberry	1 cup (8.4 oz)	230	8	33	30
Strawberry Lowfat	1 carton (8.4 oz)	210	5	35	35
Strawberry Powder	2 tbsp (0.8 oz)	90	0	22	21

FOOD	PORTION	CAL	FAT	CARB	SUG
Turkey Hill					
Cool Moos Chocolate 1% Lowfat	1 cup	180	3	32	30
Cool Moos Orange Cream 1% Lowfat	1 cup	190	3	33	32
Cool Moos Strawberry 1% Lowfat	1 cup	160	3	27	27
Cool Moos Vanilla 1% Lowfat	1 cup	160	3	26	25
MILK SUBSTITUTES					
8th Continent					
Soymilk Low Fat Chocolate	1 bottle (8 oz)	140	3	23	21
Soymilk Low Fat Vanilla	1 bottle (8 oz)	90	3	11	10
Better Than Milk					
Rice Original	2 tbsp (0.66 oz)	78	2	15	4
Rice Original Light	2 tbsp (0.66 oz)	66	0	17	4
Rice Vanilla	2 tbsp (0.66 oz)	78	2	15	5
Rice Vanilla Light	2 tbsp (0.66 oz)	66	0	17	5
Soy Carob	2 tbsp (1 oz)	90	2	18	9
Soy Chocolate	2 tbsp (1.1 oz)	112	2	21	19
Soy Light	2 tbsp (0.66 oz)	73	2	8	5
Soy Original	2 tbsp (0.8 oz)	100	3	16	5
Soy Vanilla	2 tbsp (0.7 oz)	77	2	8	6
Blue Diamond					
Almond Breeze Chocolate	8 oz	120	3	21	20
Almond Breeze Original	8 oz	60	2	8	7
Almond Breeze Vanilla	8 oz	90	3	15	15

FOOD	PORTION	CAL	FAT	CARB	SUG
Edensoy					
Extra Original	8 oz	130	4	13	7
Extra Vanilla	8 oz	150	3	23	15
Original	8 oz	130	4	13	7
Vanilla	8 oz	150	3	32	15
Galaxy					
Veggi Milk Chocolate	1 cup (8 oz)	150	2	26	20
Veggie Milk Original	1 cup (8 oz)	110	3	13	8
Harmony Farms					
Original Rice Beverage	1 cup (8 oz)	90	0	21	14
Harmony House					
Enriched Rice Beverage	1 cup (8 oz)	90	0	21	14
Enriched Soy Beverage	1 cup (8 oz)	90	0	21	14
Original Soy Beverage	1 cup (8 oz)	90	0	21	14
Health Valley					
Soo Moo	1 cup	110	0	22	17
Rice Dream					
Carob	1 box (8 oz)	150	3	32	24
Chocolate	1 box (8 oz)	170	3	36	25
Chocolate Enriched	1 box (8 oz)	170	3	36	25
Organic Original	1 box (8 oz)	120	2	25	11
Organic Original Enriched	1 box (8 oz)	120	2	25	11
Vanilla	1 box (8 oz)	130	2	28	12
Vanilla Enriched	1 box (8 oz)	130	2	28	12
Soy Dream					
Carob	8 oz	210	5	36	22
Chocolate Enriched	8 oz	210	5	35	22

FOOD	PORTION	CAL	FAT	CARB	SUG
Original	8 oz	140	5	14	8
Original Enriched	8 oz	140	5	14	8
Vanilla	8 oz	170	5	23	18
Vanilla Enriched	8 oz	140	5	23	18
White Wave					
Silk Chocolate Organic	1 cup (8.3 oz)	108	3	17	15
MILKFISH					
baked	3 oz	162	7	0	0
MILLET					
cooked	1 cup (6.1 oz)	207	2	41	—
MINERAL WATER					
(*see* WATER)					
MISO					
dried	1 oz	86	3	10	—
miso	⅓ cup	284	8	39	—
MOLASSES					
molasses	1 tbsp (0.7 oz)	53	0	14	12
Brer Rabbit					
Dark	1 tbsp	60	0	16	13
MONKFISH					
baked	3 oz	82	2	0	0
MOOSE					
roasted	3 oz	114	1	0	0
MOTH BEANS					
dried cooked	1 cup	207	1	37	—
MOUSSE **frozen**					
Sara Lee					
Chocolate	⅕ pkg (4.3 oz)	400	25	37	27

FOOD	PORTION	CAL	FAT	CARB	SUG
Weight Watchers					
Chocolate Mousse	1 (2.75 oz)	190	5	31	14

MUFFIN

FOOD	PORTION	CAL	FAT	CARB	SUG
Pepperidge Farm					
Blueberry	1 (2 oz)	180	7	28	12
Bran w/ Raisins	1 (2 oz)	180	6	30	17
Corn	1 (2 oz)	190	7	28	8
Orange Cranberry	1 (2 oz)	180	6	29	12
Sara Lee					
Blueberry	1 (2.2 oz)	220	11	27	12
Corn	1 (2.2 oz)	260	14	30	14
Weight Watchers					
Chocolate Chocolate Chip	1 (2.5 oz)	190	2	39	14
Fat Free Banana	1 (2.5 oz)	170	0	41	17
Fat Free Blueberry	1 (2.5 oz)	160	0	38	15
mix					
Betty Crocker					
Apple Cinnamon as prep	1	170	7	23	11
Apple Streusel as prep	1	210	8	33	18
Banana Nut as prep	1	170	6	27	12
Cranberry Orange as prep	1	150	5	25	12
Double Chocolate as prep	1	220	11	30	26
Golden Corn as prep	1	160	5	24	6
Lemon Poppyseed as prep	1	180	8	24	13

FOOD	PORTION	CAL	FAT	CARB	SUG
Sunkist Lemon Poppyseed as prep	1	190	7	29	14
Twice The Blueberries as prep	1	140	3	25	12
Wild Blueberry as prep	1	170	5	28	14
Gold Medal					
Corn	1	160	6	25	8
Hodgson Mill					
Bran	¼ cup (1.3 oz)	130	1	27	5
Cornbread	¼ cup (1.3 oz)	130	1	28	3
Whole Wheat	¼ cup (1.3 oz)	130	1	27	6
Robin Hood					
Apple Cinnamon	1	170	8	23	11
Banana Nut	1	170	8	21	9
Blueberry	1	160	6	24	12
Caramel Nut	1	170	7	24	11
Sweet Rewards					
Low Fat Apple Cinnamon as prep	1	140	2	26	15
ready-to-eat					
Dolly Madison					
Blueberry	1 (1.75 oz)	170	7	26	8
Mega Banana Nut	1 (5.9 oz)	620	31	78	39
Mega Blueberry	1 (5.9 oz)	590	28	78	41
Mega Chocolate Chip	1 (5.9 oz)	620	29	78	41
Mega Cranberry Orange	1 (5.9 oz)	590	28	79	41
Mega Cream Cheese	1 (5.9 oz)	620	33	73	41
Dutch Mill					
Apple Oat Bran	1 (2 oz)	180	5	31	5
Banana Walnut	1 (2 oz)	220	6	33	15
Carrot	1 (2 oz)	190	7	31	19
Corn	1 (2 oz)	190	6	31	14

FOOD	PORTION	CAL	FAT	CARB	SUG
Cranberry Orange	1 (2 oz)	170	6	26	14
Raisin Bran	1 (2 oz)	230	5	37	12
Hostess					
Banana Bran Low Fat	1 (2.7 oz)	240	3	47	24
Blueberry Low Fat	1 (2.7 oz)	230	3	47	23
Hearty Banana Nut	1 (5.9 oz)	620	31	78	39
Hearty Blueberry	1 (5.9 oz)	590	28	78	41
Hearty Chocolate Chip	1 (5.9 oz)	620	29	78	41
Hearty Cranberry Orange	1 (5.9 oz)	590	28	79	41
Hearty Cream Cheese	1 (5.9 oz)	620	33	73	41
Mini Banana Walnut	3 (1.2 oz)	160	9	16	8
Mini Blueberry	3 (1.2 oz)	150	8	18	8
Mini Chocolate Chip	3 (1.2 oz)	160	9	17	9
Mini Cinnamon Apple	3 (1.2 oz)	160	9	16	8
Mini Cinnamon Bites	3 (1.1 oz)	130	6	18	8
Mini Rocky Road	3 (1.2 oz)	160	9	17	9
Muffin Loaf Apple Spice	1 (3.7 oz)	430	18	61	41
Muffin Loaf Banana Nut	1 (3.8 oz)	460	20	63	29
Muffin Loaf Blueberry	1 (3.8 oz)	440	19	62	34
Muffin Loaf Chocolate Chocolate Chip	1 (3.8 oz)	400	17	58	32
Muffin Loaf Raspberry	1 (3.8 oz)	440	19	62	34
Oat Bran	1 (1.5 oz)	160	8	21	9
Otis Spunkmeyer					
Apple Cinnamon	1 (2 oz)	220	11	27	16
Low Fat Wild Blueberry	1 (2.25 oz)	200	4	38	24
Mayport Almond Poppy Seed	½ muffin (2 oz)	210	12	23	17
Mayport Banana Nut	1 (2.25 oz)	270	14	33	20
Mayport Cheese Streusel	½ muffin (2 oz)	220	10	30	18

FOOD	PORTION	CAL	FAT	CARB	SUG
Mayport Chocolate Chocolate Chip	1 (2.25 oz)	260	13	33	22
Mayport Chocolate Chip	½ muffin (2 oz)	240	13	28	18
Mayport Cinnamon Spice	½ muffin (2 oz)	230	13	26	16
Mayport Corn	½ muffin (2 oz)	230	13	26	14
Mayport Harvest Bran	1 (2.25 oz)	240	10	34	20
Mayport Lemon	½ muffin (2 oz)	230	13	27	15
Mayport Orange	½ muffin (2 oz)	230	13	27	16
Mayport Pineapple	½ muffin (2 oz)	210	12	25	17
Mayport Wild Blueberry	1 (2.25 oz)	230	13	27	20
Mayport Low Fat Apple Cinnamon	1 (4 oz)	380	6	75	50
Mayport Low Fat Banana Nut	1 (4 oz)	350	6	70	45
Mayport Low Fat Chocolate Chocolate Chip	1 (4 oz)	370	6	73	47
Uncle Wally's					
Fat Free Apple Cinnamon Delight	1 (1.9 oz)	110	0	28	13
Weight Watchers					
Fat Free Apple Crisp	1 (2.5 oz)	160	0	37	16
Fat Free Cranberry Orange	1 (2.5 oz)	160	0	38	14
Fat Free Double Chocolate	1 (2.5 oz)	180	0	40	26
Fat Free Wild Blueberry	1 (2.5 oz)	160	0	36	15
Low Fat Apple Cinnamon	1 (2.5 oz)	170	3	35	20
Low Fat Blueberry	1 (2.5 oz)	180	3	37	20
Low Fat Carrot	1 (2.5 oz)	160	3	34	16

FOOD	PORTION	CAL	FAT	CARB	SUG
Low Fat Chocolate Chip	1 (2.5 oz)	180	3	38	21
Low Fat Cranberry Orange	1 (2.5 oz)	180	3	38	20
Low Fat Lemon Poppy	1 (2.5 oz)	190	3	38	20
MULBERRIES					
fresh	1 cup	61	1	14	—
MULLET					
striped cooked	3 oz	127	4	0	0
MUNG BEANS					
dried cooked	1 cup	213	1	39	—
MUNGO BEANS					
dried cooked	1 cup	190	1	33	—
MUSHROOMS **canned** *BinB*					
Pieces & Stems	1 can (4.2 oz)	30	0	4	1
Sliced	1 can (4.2 oz)	30	0	4	1
Sliced With Garlic	1 can (4.2 oz)	35	1	4	1
Whole	1 can (4.2 oz)	30	0	4	1
Green Giant					
Pieces & Stems	½ cup (4.2 oz)	30	0	4	1
Sliced	½ cup (4.2 oz)	30	0	3	1
Whole	½ cup (4.2 oz)	30	0	4	1
dried					
chanterelle	1 oz	25	tr	tr	—
cloud ear	1 (5 g)	13	tr	3	—
shiitake	4 (½ oz)	44	tr	11	—
straw	1 piece (6 g)	2	tr	tr	—
tree ear	½ cup (0.4 oz)	36	tr	10	—
wood ear mok yee	½ cup (0.4 oz)	25	tr	8	—

FOOD	PORTION	CAL	FAT	CARB	SUG
fresh					
portabella	1 serv (2 oz)	14	tr	3	—
raw	1 (½ oz)	5	tr	1	—
shitake cooked	4 (2.5 oz)	40	tr	10	—
MUSKRAT					
roasted	3 oz	199	10	0	0
MUSSELS					
blue raw	1 cup	129	3	6	—
fresh blue cooked	3 oz	147	4	6	—
MUSTARD					
dry mustard	1 tsp	15	1	1	—
Boar's Head					
Delicatessen Style	1 tsp (5 g)	0	0	0	0
Honey	1 tsp (5 g)	10	0	2	1
Hunt's					
Mustard	1 tsp (5 g)	3	tr	tr	tr
Kraft					
Horseradish Mustard	1 tsp (5 g)	0	0	0	0
Mustard	1 tsp (5 g)	0	0	0	0
Luzianne					
Creole Mustard	1 tbsp	10	0	2	0
MUSTARD GREENS					
Birds Eye					
Chopped	1 cup (3 oz)	30	0	2	1
NATTO					
natto	½ cup	187	10	13	—
NAVY BEANS **dried**					
cooked	1 cup	259	1	48	—

FOOD	PORTION	CAL	FAT	CARB	SUG
Hurst					
HamBeens w/ Ham	3 tbsp (1.2 oz)	120	1	20	1

NECTARINE
Chiquita

Fresh	1 med (4.9 oz)	70	1	16	12

NEUFCHATEL
Horizon Organic

Neufchatel	2 tbsp	70	6	tr	tr
Organic Valley					
Neufchatel	1 oz	70	6	1	tr
Philadelphia					
Neufchatel	1 oz	70	6	tr	tr

NON-DAIRY CREAMERS
(*see* COFFEE WHITENERS)

NON-DAIRY WHIPPED TOPPINGS
(*see* WHIPPED TOPPINGS)

NOODLE DISHES
mix

Kraft

Noodle Classics Cheddar Cheese as prep	1 cup (7.4 oz)	400	19	47	8
Noodle Classics Savory Chicken as prep	1 cup (8.5 oz)	340	13	46	5
Lipton					
Noodles & Sauce Alfredo Broccoli as prep	1 cup (2.2 oz)	340	14	43	5
Noodles & Sauce Alfredo as prep	1 cup (2.2 oz)	330	14	42	5

FOOD	PORTION	CAL	FAT	CARB	SUG
Noodles & Sauce Beef as prep	1 cup (2.1 oz)	280	10	43	2
Noodles & Sauce Butter as prep	1 cup (2.2 oz)	310	14	41	4
Noodles & Sauce Butter & Herb as prep	1 cup (2.2 oz)	300	13	42	4
Noodles & Sauce Chicken Broccoli as prep	1 cup (2.1 oz)	310	11	44	4
Noodles & Sauce Chicken Tetrazzini as prep	1 cup (2 oz)	300	12	41	4
Noodles & Sauce Chicken as prep	1 cup (2.1 oz)	290	11	42	2
Noodles & Sauce Creamy Chicken as prep	1 cup (2.1 oz)	320	13	42	5
Noodles & Sauce Parmesan as prep	1 cup (2.1 oz)	330	15	40	5
Noodles & Sauce Sour Cream & Chives as prep	1 cup (2.2 oz)	310	14	41	4
Noodles & Sauce Stroganoff as prep	1 cup (2 oz)	300	11	40	5
shelf-stable					
Hormel					
Microcup Meals Noodles & Chicken	1 cup (7.5 oz)	200	9	20	2
NOODLES					
cellophane	1 cup	492	tr	121	—
egg cooked	1 cup (5.6 oz)	213	2	40	—
japanese soba cooked	1 cup (4 oz)	113	tr	24	—

FOOD	PORTION	CAL	FAT	CARB	SUG
japanese somen cooked	1 cup (6.2 oz)	231	tr	48	—
korean acorn noodles not prep	2 oz	195	tr	41	—
rice cooked	1 cup (6.2 oz)	192	tr	44	—
spinach/egg cooked	1 cup (5.6 oz)	211	3	39	—
Chun King					
Chow Mein	½ cup (1 oz)	137	6	19	0
Hodgson Mill					
Four Color Veggie Egg	2 oz	200	2	37	0
Whole Wheat Egg	2 oz	190	2	34	0
La Choy					
Chow Mein	½ cup (1 oz)	137	6	19	0
Chow Mein Crispy Wide	½ cup (1 oz)	148	8	16	0
Rice	½ cup (1 oz)	121	3	21	0
Manischewitz					
Fine Yolk Free	1½ cups	210	1	40	2

NOPALES

FOOD	PORTION	CAL	FAT	CARB	SUG
cooked	1 cup (5.2 oz)	23	tr	5	—

NUTMEG

FOOD	PORTION	CAL	FAT	CARB	SUG
ground	1 tsp	12	1	1	—

NUTRITION SUPPLEMENTS

(*see also* BREAKFAST DRINKS, CEREAL BARS, ENERGY BARS, ENERGY DRINKS, SPORTS DRINKS)

FOOD	PORTION	CAL	FAT	CARB	SUG
Enlive!					
Drink All Flavors	1 box (8.1 oz)	300	0	65	15
Ensure					
Supplement All Flavors	1 can (8 fl oz)	250	6	40	18
Essential					
Protein Powder	1 serv (0.6 oz)	70	tr	6	5

FOOD	PORTION	CAL	FAT	CARB	SUG
Glucerna					
Shakes All Flavors	1 can (8 oz)	220	9	29	7
Met-Rx					
Lite	1 pkg (1.6 oz)	170	1	16	3
Original	1 pkg (2.5 oz)	250	2	22	3
Protein Shake	1 can	200	3	20	1
Ultra	1 pkg (2.6 oz)	250	2	19	5
Nestle					
Additions	2⅓ tsp (0.7 oz)	100	5	9	1
NutraBalance					
EggPro	1 tbsp (7.5 g)	30	0	1	0
PermaLean					
Protein Powder Bodacious Berry	1 scoop (1 oz)	104	tr	1	3
Protein Powder Chocoholic Chocolate	1 scoop (1 oz)	104	tr	5	3
Pounds Off					
All Flavors	1 bar (2.1 oz)	210	5	32	18
NUTS MIXED					
(see also individual names)					
mixed nuts chocolate covered	¼ cup (1.5 oz)	240	17	20	17
Estee					
Fruit & Nut Mix	¼ cup	210	12	19	10
OCTOPUS					
fresh steamed	3 oz	140	2	4	—
OHELOBERRIES					
fresh	1 cup	39	tr	10	—

FOOD	PORTION	CAL	FAT	CARB	SUG
OIL					
canola	1 tbsp	124	14	0	0
corn	1 tbsp	120	14	0	0
olive	1 tbsp	119	14	0	0
safflower	1 tbsp	120	14	0	0
sesame	1 tbsp	120	14	0	0
soybean	1 tbsp	120	14	0	0
sunflower	1 tbsp	120	14	0	0
walnut	1 tbsp	120	14	0	0
Crisco					
Corn Canola	1 tbsp (0.5 fl oz)	120	14	0	0
Oil	1 tbsp (0.5 fl oz)	120	14	0	0
Eden					
Safflower	1 tbsp (0.5 oz)	120	14	0	0
Sesame	1 tbsp (0.5 oz)	140	15	0	0
House Of Tsang					
Hot Chili Sesame	1 tsp (5 g)	45	5	0	0
Mongolian Fire	1 tsp (5 g)	45	5	0	0
Pure Sesame	1 tsp (5 g)	45	5	0	0
Singapore Curry	1 tsp (5 g)	45	5	0	0
Wok Oil	1 tbsp (0.5 oz)	130	14	0	0
Italica					
Olive Oil	1 tbsp	120	9	0	0
Orville Redenbacher's					
Popping	1 tbsp (0.5 oz)	120	14	0	0
Pam					
Butter	⅓ sec spray (0.3g)	0	0	0	0
Cooking Spray	⅓ sec spray (0.3g)	0	0	0	0
Olive Oil	⅓ sec spray (0.3g)	0	0	0	0
Planters					
Peanut	1 tbsp (0.5 oz)	120	14	0	0

FOOD	PORTION	CAL	FAT	CARB	SUG
Progresso					
Olive Extra Mild	1 tbsp (0.5 oz)	120	14	0	0
Olive Extra Virgin	1 tbsp (0.5 oz)	120	14	0	0
Olive Riviera Blend	1 tbsp (0.5 oz)	120	14	0	0
Weight Watchers					
Butter Spray	⅓ sec spray	0	0	0	0
Cooking Spray	⅓ sec spray	0	0	0	0
OKRA					
fresh					
sliced cooked	8 pods	27	tr	6	—
frozen					
Birds Eye					
Cut	¾ cup (2.9 oz)	25	0	5	1
Whole	9 pods (3 oz)	25	0	5	1
OLIVES					
spanish stuffed	5 (0.5 oz)	15	1	1	0
Italia In Tavola					
Black Olives Paste	1 tbsp (0.5 oz)	20	2	tr	—
Progresso					
Olive Salad (drained)	2 tbsp (0.8 oz)	25	3	1	tr
Vlasic					
Ripe Colossal Pitted	2 (0.6 oz)	20	2	1	0
Ripe Jumbo Pitted	3 (0.6 oz)	25	2	1	0
Ripe Large Pitted	4 (0.5 oz)	25	3	1	0
Ripe Medium Pitted	5 (0.5 oz)	25	3	1	0
Ripe Sliced	¼ cup (0.5 oz)	25	3	1	0
Ripe Small Pitted	6 (0.5 oz)	25	3	1	0
ONION					
canned					
Boar's Head					
Sweet Vidalia In Sauce	1 tbsp	10	0	2	2

FOOD	PORTION	CAL	FAT	CARB	SUG
dried					
flakes	1 tbsp	16	tr	4	—
powder	1 tsp	7	tr	2	—
fresh					
raw chopped	1 tbsp	4	tr	1	—
scallions raw chopped	1 tbsp	2	tr	tr	—
Antioch Farms					
Vidalia	1 med	60	0	14	—
frozen					
Birds Eye					
Diced	⅔ cup (3 oz)	30	0	6	5
Pearl Onions In Cream Sauce	½ cup (4.4 oz)	60	2	8	6
take-out					
fried	½ cup (7.5 oz)	176	11	17	—
rings breaded & fried	8 to 9	275	16	31	—
OPOSSUM					
roasted	3 oz	188	9	0	0
ORANGE					
canned					
Dole					
FruitBowls Mandarin Oranges	1 pkg (4 oz)	70	0	18	17
fresh					
california navel	1	65	tr	16	—
california valencia	1	59	tr	14	—
florida	1	69	tr	17	—
peel	1 tbsp	6	tr	2	—
sections	1 cup	85	tr	21	—

FOOD	PORTION	CAL	FAT	CARB	SUG
ORANGE JUICE					
Big Juicy					
Drink	8 oz	110	0	28	28
Capri Sun					
Drink	1 pkg (7 oz)	100	0	25	25
Everfresh					
Juice	1 can (8 oz)	100	0	24	24
Ruby Red Orange Drink	1 can (8 oz)	130	0	33	33
Horizon Organic					
Juice Pulp Free	8 fl oz	110	0	26	22
Juicy Juice					
Punch	1 box (8.45 oz)	130	0	33	28
Punch	1 box (4.23 oz)	60	0	15	14
Kool-Aid					
Drink Mix Orange as prep	1 serv (8 oz)	60	0	16	16
Orange Drink as prep w/ sugar	1 serv (8 oz)	100	0	25	25
Minute Maid					
Simply Orange 100%	8 fl oz	110	0	26	22
Simply Orange Calcium Fortified	8 fl oz	110	0	26	22
Simply Orange Grove Made	8 fl oz	110	0	26	22
Nantucket Nectars					
100% Juice	8 oz	120	0	28	22
Ocean Spray					
100% Juice	8 oz	120	0	31	31
Shasta Plus					
Orange Drink	1 can (11.5 oz)	160	0	40	40

FOOD	PORTION	CAL	FAT	CARB	SUG
Snapple					
Orangeade	8 fl oz	120	0	29	29
Tang					
Orange Drink as prep	1 serv (8 oz)	90	0	23	23
Sugar Free Orange as prep	1 serv (8 oz)	5	0	0	0
Tropicana					
Tropical	8 oz	110	0	25	—
Turkey Hill					
Orangeade	1 cup	120	0	30	30
Veryfine					
100% Juice	1 bottle (10 oz)	150	0	37	35
Chillers Artric Orange	8 fl oz	130	0	33	32
Juice Blend	1 can (11.5 oz)	160	0	39	34
Orange Drink	1 bottle (10 oz)	160	0	41	36

OREGANO

FOOD	PORTION	CAL	FAT	CARB	SUG
ground	1 tsp	5	tr	1	—

ORGAN MEATS

(*see* BRAINS, GIBLETS, GIZZARD, HEART, KIDNEY, LIVER, SWEETBREADS)

ORIENTAL FOOD

(*see* ASIAN FOOD, EGG ROLLS, DINNER, NOODLES, RICE, SUSHI)

OYSTERS

FOOD	PORTION	CAL	FAT	CARB	SUG
canned eastern	1 cup	170	6	10	—
eastern cooked	6 med	58	2	3	—
eastern raw	6 med	58	2	3	—
pacific raw	1 med	41	1	2	—
steamed	1 med	41	1	2	—
Bumble Bee					
Fancy Whole	2 oz	70	3	3	0
Smoked	½ can (1.9 oz)	120	7	6	0

FOOD	PORTION	CAL	FAT	CARB	SUG
take-out					
breaded & fried	6 (4.9 oz)	368	18	40	—
oysters rockefeller	3 oysters	66	2	5	—
stew	1 cup	278	18	15	—
PANCAKE/WAFFLE SYRUP					
low calorie	1 tbsp	12	0	3	—
Estee					
Maple	¼ cup	80	0	20	20
Mrs. Butter-worth's					
Original	¼ cup (2 oz)	230	0	56	35
PANCAKES					
frozen					
Eggo					
Buttermilk	3 (4.1 oz)	270	8	44	10
mix					
Betty Crocker					
Buttermilk as prep	3	200	3	20	3
Original as prep	3	200	3	39	9
Bisquick					
Shake 'N Pour Blueberry as prep	3	210	4	40	8
Bruce					
Sweet Potato Pancakes	2	210	3	39	5
Estee					
Pancake Mix as prep	4 (4 in diam)	180	0	40	tr
Hodgson Mill					
Buckwheat	⅓ cup (1.8 oz)	160	1	36	2
Hungry Jack					
Potato as prep	3 (3 in diam)	90	2	16	tr
Robin Hood					
Buttermilk as prep	3	230	6	35	6

FOOD	PORTION	CAL	FAT	CARB	SUG
take-out					
blueberry	1 (4 in diam)	84	4	11	—
buckwheat	1 (4 in diam)	55	2	6	—
potato	1 (4 in diam)	78	6	4	—
w/ butter & syrup	2 (8.1 oz)	520	14	91	—
PANCREAS					
(*see* SWEETBREADS)					
PAPAYA					
fresh	1	117	tr	30	—
Sonoma					
Dried Pieces	2 pieces (2 oz)	200	4	41	35
PAPAYA JUICE					
nectar	1 cup	142	tr	36	—
Everfresh					
Premium Drink	1 can (8 oz)	140	0	35	35
Nantucket Nectars					
Cocktail	8 oz	120	0	30	27
PAPRIKA					
paprika	1 tsp	6	tr	1	—
PARSLEY					
dry	1 tsp	1	tr	tr	—
fresh chopped	½ cup	11	tr	2	—
PARSNIPS					
fresh cooked	1 (5.6 oz)	130	tr	31	—
PASSION FRUIT					
purple fresh	1	18	tr	4	—
PASSION FRUIT JUICE					
purple	1 cup	126	tr	34	—
yellow	1 cup	149	tr	36	—

FOOD	PORTION	CAL	FAT	CARB	SUG
PASTA					
dry					
corn spaghetti	2 oz	180	2	35	3
Annie Chun's					
Soba Noodles	2 oz	200	1	39	1
Barilla					
Conchiglie Rigate	1 cup (2 oz)	200	1	40	1
Gemelli as prep	1 cup (2 oz)	200	1	42	1
Cuore					
Capellini cooked	1⅓ cup (2 oz)	190	1	39	1
Fusilli cooked	1⅓ cup (2 oz)	190	1	39	1
Tortiglioni cooked	1⅓ cup (2 oz)	190	1	39	1
DeCecco					
Whole Wheat Linguine cooked	2 oz	180	2	33	1
Duc Amici					
Pasta Lite Low Carb Fusilli	2 oz	160	1	10	3
Eden					
Organic Endless Tubes	½ cup (1.9 oz)	210	1	41	2
Soba	2 oz	200	2	38	3
Somen	2 oz	200	2	38	1
Udon	2 oz	200	2	38	1
Udon Brown Rice	2 oz	200	2	38	1
Goya					
Coditos not prep	½ cup	230	1	47	2
Hodgson Mill					
Four Color Veggie Bows	2 oz	200	1	41	0
Four Color Veggie Rotini Spirals	2 oz	200	1	41	0
Four Color Veggie Wagon Wheels	2 oz	200	1	41	0

FOOD	PORTION	CAL	FAT	CARB	SUG
Pastamania! Durum Wheat Fettuccine	2 oz	200	2	38	0
Pastamania! Fettuccine Garlic & Parsley	2 oz	200	2	38	0
Pastamania! Fettuccine w/ Jerusalem Artichoke	2 oz	210	2	41	0
Pastamania! Fettuccine w/ Mushroom	2 oz	210	2	41	1
Pastamania! Fusilli Tre Colore w/ Tomato & Spinach	2 oz	200	1	40	2
Pastamania! Pesto Fettuccine	2 oz	200	2	38	0
Pastamania! Sea Shell Mix	2 oz	200	1	40	0
Pastamania! Spinach Fettuccine	2 oz	200	2	37	0
Pastamania! Thin Linguine	2 oz	200	2	38	0
Pastamania! Tomato Spinach & Durum Wheat	2 oz	210	2	40	1
Spaghetti Whole Wheat	2 oz	190	1	34	0
Lundberg					
Spaghetti Organic Brown Rice	2 oz	210	2	44	3
Ronzoni					
Lasagne	2½ pieces (2 oz)	210	1	42	2
fresh					
Di Giorno					
Angel's Hair	1 cup	160	2	31	1
Beef & Roasted Garlic Tortellini	1 cup	340	11	46	2

FOOD	PORTION	CAL	FAT	CARB	SUG
Fettuccine	1 cup	200	2	38	1
Four Cheese Raviolo	1 cup	350	15	40	1
Herb Linguine	1 cup	200	2	38	1
Italian Sausage Ravioli In Green Bell Pepper Pasta	1¼ cup	350	12	45	3
Lemon Chicken Tortellini In Cracked Black Pepper Pasta	1 cup	270	5	42	2
Light Cheese Ravioli	1 cup	280	7	40	1
Linguine	1 cup	200	2	38	1
Mozzarella Garlic Tortelloni	1 cup	300	8	42	1
Pesto Tortelloni	1 cup	320	8	46	1
Portabello Mushroom Tortelloni	1 cup	310	7	48	1
Red Bell Pepper Fettuccine	1 cup	200	2	38	1
Spinach Fettuccine	1 cup	190	2	38	tr
Sun-Dried Tomato Ravioli	1⅓ cup	380	14	48	5
Three Cheese Tortellini	¾ cup	250	7	37	2

PASTA DINNERS
canned

Chef Boyardee

FOOD	PORTION	CAL	FAT	CARB	SUG
99% Fat Free Beef Ravioli	1 cup (8.6 oz)	210	1	41	6
99% Fat Free Cheese Ravioli	1 cup (8.8 oz)	210	1	44	9
Beef Ravioli	1 cup (8.6 oz)	230	5	37	5
Beefaroni	1 cup (8.7 oz)	260	7	37	9
Macaroni & Cheese	½ can (7.5 oz)	180	2	35	0

FOOD	PORTION	CAL	FAT	CARB	SUG
Mini Ravioli	1 cup (8.8 oz)	252	6	37	5
Spaghetti & Meat Balls	1 cup (8.4 oz)	240	10	32	7
Tortellini Cheese	½ can (7 oz)	230	1	48	12
Tortellini Meat	½ can (7 oz)	260	4	48	12
Franco-American					
Beef Raviolios	1 can (7.7 oz)	250	5	39	10
Beefy Mac	1 can (7.5 oz)	228	8	30	10
Elbow Macaroni & Cheese	1 can (7.5 oz)	187	6	25	2
Spaghetti 'N Beef	1 can (7.5 oz)	226	8	30	9
Spaghetti w/ Meatballs	1 can (7.2 oz)	249	9	33	12
Kid's Kitchen					
Microwave Meals Cheezy Mac & Beef	1 cup (7.5 oz)	260	7	33	7
Microwave Meals Noodle Rings & Chicken	1 cup (7.5 oz)	150	4	17	2
Microwave Meals Spaghetti Rings & Franks	1 cup (7.5 oz)	240	9	32	11
Progresso					
Beef Ravioli	1 cup (9.1 oz)	260	5	45	9
Cheese Ravioli	1 cup (9.1 oz)	220	2	43	9
frozen					
Amy's Organic					
Macaroni & Cheese	1 pkg (9 oz)	390	14	50	6
Macaroni & Soy Cheese	1 pkg (9 oz)	360	14	42	2
Pasta Primavera	1 pkg (9.5 oz)	320	12	39	7
Ravioli w/ Sauce	1 pkg (9.5 oz)	340	12	44	7
Tofu Vegetable Lasagna	1 pkg (9.5 oz)	300	10	41	6

FOOD	PORTION	CAL	FAT	CARB	SUG
Vegetable Lasagna	1 pkg (9.5 oz)	300	10	39	7
Whole Meals Cannelloni	1 pkg (9 oz)	260	11	32	9
Banquet					
Chicken Pasta Primavera	1 meal (9.5 oz)	320	12	40	9
Family Size Egg Noodles w/ Beef & Brown Gravy	1 serv	150	5	16	1
Family Size Lasagna w/ Meat Sauce	1 cup	270	10	33	3
Family Size Macaroni & Cheese	1 cup	230	7	32	7
Fettuccine Alfredo	1 meal (9.5 oz)	350	16	40	5
Lasagna w/ Meat Sauce	1 meal (9.5 oz)	260	8	38	10
Macaroni & Cheese	1 meal (12 oz)	420	14	57	7
Birds Eye					
Easy Recipe Creations Chicken Primavera as prep	2¼ cups (8.7 oz)	260	11	31	5
Pasta Secrets Italian Pesto	2⅓ cups (6.4 oz)	240	9	32	6
Pasta Secrets Primavera	2⅓ cups (6.6 oz)	230	10	26	4
Pasta Secrets Ranch	2⅓ cups (6.6 oz)	300	15	29	8
Pasta Secrets Three Cheese	2 cups (6.1 oz)	230	8	31	8
Pasta Secrets White Cheddar	2 cups (6.3 oz)	240	10	30	7
Pasta Secrets Zesty Garlic	2 cups (5.9 oz)	240	10	31	6

FOOD	PORTION	CAL	FAT	CARB	SUG
Green Giant					
Create A Meal Creamy Alfredo as prep	1¼ cups (10 oz)	380	12	33	9
Create A Meal Creamy Cheddar as prep	1½ cups (10 oz)	290	10	29	8
Create A Meal Creamy Chicken Noodle as prep	1¼ cups (10 oz)	350	11	34	8
Pasta Accents Alfredo	2 cups (5.6 oz)	210	5	25	5
Pasta Accents Creamy Cheddar	2⅓ cups (6.7 oz)	250	8	36	6
Pasta Accents Florentine	2 cups (7.3 oz)	310	9	44	5
Pasta Accents Garden Herb Seasoning	2 cups (6.8 oz)	230	7	32	4
Pasta Accents Garlic Seasoning	2 cups (6.6 oz)	260	10	36	5
Pasta Accents Primavera	2¼ cups (7 oz)	320	12	40	5
Pasta Accents White Cheddar Sauce	1¾ cups (5.6 oz)	300	12	38	7
Healthy Choice					
Beef Macaroni	1 meal (8.5 oz)	220	4	34	9
Bowls Cheese & Chicken Tortellini	1 meal (8.7 oz)	250	5	40	5
Breaded Chicken Breast Stips w/ Macaroni & Cheese	1 meal (8 oz)	270	5	34	9
Cheese Ravioli Parmigiana	1 meal (9 oz)	260	5	44	14

FOOD	PORTION	CAL	FAT	CARB	SUG
Chicken Fettuccine Alfredo	1 meal (8.5 oz)	280	7	30	3
Fettuccine Alfredo	1 meal (8 oz)	240	5	37	4
Lasagna Roma	1 meal (13.5 oz)	420	9	59	14
Macaroni & Cheese	1 meal (9 oz)	240	5	36	8
Manicotti w/ Three Cheeses	1 meal (11 oz)	300	9	40	14
Spaghetti & Sauce w/ Seasoned Beef	1 meal (10 oz)	260	8	43	7
Stuffed Pasta Shells	1 meal (10.35 oz)	370	6	60	12
Kid Cuisine					
Magical Macaroni & Cheese	1 meal (10.6 oz)	440	13	72	25
Lean Cuisine					
Cafe Classics Bow Tie Pasta & Chicken	1 pkg (9.5 oz)	220	4	32	6
Cafe Classics Cheese Lasagna w/ Chicken Scaloppini	1 pkg (10 oz)	270	8	27	7
Cafe Classics Shrimp & Angel Hair Pasta	1 pkg (10 oz)	240	5	35	7
Everyday Favorites	1 pkg (10 oz)	270	6	40	6
Everyday Favorites Alfredo Pasta Primavera	1 pkg (10 oz)	290	7	46	6
Everyday Favorites Angel Hair Pasta	1 pkg (10 oz)	240	4	43	11
Everyday Favorites Cheese Cannelloni	1 pkg (9.1 oz)	230	4	28	8
Everyday Favorites Cheese Ravioli	1 pkg (8.5 oz)	260	7	38	8
Everyday Favorites Chicken Lasagna	1 pkg (10 oz)	280	7	34	6

FOOD	PORTION	CAL	FAT	CARB	SUG
Everyday Favorites Classic Cheese Lasagna	1 pkg (11.5 oz)	290	6	38	9
Everyday Favorites Fettucini Alfredo	1 pkg (9.25 oz)	280	7	42	6
Everyday Favorites Fettucini Primavera	1 pkg (10 oz)	270	7	38	8
Everyday Favorites Lasagna w/ Meat Sauce	1 pkg (10.5 oz)	300	8	35	7
Everyday Favorites Macaroni & Cheese	1 pkg (10 oz)	290	7	42	5
Everyday Favorites Macaroni & Beef	1 pkg (10 oz)	270	4	43	9
Everyday Favorites Penne Pasta	1 pkg (10 oz)	260	4	47	13
Everyday Favorites Spaghetti w/ Meat Sauce	1 pkg (11.5 oz)	290	5	50	10
Everyday Favorites Spaghetti w/ Meatballs	1 pkg (9.5 oz)	270	6	37	6
Everyday Favorties	1 pkg (9.25 oz)	270	6	33	5
Family Style Favorites Five Cheese Lasagna	1 serv (8 oz)	210	5	27	6
Skillet Sensations Chicken Alfredo	1 serv	280	6	36	6
Marie Callender's					
Cheese Ravioli In Marinara Sauce w/ Spirals & Garlic Bread	1 meal (16 oz)	750	29	96	18
Extra Cheese Lasagna	1 meal (15 oz)	590	27	61	19

FOOD	PORTION	CAL	FAT	CARB	SUG
Fettuccine Alfredo & Garlic Bread	1 meal (14 oz)	920	55	62	5
Fettuccine Alfredo Supreme	1 meal (13 oz)	450	27	35	1
Fettuccine Primavera w/ Tortellini	1 meal (14 oz)	750	49	57	10
Fettuccine w/ Broccoli & Chicken	1 meal (13 oz)	710	43	53	7
Lasagna w/ Meat Sauce	1 meal (15 oz)	630	31	59	24
Macaroni & Cheese	1 meal (12 oz)	540	24	55	12
Skillet Meal Chicken Alfredo	½ pkg	490	29	32	5
Skillet Meal Penne Pasta & Meatballs	½ pkg	600	31	53	4
Skillet Meal Rigatoni Vegetables In Cheese Sauce	1 cup	290	12	32	16
Spaghetti w/ Meat Sauce & Garlic Bread	1 meal (17 oz)	670	25	65	20
Stuffed Pasta Trio	1 meal (10.5 oz)	380	16	40	26
Morton					
Macaroni & Cheese	1 serv (8 oz)	240	8	34	10
Spaghetti w/ Meat Sauce	1 meal (8.5 oz)	200	6	30	13
Quorn					
Fettuccine Alfredo	1 pkg (10.5 oz)	360	16	40	5
Lasagna	1 pkg (10.5 oz)	360	12	43	13
Stouffer's					
Cheddar Pasta w/ Beef & Tomatoes	1 pkg (11 oz)	450	19	45	7
Cheese Manicotti	1 pkg (9 oz)	380	17	38	10

FOOD	PORTION	CAL	FAT	CARB	SUG
Cheese Ravioli	1 pkg (10.6 oz)	380	13	51	11
Chicken Lasagna	1 serv (7.8 oz)	320	17	29	5
Fettucini Alfredo	1 pkg (10 oz)	520	28	17	5
Fettucini Primavera	1 pkg (10 oz)	430	20	49	6
Five Cheese Lasagna	1 pkg (10.75 oz)	360	13	40	10
Grilled Chicken & Angel Hair Pasta	1 pkg (10.9 oz)	380	13	40	6
Homestyle Chicken Fettucini	1 pkg (10.5 oz)	390	15	32	8
Homestyle Chicken Parmigiana w/ Spaghetti	1 pkg (12 oz)	460	16	54	9
Homestyle Veal Parmigiana w/ Spaghetti	1 pkg (11.9 oz)	430	17	49	10
Lasagna Bake	1 pkg (10.25 oz)	370	12	47	9
Lasagna w/ Meat Sauce	1 pkg (10.5 oz)	370	14	39	6
Macaroni & Cheese	1 cup (6 oz)	320	16	31	5
Macaroni & Cheese w/ Broccoli	1 pkg (10.5 oz)	360	17	37	7
Macaroni & Beef	1 pkg (11.5 oz)	420	20	40	12
Noodles Romanoff	1 pkg (12 oz)	490	25	48	7
Pasta Shells w/ American Cheese	1 cup (6 oz)	260	10	31	8
Salisbury Steak w/ Macaroni & Cheese	1 serv (11.3 oz)	410	19	34	4
Spaghetti w/ Meat Sauce	1 pkg (10 oz)	350	12	46	7
Spaghetti w/ Meatballs	1 pkg (12.6 oz)	440	15	56	8
Tuna Noodle Casserole	1 pkg (10 oz)	320	10	37	7
Turkey Tettrazini	1 pkg (10 oz)	360	17	33	5
Vegetable Lasagna	1 pkg (10.5 oz)	440	20	43	9

FOOD	PORTION	CAL	FAT	CARB	SUG
Weight Watchers					
Garden Lasagna	1 pkg (11 oz)	270	7	36	6
Homestyle Macaroni & Cheese	1 pkg (9 oz)	290	7	45	2
Smart Ones Angel Hair Pasta	1 pkg (9 oz)	180	2	32	4
Smart Ones Bowtie Pasta & Mushrooms Marsala	1 pkg (9.65 oz)	270	7	40	3
Smart Ones Chicken Fettucini	1 pkg (10 oz)	300	7	39	4
Smart Ones Creamy Rigatoni w/ Broccoli & Chicken	1 pkg (9 oz)	230	2	40	5
Smart Ones Fettucini Alfredo w/ Broccoli	1 pkg (8.5 oz)	230	6	32	8
Smart Ones Lasagna Florentine	1 pkg (10 oz)	200	2	33	5
Smart Ones Lasagna Alfredo	1 pkg (9 oz)	300	7	46	6
Smart Ones Lasagna w/ Meat Sauce	1 pkg (10.25 oz)	270	6	36	8
Smart Ones Lasagna w/ Meat Sauce	1 pkg (9 oz)	240	2	43	5
Smart Ones Macaroni & Cheese	1 pkg (9 oz)	220	2	42	5
Smart Ones Pasta & Spinach Romano	1 pkg (10.4 oz)	260	8	35	7
Smart Ones Pasta w/ Tomato Basil Sauce	1 pkg (9.6 oz)	260	7	40	4
Smart Ones Penne Pasta w/ Sun-Dried Tomatoes	1 pkg (10 oz)	280	8	40	5

FOOD	PORTION	CAL	FAT	CARB	SUG
Smart Ones Penne Pollo	1 pkg (10 oz)	290	6	38	5
Smart Ones Ravioli Florentine	1 pkg (8.5 oz)	220	2	43	5
Smart Ones Spaghetti Marinara	1 pkg (9 oz)	280	7	46	7
Smart Ones Spaghetti w/ Meat Sauce	1 pkg (10 oz)	280	6	41	8
Smart Ones Spicy Penne & Ricotta	1 pkg (10.2 oz)	280	6	45	5
Smart Ones Tuna Noodle Casserole	1 pkg (9.5 oz)	270	7	38	6
Smart Ones Zita Mozzarella	1 pkg (9 oz)	290	7	47	5
Yves					
Veggie Lasagna	1 pkg (10.5 oz)	300	3	51	9
Veggie Macaroni	1 pkg (10.5 oz)	230	2	38	6
Veggie Penne	1 pkg (10.5 oz)	220	2	36	7
mix					
Hamburger Helper					
Ravioli as prep	1 cup	280	10	30	5
Ravioli w/ White Cheese Topping as prep	1 cup	310	10	34	7
Kraft					
Deluxe Macaroni & Cheese Four Cheese Blend as prep	1 cup (6.2 oz)	320	10	44	4
Deluxe Macaroni & Cheese Original as prep	1 cup (6.1 oz)	320	10	44	4

FOOD	PORTION	CAL	FAT	CARB	SUG
Light Deluxe Macaroni & Cheese as prep	1 cup (6.5 oz)	290	5	48	7
Macaroni & Cheese All Shapes as prep	1 cup (6.9 oz)	410	18	49	8
Macaroni & Cheese Original as prep	1 cup (6.9 oz)	410	18	49	8
Macaroni & Cheese Original as prep light recipe	1 cup (6.4 oz)	290	6	48	8
Premium Macaroni & Cheese Cheesy Alfredo as prep	1 cup (6.9 oz)	410	19	49	8
Premium Macaroni & Cheese Mild White Cheddar as prep	1 cup (6.8 oz)	410	19	49	8
Premium Macaroni & Cheese Thick 'N Creamy as prep	1 cup (7.6 oz)	420	19	50	9
Premium Macaroni & Cheese Three Cheese as prep	1 cup (6.9 oz)	410	18	49	8
Spaghetti Classics Mild Italian as prep	1 cup (9.1 oz)	240	3	46	9
Spaghetti Classics Tangy Italian as prep	1 cup (8.9 oz)	240	2	46	7
Spaghetti Classics Zesty Cheese as prep	1 cup (8.6 oz)	240	2	46	9

FOOD	PORTION	CAL	FAT	CARB	SUG
Spaghetti Classics w/ Meat Sauce as prep	1 cup (8.2 oz)	330	10	47	7
Lipton					
Pasta & Sauce Angel Hair Chicken Broccoli as prep	1 cup	260	8	43	2
Pasta & Sauce Angel Hair Parmesan as prep	1 cup	280	11	41	3
Pasta & Sauce Bow Tie Chicken Primavera as prep	1 cup	290	10	43	6
Pasta & Sauce Bow Tie Italian Cheese as prep	1 cup	300	12	41	4
Pasta & Sauce Butter & Herbs as prep	1 cup	270	10	40	3
Pasta & Sauce Cheddar Broccoli as prep	1 cup	340	11	49	7
Pasta & Sauce Chicken Herb Parmesan as prep	1 cup	80	9	43	3
Pasta & Sauce Chicken Stir-Fry as prep	1 cup	270	8	43	3
Pasta & Sauce Creamy Garlic as prep	1 cup	350	13	50	6

FOOD	PORTION	CAL	FAT	CARB	SUG
Pasta & Sauce Creamy Mushroom as prep	1 cup	320	11	46	4
Pasta & Sauce Garlic & Butter Linguine as prep	1 cup	260	9	40	3
Pasta & Sauce Mild Cheddar Cheese as prep	1 cup	290	10	41	4
Pasta & Sauce Roasted Garlic Chicken as prep	1 cup	290	10	43	3
Pasta & Sauce Roasted Garlic & Olive Oil w/ Tomato as prep	1 cup	270	9	42	3
Pasta & Sauce Rotini Primavera as prep	1 cup	320	12	45	4
Pasta & Sauce Savory Herb w/ Garlic as prep	1 cup	280	9	52	3
Pasta & Sauce Three Cheese Rotini as prep	1 cup	320	10	44	5
Melting Pot					
Terrazza Black Beans & Penne	1 cup	180	1	36	5
Terrazza Florentine Red Beans & Fusilli	1 cup	220	1	43	6
Terrazza Red Lentils & Bow Ties	1 cup	240	2	42	7
Terrazza Tuscan White Beans & Gemell	1 cup	220	1	44	6

FOOD	PORTION	CAL	FAT	CARB	SUG
Velveeta					
Rotini & Cheese w/ Broccoli as prep	1 cup (7.2 oz)	400	16	47	5
Shells & Cheese Bacon as prep	1 cup (6.8 oz)	360	14	43	4
Shells & Cheese Original as prep	1 cup (6.6 oz)	360	13	44	4
Shells & Cheese Salsa as prep	1 cup (7.5 oz)	380	14	47	5
ready-to-eat					
Tyson					
Rosemary Penne	1 pkg (12.5 oz)	330	5	45	2
shelf-stable					
Hormel					
Microcup Meals Lasagna	1 cup (7.5 oz)	250	14	24	6
Microcup Meals Macaroni & Cheese	1 cup (7.5 oz)	260	11	30	3
Microcup Meals Ravioli w/ Tomato Sauce	1 cup (7.5 oz)	220	6	34	12
Microcup Meals Spaghetti & Meatballs	1 cup (7.5 oz)	220	7	28	10
Kid's Kitchen					
Microwave Meals Beefy Macaroni	1 cup (7.5 oz)	190	6	23	4
Microwave Meals Macaroni & Cheese	1 cup (7.5 oz)	260	11	30	3
Microwave Meals Mini Ravioli	1 cup (7.5 oz)	240	7	34	6
Microwave Meals Spaghetti & Meatballs	1 cup (7.5 oz)	220	7	28	10

FOOD	PORTION	CAL	FAT	CARB	SUG
Microwave Meals Spaghetti Ring & Meatballs	1 cup (7.5 oz)	250	7	35	12
Lunch Bucket					
Beef Ravioli In Tomato Sauce	1 pkg (7.5 oz)	180	4	32	8
Italian Pasta w/ Chicken	1 pkg (7.5 oz)	130	2	24	7
Lasagna 'n Meatsauce	1 pkg (7.5 oz)	160	3	29	9
Macaroni 'n Beef in Meatsauce	1 pkg (7.5 oz)	180	5	10	0
Macaroni 'n Cheese	1 pkg (7.5 oz)	190	7	24	0
Pasta'n Chicken	1 pkg (7.5 oz)	150	5	22	1
Spaghetti 'n Meatsauce	1 pkg (7.5 oz)	160	3	29	9
take-out					
lasagna	1 piece (2.5 in x 2.5 in)	374	21	25	—
macaroni & cheese	1 cup	230	10	26	—
manicotti	¾ cup (6.4 oz)	273	12	28	—
rigatoni w/ sausage sauce	¾ cup	260	12	28	—
spaghetti w/ meatballs & cheese	1 cup	407	19	30	—

PASTA SALAD
mix

Kraft

FOOD	PORTION	CAL	FAT	CARB	SUG
Herb & Garlic as prep	¾ cup (4.9 oz)	280	14	34	5
Pasta Salad Classic Ranch w/ Bacon as prep	¾ cup (4.7 oz)	350	22	32	3
Pasta Salad Creamy Ceasar as prep	¾ cup (4.8 oz)	340	21	31	5
Pasta Salad Garden Primavera as prep	¾ cup (5 oz)	240	8	35	3

FOOD	PORTION	CAL	FAT	CARB	SUG
Pasta Salad Italian 97% Fat Free as prep	¾ cup (4.9 oz)	190	2	34	5
Pasta Salad Parmesan Peppercorn as prep	¾ cup (4.9 oz)	360	23	29	3
Suddenly Salad					
Classic Pasta	¾ cup	250	8	38	5
Classic Pasta Reduced Fat Recipe	¾ cup	210	4	38	5
Garden Italian 98% Fat Free	¾ cup	140	1	28	4
take-out					
elbow macaroni salad	3.5 oz	160	5	26	—
italian style pasta salad	3.5 oz	140	7	15	—
mustard macaroni salad	3.5 oz	190	10	23	—
pasta salad w/ vegetables	3.5 oz	140	4	21	—

PASTRY

(*see* BROWNIE, CAKE, DANISH PASTRY)

PATE

antipasto pate	1 can (2.25 oz)	110	9	3	1
duck pate	1 oz	96	8	1	tr
mushroom anchovy pate	1 can (2.25 oz)	130	11	7	1
pork pate	1 oz	107	10	1	1
pork pate en croute	1 oz	91	7	3	tr
salmon pate	1 can (2.25 oz)	140	10	6	1
shrimp	1 can (2.25 oz)	140	10	7	1
smoked turkey	1 can (2.25 oz)	170	13	7	1

FOOD	PORTION	CAL	FAT	CARB	SUG
PEACH					
canned					
Del Monte					
Fruit Pleasures Raspberry Flavored Peaches	½ cup (4.5 oz)	80	0	20	19
Sliced Cling Fruit Naturals	½ cup (4.4 oz)	60	0	15	14
fresh					
Chiquita					
Peach	1 med (3.4 oz)	40	0	10	9
PEACH JUICE					
Nantucket Nectars					
The Original	8 oz	120	0	30	26
PEANUT BUTTER					
Estee					
Creamy Low Sodium	2 tbsp (1 oz)	190	15	7	2
Jif					
Apple Cinnamon	2 tbsp (1.3 oz)	200	16	11	8
Berry Blend	2 tbsp (1.2 oz)	200	17	10	7
Chocolate Silk	2 tbsp (1.0 oz)	100	16	11	12
Creamy	2 tbsp (1.1 oz)	190	16	7	3
Extra Crunchy	2 tbsp (1.1 oz)	190	16	7	3
Reduced Fat Creamy	2 tbsp (1.3 oz)	190	12	15	4
Reduced Fat Crunchy	2 tbsp (1.3 oz)	190	12	15	4
Simply	2 tbsp (1.1 oz)	190	16	6	2
Tree Of Life					
Peanut Wonder	2 tbsp (1.1 oz)	100	3	13	5
PEANUTS					
dry roasted w/ salt	30 nuts (1 oz)	170	14	6	2

FOOD	PORTION	CAL	FAT	CARB	SUG
Estee					
Candy Coated	¼ cup	200	9	23	6
Frito Lay					
Honey Roasted	1 serv (1.5 oz)	270	21	10	5
Hot	1 serv (1.1 oz)	190	16	6	2
Salted	1 oz	200	16	5	1
Lance					
Honey Toasted	1 pkg (1.38 oz)	220	15	13	5
Roasted	1 pkg (1.75 oz)	190	14	6	1
Salted	1 pkg (1.13 oz)	200	15	6	0
Salted Long Tube	¼ cup (1 oz)	180	14	5	0
Little Debbie					
Salted	¼ cup (1 oz)	160	14	5	1
Pennant					
Oil Roasted	1 oz	170	14	6	1
Tom's					
Double Coated	1 pkg (1.35 oz)	220	15	15	10
Toasted	1 pkg (1.4 oz)	240	19	7	1
Weight Watchers					
Honey Roasted	1 pkg (0.7 oz)	100	5	7	3

PEAR
fresh

asian	1 (4.3 oz)	51	tr	13	—
Chiquita					
Pear	1 med (5.8 oz)	100	1	25	17

PEAS
canned

Green Giant					
Sweet	½ cup (4.3 oz)	60	0	11	3
Sweet 50% Less Sodium	½ cup (4.3 oz)	60	0	11	2

FOOD	PORTION	CAL	FAT	CARB	SUG
LeSueur					
Early Peas	½ cup (4.2 oz)	60	0	12	4
Early Peas 50% Less Sodium	½ cup (4.2 oz)	60	0	11	3
Sweet	½ cup (4.2 oz)	60	0	12	4
Sweet 50% Less Sodium	½ cup (4.2 oz)	60	0	11	3
dried					
Hurst					
HamBeens Green Split Peas w/ Ham	1 serv	120	1	21	1
fresh					
green cooked	½ cup	67	tr	13	—
green raw	½ cup	58	tr	11	—
snap peas cooked	½ cup	34	tr	6	—
frozen					
Birds Eye					
Butter Peas	⅓ cup (2.7 oz)	110	1	20	1
Crowder	½ cup (3 oz)	120	1	22	1
Field Peas w/ Snaps	⅔ cup (3.4 oz)	130	1	24	1
Purple Hull Peas	½ cup (2.8 oz)	110	1	21	1
Green Giant					
Butter Sauce	¾ cup (4 oz)	100	2	16	4
Butter Sauce LeSueur Baby Peas	¾ cup (4 oz)	100	2	16	4
Harvest Fresh LeSueur Baby	⅔ cup (3.2 oz)	70	0	13	4
Harvest Fresh Sugar Snap	⅔ cup (3.2 oz)	50	0	10	5
Harvest Fresh Sweet	⅔ cup (3.3 oz)	60	0	12	6
LaSueur Baby Sweet	⅔ cup (2.8 oz)	60	0	11	3
LaSueur Early June	⅔ cup (2.8 oz)	80	0	11	3

FOOD	PORTION	CAL	FAT	CARB	SUG
LaSueur Early June w/ Mushrooms	¾ cup (3 oz)	60	0	10	2
Select Sugar Snap	¾ cup (2.8 oz)	35	0	7	3
Sweet	⅝ cup (3.1 oz)	70	0	13	2
La Choy					
Snow Pea Pods	½ pkg (3 oz)	35	2	4	2
take-out					
pea & potato curry	1 serv (7 oz)	284	22	19	—
pea curry	1 serv (4.4 oz)	438	42	11	—
PECANS					
halves dry roasted w/ salt	20 (1 oz)	200	21	4	1
Planters					
Halves	1 oz	190	20	4	tr
PECTIN					
Sure Jell					
For Lower Sugar Recipes	1 tsp (2.8 g)	20	0	4	4
Fruit Pectin	1 tsp (3.6 g)	20	0	4	4
PEPEAO					
dried	½ cup	36	tr	10	—
PEPPER					
black	1 tsp	5	tr	1	—
cayenne	1 tsp	6	tr	1	—
red	1 tsp	6	tr	1	—
white	1 tsp	7	tr	2	—
PEPPERS **canned**					
Chi-Chi's					
Chilies Diced Green	2 tbsp (1.2 oz)	10	0	1	0
Chilies Green Whole	¾ pepper (1 oz)	10	0	1	0

FOOD	PORTION	CAL	FAT	CARB	SUG
Progresso					
Cherry Sliced & So Hot	2 tbsp (1 oz)	25	2	2	1
Hot Cherry	1 (1 oz)	10	0	2	0
Pepper Salad (drained)	2 tbsp (1 oz)	15	1	1	tr
Roasted	1 piece (1 oz)	10	0	3	tr
Sweet Fried w/ Onions	2 tbsp (0.9 oz)	20	2	2	1
Tuscan	3 (1 oz)	10	0	2	0
Rosarita					
Chilies Diced Green	2 tbsp (1 oz)	6	tr	1	tr
Chilies Green Strips	¼ cup (1.2 oz)	5	tr	1	1
Chilies Whole Green	2 tbsp (1.2 oz)	5	tr	1	1
Jalapeno Whole w/ Escabeche	¼ cup (1.2 oz)	8	tr	1	tr
Jalapenos Diced	2 tbsp (1 oz)	5	tr	1	tr
Jalapenos Nacho Sliced	2 tbsp (1 oz)	2	tr	1	tr
Vlasic					
Hot Sliced Cherry	1 oz	5	0	1	1
Jalapeno Sliced	1 oz	10	0	2	2
Mild Cherry	1 oz	5	0	1	1
Pepper Rings Hot	1 oz	5	0	1	1
Pepper Rings Mild	1 oz	5	0	1	1
dried					
ancho	1 (0.6 oz)	48	1	9	—
pasilla	1 (7 g)	24	1	4	—
red	1 tbsp	1	tr	tr	—
fresh					
banana fresh	1 (4 in) (1.2 oz)	9	tr	2	—
chili green hot fresh chopped	½ cup	30	tr	7	—
chili red fresh chopped	½ cup	30	tr	7	—

FOOD	PORTION	CAL	FAT	CARB	SUG
green fresh	1 (2.6 oz)	20	tr	5	—
habanero chile	1 tsp	9	tr	2	—
jalapeno fresh	1 (0.5 oz)	4	tr	1	—
red fresh	1 (2.6 oz)	20	tr	5	—
yellow fresh	1 (6.5 oz)	50	tr	12	—
Chiquita					
Pepper	1 med (5.2 oz)	30	0	7	4
frozen					
Birds Eye					
Diced Green	¾ cup (2.9 oz)	20	0	4	3
PERCH					
fresh					
cooked	3 oz	99	1	0	0
PERSIMMONS					
fresh	1	32	tr	8	—
fresh japanese	1	118	tr	31	—
Sonoma					
Dried	6–8 pieces (1.4 oz)	140	0	35	26
PHEASANT					
roasted	3.5 oz	215	9	0	0
PICANTE					
(*see* SALSA)					
PICKLES					
Claussen					
Bread 'N Butter Chips	4 slices (1 oz)	20	0	4	3
Deli Style Hearty Garlic Whole	½ (1 oz)	5	0	1	tr
Kosher Dill Spears	1 spear (1.2 oz)	5	0	1	0
Kosher Dills Halves	1 half (1 oz)	5	0	1	0
Kosher Dills Mini	1 (0.8 oz)	5	0	1	0

FOOD	PORTION	CAL	FAT	CARB	SUG
Kosher Dills Whole	½ (1 oz)	5	0	1	0
New York Deli Style Half Sours Whole	½ (1 oz)	5	0	1	tr
Sandwich Slices Bread 'N Butter	2 (1.2 oz)	25	0	5	3
Sandwich Slices Deli Style Hearty Garlic	2 (1.2 oz)	5	0	1	tr
Sandwich Slices Kosher Dills	2 (1.2 oz)	5	0	1	tr
Super Slices For Burgers	1 (0.8 oz)	5	0	1	0
Vlasic					
Hamburger Dill Chips	1 oz	5	0	1	1
Kosher Cross Cuts	1 oz	5	0	1	1
Kosher Spears	1 oz	5	0	1	1
Kosher Whole	1 oz	5	0	1	1
Sweet Butter Chips	1 oz	30	0	7	7
Sweet Gerkins	1 oz	35	0	9	9
Whole Dills	1 oz	5	0	1	1

PIE
frozen

Mrs. Smith's

FOOD	PORTION	CAL	FAT	CARB	SUG
Apple	1 slice (4.3 oz)	350	19	41	8
Blueberry	1 slice (4.6 oz)	330	17	43	16
Cappuccino	1 slice (4.2 oz)	300	13	45	27
Cherry	1 slice (4.3 oz)	320	17	41	7
Cherry Crumb	1 slice (4.2 oz)	320	12	52	28
Chocolate Cream	1 slice (4.6 oz)	340	18	43	25
Chocolate Mint Cream	1 slice (4.3 oz)	360	15	53	32
Coconut Custard	1 slice (4.4 oz)	260	14	28	16
Cookies 'N Cream	1 slice (4.3 oz)	360	16	52	32
Dutch Apple	1 slice (4.4 oz)	330	13	50	25

FOOD	PORTION	CAL	FAT	CARB	SUG
French Silk	1 slice (4.4 oz)	560	40	48	34
Key West Line	1 slice (4.3 oz)	430	18	62	49
Lemon Cream	1 slice (5 oz)	440	26	49	32
Lemonade	1 slice (4.3 oz)	340	15	51	31
Mince	1 slice (4.6 oz)	380	17	53	26
Mixed Berry	1 slice (4.2 oz)	300	13	44	24
Peach	1 slice (4.6 oz)	320	17	40	16
Peach Lattice	1 slice (4.2 oz)	290	13	42	23
Peanut Butter Silk	1 slice (4.6 oz)	600	41	51	36
Pecan	1 slice (4.8 oz)	560	27	75	33
Pumpkin Custard	1 slice (4.6 oz)	270	13	35	18
Raspberry	1 slice (4.6 oz)	330	17	44	18
S'Mores Cream	1 slice (4.3 oz)	360	16	53	32
Strawberry Banana	1 slice (4.3 oz)	330	15	48	27
Sweet Potato Custard	1 slice (4.6 oz)	340	17	44	25
Sara Lee					
Apple 45% Reduced Fat	⅙ pie (4.5 oz)	290	8	51	16
Chocolate Silk	⅕ pie (4.8 oz)	500	32	49	35
Coconut Cream	⅕ pie (4.8 oz)	480	31	47	35
Homestyle Apple	⅛ pie (4.6 oz)	340	16	46	26
Homestyle Blueberry	⅛ pie (4.6 oz)	360	15	54	26
Homestyle Cherry	⅛ pie (4.6 oz)	320	16	42	27
Homestyle Dutch Apple	⅛ pie (4.6 oz)	350	15	53	30
Homestyle Mince	⅛ pie (4.6 oz)	390	17	56	30
Homestyle Peach	⅛ pie (4.6 oz)	320	14	46	30
Homestyle Pecan	⅛ pie (4.2 oz)	520	24	70	28
Homestyle Pumpkin	⅛ pie (4.6 oz)	260	11	37	18
Homestyle Raspberry	⅛ pie (4.6 oz)	380	19	48	20
Lemon Meringue	⅙ pie (5 oz)	350	11	59	42
Weight Watchers					
Mississippi Mud	1 piece (2.45 oz)	160	5	26	16

FOOD	PORTION	CAL	FAT	CARB	SUG
mix					
Jell-O					
No Bake Chocolate Silk as prep	⅛ pie (4.4 oz)	320	16	37	20
snack					
Dolly Madison					
Apple	1 (4.5 oz)	480	22	67	36
Blueberry	1 (4.5 oz)	480	21	70	31
Cherry	1 (4.5 oz)	470	22	65	35
Chocolate Pudding	1 (4.5 oz)	530	25	71	31
Lemon	1 (4.5 oz)	500	24	66	46
Peach	1 (4.5 oz)	480	21	66	30
Pecan	1 (3 oz)	360	19	44	19
Pecan Fried	1 (4.5 oz)	530	21	80	32
Pineapple	1 (4.5 oz)	460	21	62	29
Hostess					
Apple	1 (4.5 oz)	480	22	67	36
Blackberry	1 (4.5 oz)	520	21	79	29
Blueberry	1 (4.5 oz)	480	21	70	31
Cherry	1 (4.5 oz)	470	22	65	35
French Apple	1 (4.5 oz)	480	22	67	30
Lemon	1 (4.5 oz)	500	24	66	46
Peach	1 (4.5 oz)	480	21	68	30
Pineapple	1 (4.5 oz)	460	21	62	29
Strawberry	1 (4.5 oz)	510	23	71	35
Lance					
Pecan	1 (3 oz)	350	17	46	35
Tastykake					
Apple	1 (4 oz)	270	11	41	20
Blueberry	1 (4 oz)	300	11	49	23
Cherry	1 (4 oz)	290	11	46	16

FOOD	PORTION	CAL	FAT	CARB	SUG
Coconut Creme	1 (4 oz)	370	21	42	21
French Apple	1 (4.2 oz)	310	11	52	30
Lemon	1 (4 oz)	300	13	44	24
Peach	1 (4 oz)	280	11	43	21
Pineapple	1 (4 oz)	290	12	45	24
Pineapple Cheese	1 (4 oz)	320	12	50	26
Pumpkin	1 (4 oz)	340	14	47	22
Strawberry	1 (3.5 oz)	320	12	51	29
Tastyklair	1 (4 oz)	400	20	50	26
Tom's					
Apple	1 pkg (3 oz)	330	17	42	21
Banana Marshmallow	1 pkg (2.75 oz)	320	11	54	33
Cherry	1 pkg (3 oz)	320	18	37	24
Chocolate Marshmallow	1 pkg (2.75 oz)	320	11	53	32

PIE CRUST
frozen

Pepperidge Farm

FOOD	PORTION	CAL	FAT	CARB	SUG
Puff Pastry Sheets	⅙ sheet (1.4 oz)	170	11	14	1
Puff Pastry Shell	1 (1.6 oz)	190	13	16	2
Puff Pastry Squares	1 sq (2 oz)	240	16	19	2
Pet-Ritz					
Deep Dish	⅛ pie (0.7 oz)	90	5	11	1
Regular	⅛ pie (0.6 oz)	80	5	9	tr
Tart Shells	1 (1 oz)	130	8	13	0

ready-to-eat

Keebler

FOOD	PORTION	CAL	FAT	CARB	SUG
Graham Single Serve	1 (0.8 oz)	120	6	15	6
Reduced Fat Graham	⅛ pie (0.7 oz)	90	4	14	6

refrigerated

All Ready

FOOD	PORTION	CAL	FAT	CARB	SUG
Crust	⅛ pie (0.9 oz)	120	7	13	tr

FOOD	PORTION	CAL	FAT	CARB	SUG
PIE FILLING					
apple	⅛ can (2.6 oz)	74	tr	19	18
apple	1 can (21 oz)	599	1	156	143
Comstock					
MoreFruit Light Cherry	⅓ cup (2.9 oz)	60	0	13	11
Red Ruby Cherry	⅓ cup (3.1 oz)	90	0	23	19
Libby					
Pumpkin Pie Mix	⅓ cup	90	1	20	17
Smucker's					
Pie Glaze Strawberry	2 oz	80	0	21	20
PIEROGI					
Health Is Wealth					
Potato & Cheddar	2 (2.8 oz)	140	2	27	1
Potato & Onion	2 (2.8 oz)	140	2	27	1
Mrs. T's					
Jalapeno & Cheddar	3 (4.2 oz)	190	3	35	3
Potato & Cheddar	3 (4.2 oz)	180	3	34	3
Potato & Onion	3 (4.2 oz)	180	2	34	2
Sweet Potato	3 (4.2 oz)	300	0	35	16
PIG'S EARS AND FEET					
ear simmered	1	184	12	tr	—
feet simmered	3 oz	165	11	0	0
Hormel					
Pickled Feet	2 oz	80	6	0	0
Pickled Hocks	2 oz	110	8	0	0
PIGEON					
w/ skin & bone	3.5 oz	169	10	0	0
PIGEON PEAS					
dried cooked	½ cup	102	tr	20	—

FOOD	PORTION	CAL	FAT	CARB	SUG
PIGNOLIA					
(*see* PINE NUTS)					
PIKE					
northern cooked	3 oz	96	1	0	0
PILLNUTS					
canarytree dried	1 oz	204	23	1	—
PIMIENTOS					
Dromedary					
Peeled	½ tsp (4 g)	0	0	0	0
Unpeeled	½ tsp (4 g)	0	0	0	0
PINE NUTS					
Progresso					
Pignoli	1 jar (1 oz)	170	13	2	0
PINEAPPLE					
canned					
Dole					
Chunks Juice Pack	½ cup	60	0	15	13
dried					
Sonoma					
Pieces	2 pieces (1.4 oz)	140	2	30	26
fresh					
Bonita Hill					
Golden Extra Sweet	2 slices (3.9 oz)	60	0	16	13
PINK BEANS					
dried					
cooked	1 cup	252	1	47	—
PINTO BEANS					
canned					
pinto	1 cup	186	1	35	—
Chi-Chi's					
Pinto Beans	½ cup (4.3 oz)	100	1	18	1

FOOD	PORTION	CAL	FAT	CARB	SUG
Eden					
Organic	½ cup (4.6 oz)	100	0	18	—
Organic Spicy w/ Jalapeno & Red Peppers	½ cup (4.6 oz)	125	0	24	2
Green Giant					
Pinto Beans	½ cup (4.4 oz)	110	1	20	2
Progresso					
Pinto Beans	½ cup (4.6 oz)	110	1	18	tr
dried					
cooked	1 cup	235	1	44	—
Hurst					
HamBeens w/ Ham	3 tbsp (1.2 oz)	120	1	20	1
frozen					
cooked	3 oz	152	tr	29	—
PINYON					
(*see* PINE NUTS)					
PISTACHIOS					
dried	1 cup	739	62	32	—
dry roasted	1 oz	172	15	8	—
dry roasted salted	1 cup	776	68	35	—
dry roasted salted	1 oz	172	15	8	—
dry roasted w/ salt	47 nuts (1 oz)	160	13	8	2
Lance					
Pistachios	1 pkg (1⅛ oz)	90	7	4	0
Sonoma					
Salted Shelled	¼ cup (1 oz)	190	14	9	3
PITANGA					
fresh	1	2	tr	1	—
fresh	1 cup	57	1	13	—

FOOD	PORTION	CAL	FAT	CARB	SUG
PIZZA					
Amy's Organic					
Cheese	1 (13 oz)	310	11	39	5
Pocket Sandwich Cheese Pizza	1 (4.5 oz)	290	9	38	4
Pocket Sandwich Veggie Pepperoni Pizza	1 (4.5 oz)	220	7	28	5
Roasted Vegetable	1 (12 oz)	270	8	43	5
Spinach	1 (14 oz)	320	11	40	5
Appian Way					
Pizza Mix Thick Crust	⅓ pie (4.2 oz)	290	5	51	4
Pizza Mix	⅓ pie (4.1 oz)	250	3	48	4
Thin Crust					
Banquet					
Pepperoni	1 pie (6.75 oz)	490	23	56	30
Pizza Snack Cheese	6 pieces (7.5 oz)	200	8	24	4
Pizza Snack Pepperoni	6 pieces (7.5 oz)	230	11	23	4
Pizza Snack Pepperoni & Sausage	6 pieces (7.5 oz)	210	9	24	4
Di Giorno					
Rising Crust 12 inch Four Cheese	⅙ pie (4.9 oz)	320	11	39	6
Rising Crust 12 inch Italian Sausage	⅙ pie (5.3 oz)	360	14	40	6
Rising Crust 12 inch Pepperoni	⅙ pie (5.2 oz)	370	16	40	6
Rising Crust 12 inch Supreme	⅙ pie (5.8 oz)	380	17	40	7
Rising Crust 12 inch Three Meat	⅙ pie (5.4 oz)	380	16	40	6
Rising Crust 12 inch Vegetable	⅙ pie (5.6 oz)	310	10	41	7

FOOD	PORTION	CAL	FAT	CARB	SUG
Rising Crust 8 inch Chicken Supreme	⅛ pie (4.8 oz)	270	9	33	5
Rising Crust 8 inch Four Cheese	⅛ pie (4 oz)	260	9	33	5
Rising Crust 8 inch Italian Sausage	⅛ pie (4.4 oz)	300	12	33	5
Rising Crust 8 inch Pepperoni	⅛ pie (4.2 oz)	300	13	33	5
Rising Crust 8 inch Spinach	⅛ pie (4.3 oz)	250	8	33	5
Rising Crust 8 inch Supreme	⅛ pie (4.7 oz)	310	14	34	5
Rising Crust 8 inch Three Meat	⅛ pie (4.4 oz)	310	13	34	5
Rising Crust 8 inch Vegetable	⅛ pie (4.6 oz)	250	8	33	6
Health Is Wealth					
Pizza Munchees	6 (3 oz)	190	5	9	0
Healthy Choice					
French Bread Cheese	1 piece (6 oz)	340	5	51	9
French Bread Pepperoni	1 piece (6 oz)	340	5	49	6
French Bread Sausage	1 piece (6 oz)	320	5	48	9
French Bread Supreme	1 piece (6.35 oz)	330	5	51	7
French Bread Vegetable	1 piece (6 oz)	280	4	44	8
Jack's					
Great Combinations 12 inch Bacon Cheeseburger	¼ pie (4.7 oz)	360	18	31	4
Great Combinations 12 inch Double Cheese	¼ pie (4.9 oz)	380	19	32	5

FOOD	PORTION	CAL	FAT	CARB	SUG
Great Combinations 12 inch Pepperoni	¼ pie (5.2 oz)	410	19	42	5
Great Combinations 12 inch Pepperoni & Mushrooms	¼ pie (4.8 oz)	340	16	32	5
Great Combinations 12 inch Sausage	¼ pie (5.4 oz)	390	18	40	5
Great Combinations 12 inch Sausage & Mushroom	¼ pie (4.9 oz)	310	15	29	5
Great Combinations 12 inch Sausage & Pepperoni	¼ pie (4.8 oz)	350	19	29	4
Great Combinations 12 inch Supreme	¼ pie (5.2 oz)	350	18	30	3
Great Combinations 9 inch Double Cheese	½ pie (5.5 oz)	430	21	38	5
Great Combinations 9 inch Pepperoni & Sausage	½ pie (5.1 oz)	380	18	36	5
Naturally Rising 12 inch Bacon Cheeseburger	⅙ pie (5 oz)	350	15	35	7
Naturally Rising 12 inch Canadian Bacon	⅙ pie (4.9 oz)	280	9	34	7
Naturally Rising 12 inch Cheese	⅙ pie (4.5 oz)	290	10	35	7
Naturally Rising 12 inch Combination w/ Sausage & Pepperoni	⅙ pie (5.2 oz)	360	17	34	7
Naturally Rising 12 inch Pepperoni	⅙ pie (4.9 oz)	350	16	35	7

FOOD	PORTION	CAL	FAT	CARB	SUG
Naturally Rising 12 inch Pepperoni Supreme	⅙ pie (5.1 oz)	340	16	34	11
Naturally Rising 12 inch Sausage	⅙ pie (5.1 oz)	340	15	34	7
Naturally Rising 12 inch Spicy Italian Sausage	⅙ pie (5.1 oz)	330	14	34	11
Naturally Rising 12 inch The Works	⅙ pie (5.3 oz)	330	14	34	7
Naturally Rising 9 inch Cheese	⅓ pie (4.7 oz)	300	10	38	7
Naturally Rising 9 inch Combination w/ Sausage & Pepperoni	¼ pie (4.2 oz)	300	14	29	5
Naturally Rising 9 inch Pepperoni	⅓ pie (5.2 oz)	360	16	38	7
Naturally Rising 9 inch Sausage	⅓ pie (5.4 oz)	360	16	38	7
Naturally Rising 9 inch The Works	¼ pie (4.5 oz)	280	12	29	6
Original 12 inch Canadian Bacon	¼ pie (4.4 oz)	280	10	31	5
Original 12 inch Cheese	⅓ pie (5 oz)	360	13	41	6
Original 12 inch Hamburger	¼ pie (4.4 oz)	300	14	28	4
Original 12 inch Pepperoni	¼ pie (4.3 oz)	330	15	31	4
Original 12 inch Sausage	¼ pie (4.3 oz)	300	14	28	4
Original 12 inch Spicy Italian Sausage	¼ pie (4.3 oz)	290	13	29	5

FOOD	PORTION	CAL	FAT	CARB	SUG
Original 9 inch Pepperoni	½ pie (5 oz)	380	18	37	5
Original 9 inch Sausage	½ pie (5.1 oz)	360	16	36	5
Pizza Bursts Combination Sausage & Pepperoni	6 pieces (3 oz)	250	12	26	3
Pizza Bursts Pepperoni	6 pieces (3 oz)	260	14	25	3
Pizza Bursts Sausage	6 pieces (3 oz)	250	12	25	3
Pizza Bursts Supercheese	6 pieces (3 oz)	250	12	25	3
Pizza Bursts Supreme	6 pieces (3 oz)	250	13	26	3
Kid Cuisine					
Backpacking Pizza Snack	6 pieces	230	11	23	4
Big League Hamburger	1 meal (8.3 oz)	400	11	61	32
Fire Chief Cheese	1 pie (5.2 oz)	340	10	44	7
Pirate Pizza w/ Cheese	1 meal (8 oz)	430	11	71	34
Poolside Pepperoni	1 (5.2 oz)	380	14	44	7
Lean Cuisine					
Everyday Favorites French Bread Cheese	1 pkg (6 oz)	320	7	48	6
Everyday Favorites French Bread Deluxe	1 pkg (6.1 oz)	290	6	43	5
Everyday Favorites French Bread Pepperoni	1 pkg (5.25 oz)	300	8	43	6
Everyday Favorites French Bread Sun Dried Tomatoes	1 serv (6 oz)	340	8	48	8
Marie Callender's					
French Bread Cheese	1 (7.2 oz)	530	24	50	5

FOOD	PORTION	CAL	FAT	CARB	SUG
French Bread Pepperoni	1 (7.5 oz)	570	28	50	5
French Bread Supreme	1 (7.5 oz)	510	23	50	5
Pepperidge Farm					
Gourmet Crust Cheese	1 (4.4 oz)	390	20	39	11
Gourmet Crust Pepperoni	1 (4.5 oz)	420	23	39	8
Stouffer's					
French Bread Bacon Cheddar	1 piece (5.7 oz)	430	21	46	4
French Bread Cheese	1 piece (5.2 oz)	370	16	43	4
French Bread Cheeseburger	1 piece (6 oz)	420	20	44	3
French Bread Deluxe	1 piece (6.2 oz)	430	21	49	5
French Bread Double Cheese	1 piece (5.9 oz)	400	16	49	4
French Bread Pepperoni	1 piece (5.6 oz)	430	20	46	5
French Bread Pepperoni & Mushroom	1 piece (6.1 oz)	440	20	49	4
French Bread Sausage	1 piece (6 oz)	420	18	48	5
French Bread Sausage & Pepperoni	1 piece (6.25 oz)	470	23	47	4
French Bread Three Meat	1 piece (6.25 oz)	460	21	48	4
French Bread Vegetable Deluxe	1 piece (6.4 oz)	380	16	46	4
French Bread White Pizza	1 piece (5.1 oz)	460	23	45	1
Tombstone					
Double Top Pepperoni	⅛ pie (4.5 oz)	340	19	24	5
Double Top Sausage	⅛ pie (4.6 oz)	320	17	25	6

FOOD	PORTION	CAL	FAT	CARB	SUG
Double Top Sausage & Pepperoni	⅙ pie (4.6 oz)	340	19	25	5
Double Top Supreme	⅙ pie (4.7 oz)	330	18	25	5
Double Top Two Cheese	⅙ pie (5.2 oz)	380	19	29	6
For One ½ Less Fat Cheese	1 pie (6.5 oz)	460	10	43	8
For One ½ Less Fat Vegetable	1 pie (7.2 oz)	360	9	48	11
For One Extra Cheese	1 pie (6.9 oz)	520	28	47	8
For One Pepperoni	1 pie (6.9 oz)	550	32	41	8
For One Supreme	1 pie (7.5 oz)	550	32	42	8
Light Supreme	⅕ pie (4.8 oz)	270	9	30	6
Light Vegetable	⅕ pie (4.6 oz)	240	7	31	5
Original 12 inch Canadian Bacon	¼ pie (5.5 oz)	350	14	36	7
Original 12 inch Deluxe	⅕ pie (4.8 oz)	310	14	29	6
Original 12 inch Extra Cheese	¼ pie (5.1 oz)	350	15	35	7
Original 12 inch Hamburger	⅕ pie (4.4 oz)	310	15	29	5
Original 12 Inch Pepperoni	¼ pie (5.3 oz)	400	21	35	7
Original 12 inch Sausage	⅕ pie (4.4 oz)	300	14	29	6
Original 12 inch Sausage & Mushroom	⅕ pie (4.6 oz)	300	14	29	6
Original 12 inch Sausage & Pepperoni	⅕ pie (4.4 oz)	320	16	29	6
Original 12 inch Supreme	⅕ pie (5.1 oz)	320	16	29	6

FOOD	PORTION	CAL	FAT	CARB	SUG
Original 9 inch Deluxe	⅓ pie (4.4 oz)	280	13	27	5
Original 9 inch Extra Cheese	½ pie (5.6 oz)	380	19	40	8
Original 9 inch Hamburger	⅓ pie (4 oz)	280	13	27	5
Original 9 inch Pepperoni	⅓ pie (4 oz)	300	15	27	5
Original 9 inch Pepperoni & Sausage	⅓ pie (4.1 oz)	300	15	27	5
Original 9 inch Sausage	⅓ pie (4 oz)	280	13	27	5
Original 9 inch Supreme	⅓ pie (4.4 oz)	310	16	27	5
Oven Rising Italian Sausage	⅙ pie (5.1 oz)	320	13	35	12
Oven Rising Pepperoni	⅙ pie (4.9 oz)	340	15	34	7
Oven Rising Supreme	⅙ pie (5.1 oz)	320	14	34	8
Oven Rising Three Cheese	⅙ pie (4.8 oz)	320	13	34	7
Oven Rising Three Meat	⅙ pie (5.1 oz)	340	15	34	7
Thin Crust Four Meat Combo	¼ pie (5 oz)	380	23	26	5
Thin Crust Italian Sausage	¼ pie (5 oz)	370	22	26	5
Thin Crust Pepperoni	¼ pie (4.8 oz)	400	25	25	5
Thin Crust Supreme	¼ pie (5 oz)	380	22	26	5
Thin Crust Supreme Taco	¼ pie (5.1 oz)	370	23	27	5
Thin Crust Three Cheese	¼ pie (4.7 oz)	360	21	25	5

FOOD	PORTION	CAL	FAT	CARB	SUG
Weight Watchers					
Smart Ones Deluxe Combo	1 (6.57 oz)	380	11	47	3
Smart Ones Pepperoni	1 (5.56 oz)	390	12	46	3
take-out					
cheese	12 in pie	1121	26	164	—
cheese	⅛ of 12 in pie	140	3	21	—
cheese deep dish individual	1 (5.5 oz)	460	24	47	4
cheese meat & vegetables	12 in pie	1472	43	170	—
cheese meat & vegetables	⅛ of 12 in pie	184	5	21	—
pepperoni	12 in pie	1445	56	157	—
pepperoni	⅛ of 12 in pie	181	7	20	—
PIZZA DOUGH					
crust	1 slice (1.7 oz)	130	2	25	1
Betty Crocker					
Italian Herb Crust Mix	¼ crust (1.6 oz)	180	2	32	1
Boboli					
Thin Crust	⅛ crust (2 oz)	160	4	24	1
Pillsbury					
Crust	⅕ crust (2 oz)	150	2	27	3
Robin Hood					
Crust	¼ crust	160	2	33	1
PIZZA SAUCE					
Hunt's					
Fully Prepared	¼ cup (2.2 oz)	21	1	4	3
Pizza Sauce	¼ cup (2.2 oz)	27	1	5	2
Prima Choice Supper Heavy	¼ cup (2.2 oz)	28	1	6	3

FOOD	PORTION	CAL	FAT	CARB	SUG
Muir Glen					
Organic	¼ cup (2.2 oz)	40	0	6	3
Progresso					
Pizza Sauce	¼ cup (2.1 oz)	20	0	4	2
PLANTAINS					
fresh uncooked	1 (6.3 oz)	218	1	57	—
sliced cooked	½ cup	89	tr	24	—
take-out					
ripe fried	2.8 oz	214	7	38	—
PLUMS					
canned					
purple in heavy syrup	3	119	tr	31	—
purple in heavy syrup	1 cup	320	tr	60	—
purple in light syrup	3	83	tr	22	—
purple in light syrup	1 cup	158	tr	41	—
purple juice pack	3	55	tr	14	—
purple juice pack	1 cup	146	tr	38	—
purple water pack	1 cup	102	tr	27	—
purple water pack	3	39	tr	10	—
fresh					
plum	1	36	tr	9	—
sliced	1 cup	91	1	21	—
Chiquita					
Purple	2 med (4.6 oz)	80	1	19	10
POI					
poi	½ cup	134	tr	33	—
POKEBERRY SHOOTS					
cooked	½ cup	16	tr	3	—
raw	½ cup	18	tr	3	—

FOOD	PORTION	CAL	FAT	CARB	SUG
POLENTA					
Frieda's					
Dried Tomato	4 oz	80	0	17	1
Italian Herb	4 oz	80	0	17	0
Mexicana	4 oz	80	0	17	0
Original	4 oz	80	0	16	0
Wild Mushroom	4 oz	80	0	17	0
Melissa's					
Original	4 oz	80	0	16	0
POLLACK					
altantic fillet baked	5.3 oz	178	2	0	0
atlantic baked	3 oz	100	1	0	0
Mrs. Paul's					
Fillets Light frozen	1 fillet (4.5 oz)	240	11	18	—
POMEGRANATE					
fresh	1	104	tr	26	—
Cortas					
Concentrated Juice	1 tbsp (0.6 oz)	40	0	9	7
POMPANO					
florida cooked	3 oz	179	10	0	0
florida raw	3 oz	140	8	0	0
POPCORN					
air-popped	1 cup (0.3 oz)	31	tr	6	—
air-popped	1 oz	108	1	22	—
caramel coated	1 oz	122	4	22	11
caramel coated	1 cup (1.2 oz)	152	5	28	14
carmel coated w/ peanuts	⅔ cup (1 oz)	114	2	23	11
cheese	1 oz	149	9	15	—
cheese	1 cup (0.4 oz)	58	4	6	—

FOOD	PORTION	CAL	FAT	CARB	SUG
oil popped	1 oz	142	8	16	tr
oil popped	1 cup (0.4 oz)	55	3	6	tr
Chester's					
Butter	3 cups	160	12	15	0
Caramel Craze	¾ cup	130	2	27	18
Cheddar Cheese	3 cups	190	13	17	2
Microwave Butter	5 cups	200	12	22	tr
Cracker Jack					
Fat Free Butter Toffee	¾ cup	110	0	26	17
Fat Free Caramel	¾ cup	110	0	26	17
Original	½ cup (1 oz)	120	2	23	15
Estee					
Caramel	1 cup	120	2	26	1
Herr's					
Regular	3 cups (1 oz)	140	11	11	1
Jolly Time					
America's Best 94% Fat Free	1 cup	20	0	5	0
Blast O Butter	1 cup	45	3	5	0
Blast O Butter Light	1 cup	30	2	4	0
Butter Licious	1 cup	35	2	4	0
Butter Licious Light	1 cup	30	2	4	0
Crispy & White	1 cup	40	3	4	0
Crispy & White Light	1 cup	25	1	4	0
Healthy Pop 94% Fat Free	1 cup	20	0	5	0
White Air Popped	5 cups	100	1	24	0
Yellow Air Popped	5 cups	100	1	24	tr
Lance					
Cheese	1 pkg (0.6 oz)	90	5	9	0
Plain	1 pkg (0.5 oz)	70	3	10	0

FOOD	PORTION	CAL	FAT	CARB	SUG
White Cheddar	1 pkg (0.6 oz)	100	8	7	1
White Cheddar	1 pkg (0.9 oz)	150	11	10	1
Newman's Own					
Microwave Butter Flavor	3½ cups	170	11	16	0
Microwave Light Butter	3½ cups	110	3	20	0
Microwave Light Natural	3½ cups	110	3	20	0
Microwave Natural	3½ cups	170	11	16	0
Popcorn unpopped	3 tbsp	110	2	27	0
Orville Redenbacher's					
Gourmet Original	3 cups	92	1	22	0
Hot Air	3 cups	92	1	22	0
Microwave Butter	3 cups	168	13	15	0
Microwave Butter No Salt Added	3 cups	176	12	19	0
Microwave Butter Light	3 cups	122	6	20	0
Microwave Caramel	1 serv	179	10	23	12
Microwave Golden Cheddar	1 serv	169	13	15	0
Microwave Natural	3 cups	164	11	18	0
Microwave Natural No Salt Added	3 cups	174	12	19	0
Microwave Natural Light	3 cups	118	5	19	0
Microwave Smartpop	1 serv	96	3	20	0
Microwave Smartpop Butter Snack Size	1 bag	155	4	34	6
Microwave Snack Size Butter	1 bag	287	22	25	0

FOOD	PORTION	CAL	FAT	CARB	SUG
Microwave Snack Size Butter Light	1 bag	183	8	30	0
Microwave White Cheddar	1 serv	169	13	15	0
Redenbudders Microwave Herb & Garlic	1 serv	176	13	16	0
Redenbudders Microwave Zesty Butter	1 serv	177	13	16	0
Redenbudders Movie Theater Butter Light	1 serv	113	5	20	0
Redenbudders Movie Theater Microwave Butter	1 serv	176	13	16	0
Smart Pop Movie Theater Butter	1 serv	92	2	20	0
White	3 cups	92	1	22	0
Planters					
Fiddle Faddle Caramel Fat Free	1 cup (1 oz)	110	0	28	16
Pop Secret					
94% Fat Free Butter	1 cup (5 g)	20	0	4	0
94% Fat Free Natural	1 cup (5 g)	20	0	4	0
Butter	1 cup (7 g)	35	3	4	0
Cheddar Cheese	1 cup (6 g)	30	2	3	0
Jumbo Pop Butter	1 cup (7 g)	40	3	4	0
Jumbo Pop Movie Theater Butter	1 cup (7 g)	40	3	4	0
Light Butter	1 cup (5 g)	20	1	4	0
Light Movie Theater Butter	1 cup (5 g)	25	1	4	0
Light Natural	1 cup (5 g)	25	1	4	0

FOOD	PORTION	CAL	FAT	CARB	SUG
Movie Theater Butter	1 cup (7 g)	40	3	3	0
Nacho Cheese	1 cup (6 g)	30	2	3	0
Natural	1 cup (7 g)	35	3	4	0
Real Butter	1 cup (7 g)	35	3	4	0
Smartfood					
Butter	3 cups	150	9	15	2
Low Fat Toffee Crunch	¾ cup	110	1	25	19
Reduced Fat Golden Butter	3⅓ cups	130	4	21	0
Reduced Fat White Cheddar	3 cups	140	6	19	1
White Cheddar	2 cups	190	12	17	5
Snyder's Of Hanover					
Butter	⅝ oz	110	10	6	0
Tom's					
Caramel Corn	1 pkg (1.6 oz)	180	3	39	23
Utz					
Au Natural	3 cups (1 oz)	120	1	25	0
Butter	2 cups (1 oz)	170	12	13	tr
Cheese	2 cups (1 oz)	150	10	14	1
Hulless Puff'N Corn	2 cups (1 oz)	180	15	11	0
Hulless Puff'N Corn Hot Cheese	1 pkg (1.75 oz)	290	22	21	3
Hulless Pull'N Corn Cheese	2 cups (1 oz)	170	12	13	0
White Cheddar	2 cups (1 oz)	150	9	15	3
Weight Watchers					
Butter	1 pkg (0.66 oz)	90	3	14	0
Butter Toffee	1 pkg (0.9 oz)	110	3	21	11
Caramel	1 pkg (0.9 oz)	100	1	22	11
Microwave	1 pkg (1 oz)	100	1	20	0
White Cheddar Cheese	1 pkg (0.66 oz)	90	4	12	0

FOOD	PORTION	CAL	FAT	CARB	SUG
POPCORN CAKES					
popcorn cake	1 (0.3 oz)	38	tr	8	—
Orville Redenbacher's					
BBQ Mini	8 (0.5 oz)	55	1	12	1
Butter	2 (0.6 oz)	134	1	13	1
Butter Mini	8 (0.5 oz)	56	1	11	tr
Caramel	1 (0.4 oz)	34	tr	8	2
Caramel Mini	7 (0.5 oz)	50	tr	12	3
Nacho Cheese Mini	8 (0.5 oz)	56	1	11	tr
Peanut Crunch Mini	7 (0.5 oz)	55	1	11	3
White Cheddar	2 (0.6 oz)	63	1	13	tr
White Cheddar Mini	8 (0.5 oz)	56	1	12	tr
POPOVER					
mix as prep	1 (1.2 oz)	67	2	10	—
POPPY SEEDS					
poppy seeds	1 tsp	15	1	1	—
PORGY					
fresh	3 oz	77	tr	0	0
PORK					
canned					
Hormel					
Pickled Tidbits	2 oz	100	8	0	0
fresh					
boston blade roast lean & fat cooked	3 oz	229	16	0	0
boston blade steak lean & fat cooked	3 oz	220	14	0	0
center loin roast lean bone in cooked	3 oz	169	8	0	0

FOOD	PORTION	CAL	FAT	CARB	SUG
center loin chop lean bone in cooked	3 oz	172	7	0	0
center rib chop lean & fat bone in cooked	3 oz	213	13	0	0
center rib roast lean & fat bone in cooked	3 oz	217	13	0	0
fresh ham rump lean roasted	3 oz	175	7	0	0
fresh ham rump lean & fat roasted	3 oz	214	12	0	0
fresh ham shank lean roasted	3 oz	183	9	0	0
fresh ham shank lean & fat roasted	3 oz	246	17	0	0
fresh ham whole lean roasted	3 oz	179	8	0	0
fresh ham whole lean roasted diced	1 cup	285	13	0	0
fresh ham whole lean & fat roasted	3 oz	232	15	0	0
fresh ham whole lean & fat roasted diced	1 cup	369	24	0	0
ground cooked	3 oz	252	18	0	0
loin chop lean bone in braised	3 oz	191	11	0	0
loin chop lean bone in broiled	3 oz	199	12	0	0
loin roast lean bone in roasted	3 oz	210	13	0	0
loin whole lean & fat braised	3 oz	203	12	0	0

FOOD	PORTION	CAL	FAT	CARB	SUG
loin whole lean & fat broiled	3 oz	206	12	0	0
loin whole lean & fat roasted	3 oz	211	12	0	0
lungs braised	3 oz	84	3	0	0
pancreas cooked	3 oz	186	9	0	0
ribs country style lean & fat braised	3 oz	252	18	0	0
shoulder arm picnic lean & fat roasted	3 oz	269	20	0	0
shoulder whole lean & fat roasted	3 oz	248	18	0	0
shoulder whole lean & fat roasted diced	1 cup	394	29	0	0
shoulder whole lean roasted	3 oz	196	12	0	0
shoulder whole lean roasted diced	1 cup	311	18	0	0
sirloin chop lean & fat bone in braised	3 oz	208	13	0	0
sirloin roast lean & fat bone in cooked	3 oz	222	14	0	0
spareribs braised	3 oz	338	26	0	0
spleen braised	3 oz	127	3	0	0
tail simmered	3 oz	336	30	0	0
tenderloin lean roasted	3 oz	139	4	0	0
top loin chop boneless lean & fat cooked	3 oz	198	11	0	0

FOOD	PORTION	CAL	FAT	CARB	SUG
top loin roast boneless lean & fat cooked	3 oz	192	10	0	0
Oscar Mayer					
Sweet Morsel Smoked Boneless Pork Shoulder Butt	3 oz	180	15	0	0
ready-to-eat					
Tyson					
Pork Pattie	1 (3.8 oz)	200	11	9	7
take-out					
chicharrones pork cracklings fried	1 cup	844	72	22	—
PORK DISHES					
pork roast	2 oz	70	3	0	0
tourtiere	1 piece (4.9 oz)	451	34	21	—
POSOLE					
(*see* HOMINY)					
POT PIE					
Amy's Organic					
Broccoli	1 (7.5 oz)	430	22	46	3
Country Vegetable	1 (7.5 oz)	370	16	47	5
Shepard's	1 (8 oz)	160	4	27	5
Vegetable	1 (7.5 oz)	360	18	44	3
Vegetable Non-Dairy	1 (7.5 oz)	320	9	50	3
Banquet					
Beef	1 (7 oz)	400	23	38	8
Cheesy Potato & Broccoli w/ Ham	1 (7 oz)	410	23	40	8
Chicken	1 (7 oz)	380	22	36	6
Chicken & Broccoli	1 (7 oz)	350	20	32	9

FOOD	PORTION	CAL	FAT	CARB	SUG
Family Size Hearty Chicken	1 cup	460	29	39	14
Macaroni & Cheese	1 pkg (6.5 oz)	210	5	34	10
Turkey	1 (7 oz)	370	20	38	6
Vegetable Cheese	1 (7 oz)	340	17	39	19
Healthy Choice					
Colonial Chicken	1 (9.5 oz)	310	7	40	15
Lean Cuisine					
Everyday Favorites Chicken Pie	1 pkg (9.5 oz)	300	8	38	14
Everyday Favorites Vegetable Eggroll	1 pkg (9 oz)	300	5	57	16
Marie Callender's					
Beef	1 (9.5 oz)	680	42	53	7
Chicken	1 (9.5 oz)	680	48	53	9
Chicken & Broccoli	1 (9.5 oz)	670	43	54	11
Chicken Au Gratin	1 (9.5 oz)	690	46	50	3
Turkey	1 (9.5 oz)	680	46	56	10
Morton					
Macaroni & Cheese	1 (6.5 oz)	210	5	34	10
Vegetable w/ Beef	1 (7 oz)	340	21	33	8
Vegetable w/ Chicken	1 (7 oz)	320	18	32	7
Vegetable w/ Turkey	1 (7 oz)	310	18	29	8
Mrs. Paterson's					
Aussie Pie Chicken	1 (5.5 oz)	460	25	45	3
Aussie Pie Chicken Low Fat	1 (5.5 oz)	380	17	44	3
Aussie Pie Philly Steak	1 (5.5 oz)	420	24	39	3
Stouffer's					
Beef Pie	1 pkg (10 oz)	450	26	36	10
Chicken Pie	1 pkg (10 oz)	540	33	38	11
Turkey	1 pkg (10 oz)	530	33	36	11

FOOD	PORTION	CAL	FAT	CARB	SUG
Swanson					
Beef	1 (7 oz)	376	19	39	4
Chicken	1 (7 oz)	416	22	45	5
Turkey	1 (7 oz)	440	24	44	5
take-out					
beef	⅛ of 9 in pie (7.4 oz)	515	30	39	—
chicken	⅛ of 9 in pie (8.1 oz)	545	31	42	—
POTATO					
canned					
potatoes	½ cup	54	tr	12	—
Hormel					
Au Gratin & Bacon	1 can (7.5 oz)	250	14	23	1
fresh					
baked skin only	1 skin (2 oz)	115	tr	27	—
baked w/ skin	1 (6.5 oz)	220	tr	51	—
baked w/o skin	1 (5 oz)	145	tr	34	—
baked w/o skin	½ cup	57	tr	13	—
boiled	½ cup	68	tr	16	—
microwaved	1 (7 oz)	212	tr	49	—
microwaved w/o skin	½ cup	78	tr	18	—
raw w/o skin	1 (3.9 oz)	88	tr	20	—
PurelyIdaho					
Oven Roasts	1 serv (3 oz)	70	0	17	1
frozen					
french fries	10 strips	111	4	17	—
french fries thick cut	10 strips	109	4	17	—
hashed brown	½ cup	170	9	22	—
potato puffs	½ cup	138	7	19	—
potato puffs as prep	1	16	1	2	—
Birds Eye					
Baby Gourmet	7 (4 oz)	100	0	21	0
Whole	3 (2.6 oz)	50	0	13	0

FOOD	PORTION	CAL	FAT	CARB	SUG
Healthy Choice					
Cheddar Broccoli Potatoes	1 meal (10.5 oz)	330	7	53	8
Lean Cuisine					
Everyday Favorites Deluxe Cheddar Potato	1 pkg (10.4 oz)	250	6	37	6
Oh Boy!					
Stuffed With Cheddar Cheese	1 (5 oz)	130	4	22	0
Stouffer's					
Au Gratin	½ cup (5.75 oz)	130	6	15	3
Scalloped	½ cup (5.75 oz)	140	6	17	3
Weight Watchers					
Smart Ones Baked Broccoli & Cheese	1 pkg (10 oz)	250	6	39	9
mix					
au gratin as prep	4½ oz	127	6	18	—
instant mashed flakes as prep w/ whole milk & butter	½ cup	118	6	16	—
instant mashed flakes not prep	½ cup	78	tr	18	—
instant mashed granules as prep w/ whole milk & butter	½ cup	114	5	15	—
instant mashed granules not prep	½ cup	372	1	86	—
scalloped as prep	4½ oz	127	6	18	—
Barbara's					
Mashed not prep	⅓ cup (0.8 oz)	70	0	17	0

FOOD	PORTION	CAL	FAT	CARB	SUG
Betty Crocker					
Au Gratin Low Fat Recipe	½ cup	110	1	22	3
Au Gratin as prep	½ cup	150	6	22	3
Cheddar & Bacon	½ cup	150	6	21	2
Cheddar & Bacon Low Fat Recipe	½ cup	120	3	21	2
Cheddar & Sour Cream	½ cup	130	3	25	3
Chicken & Vegetable	⅔ cup	140	4	23	4
Chicken & Vegetable Low Fat Recipe	⅔ cup	120	3	23	4
Hash Browns	½ cup	190	8	30	0
Homestyle Broccoli Au Gratin	½ cup	140	6	21	6
Homestyle Broccoli Au Gratin Low Fat Recipe	½ cup	110	3	21	6
Homestyle Cheddar Cheese	½ cup	120	3	21	2
Homestyle Cheddar Cheese Stove Top Recipe	½ cup	140	5	21	2
Homestyle Cheesy Scalloped	½ cup	140	6	21	5
Homestyle Cheesy Scalloped Low Fat Recipe	½ cup	110	3	21	5
Julienne	½ cup	150	6	21	5
Mashed Butter & Herb	½ cup	160	8	20	2
Mashed Butter & Herb Reduced Fat Recipe	½ cup	130	5	20	2
Mashed Chicken & Herb	½ cup	150	7	21	2

FOOD	PORTION	CAL	FAT	CARB	SUG
Mashed Chicken & Herb Reduced Fat Recipe	½ cup	120	4	21	2
Mashed Four Cheese	½ cup	150	7	20	3
Mashed Four Cheese Reduced Fat Recipe	½ cup	120	4	20	3
Mashed Potato Buds	⅔ cup	160	8	19	2
Mashed Potato Buds Reduced Fat Recipe	⅔ cup	120	4	19	2
Mashed Roasted Garlic	½ cup	150	8	19	2
Mashed Roasted Garlic Reduced Fat Recipe	½ cup	130	5	19	2
Mashed Sour Cream & Chives	½ cup	150	7	21	3
Mashed Sour Cream & Chives Reduced Fat Recipe	½ cup	120	4	21	3
Potato Shakers Original	⅔ cup	140	4	23	2
Potato Shakers Original Low Fat Recipe	⅔ cup	120	2	23	2
Ranch	½ cup	160	6	25	4
Scalloped	½ cup	150	6	23	3
Scalloped Low Fat Recipe	⅔ cup	110	1	23	3
Sour Cream'n Chive	½ cup	160	7	22	5
Three Cheese	½ cup	150	6	23	3
Twice Baked Cheddar & Bacon Low Fat Recipe	⅔ cup	130	3	22	4
Twice Baked Cheddar & Bacon as prep	⅔ cup	210	11	22	4
Hungry Jack					
Au Gratin as prep	½ cup	150	5	24	3

FOOD	PORTION	CAL	FAT	CARB	SUG
Cheddar & Bacon as prep	½ cup	150	5	24	3
Chessy Scalloped as prep	½ cup	150	5	24	3
Creamy Scalloped as prep	½ cup	150	5	24	3
Mashed Butter Flavored as prep	½ cup	150	7	19	2
Mashed Flakes as prep	½ cup	160	7	20	2
Mashed Garlic Flavored as prep	½ cup	150	7	19	2
Mashed Parsley Butter as prep	½ cup	150	7	19	2
Mashed Sour Cream 'n Chives as prep	½ cup	150	7	19	2
Sour Cream & Chives as prep	½ cup	160	6	23	3
Idaho					
Mashed Potato Flakes as prep	½ cup	150	6	20	2
Mashed Potato Granules as prep	½ cup	160	7	22	2
Shake 'N Bake					
Perfect Potatoes Crispy Cheddar	⅛ pkg (7 g)	30	2	2	tr
Perfect Potatoes Herb & Garlic	⅛ pkg (7 g)	20	0	5	1
Perfect Potatoes Home Fries	⅛ pkg (7 g)	20	0	5	1
Perfect Potatoes Parmesan Peppercorn	⅛ pkg (7 g)	25	1	3	1
Perfect Potatoes Savory Onion	⅛ pkg (7 g)	20	0	5	1

FOOD	PORTION	CAL	FAT	CARB	SUG
shelf-stable					
Lunch Bucket					
Scalloped w/ Ham Chunks	1 pkg (7.5 oz)	170	7	24	tr
Micro Cup Meals					
Microcup Meals Scalloped Potatoes w/ Ham	1 cup (7.5 oz)	240	14	20	1
take-out					
au gratin w/ cheese	½ cup	178	10	17	—
baked topped w/ cheese sauce	1	475	29	47	—
baked topped w/ cheese sauce & bacon	1	451	26	44	—
baked topped w/ cheese sauce & broccoli	1	402	14	47	—
baked topped w/ cheese sauce & chili	1	481	22	56	—
baked topped w/ sour cream & chives	1	394	22	50	—
curry	1 serv (6 oz)	292	16	36	—
french fries	1 reg	235	12	29	—
french fries	1 lg	355	19	44	—
hash brown	½ cup (2.5 oz)	151	9	16	—
indian yogurt potatoes	1 serv	315	9	52	—
mashed	½ cup	111	4	18	—
mustard potato salad	3.5 oz	120	6	16	—
o'brien	1 cup	157	3	30	—
potato dumpling	3.5 oz	334	1	74	—

FOOD	PORTION	CAL	FAT	CARB	SUG
potato pancakes	1 (1.3 oz)	101	7	11	—
potato salad	½ cup	179	10	14	—
scalloped	½ cup	127	5	18	—

POTATO STARCH

potato starch	1 oz	96	tr	24	—

POUT

ocean baked	3 oz	86	1	0	0

PRESERVE

(*see* JAM/JELLY/PRESERVES)

PRETZELS

chocolate covered	1 (0.4 oz)	50	2	8	—
Bachman					
Thin'n Right	12 (1 oz)	120	1	23	tr
Estee					
Chocolate Covered	7	130	6	19	0
Dutch	2 (1.1 oz)	130	1	26	tr
Unsalted	23 (1 oz)	120	1	25	tr
Gardetto's					
Mustard	1 pkg (0.5 oz)	50	1	10	0
Herr's					
Hard Sourdough	1 (1 oz)	100	0	23	0
Lance					
Pretzels	1 pkg (1.25 oz)	140	1	28	1
Little Debbie					
Mini Twists	1 pkg (1.2 oz)	140	1	28	tr
Nabisco					
Air Crisps Fat Free	23 pieces (1 oz)	110	0	23	2
Nestle					
Flipz Milk Chocolate Covered	9 pieces (1 oz)	130	5	19	10

FOOD	PORTION	CAL	FAT	CARB	SUG
Flipz White Fudge Covered	9 pieces (1 oz)	130	6	19	11
Newman's Own					
Salted Rounds Organic	1 pkg (1.4 oz)	150	2	31	2
Rold Gold					
Crispy's Thins	4 (1 oz)	110	2	22	1
Fat Free Cheddar Cheese	17 (1 oz)	110	0	23	2
Fat Free Honey Mustard	17 (1 oz)	110	0	23	2
Fat Free Sticks	48 (1 oz)	110	0	23	1
Fat Free Thins	12 pieces (1 oz)	110	0	24	tr
Fat Free Tiny Twists	18 pieces (1 oz)	110	0	23	tr
Honey Mustard	16 (1 oz)	110	1	22	1
Rods	3 (1 oz)	110	1	22	1
Sour Dough Nuggets	11 (1 oz)	110	0	24	1
Snyder's Of Hanover					
Dips White Fudge	1 oz	130	6	19	12
Hard Sourdough	1 oz	100	0	22	0
Hard Sourdough Unsalted	1 oz	100	0	22	0
Logs	1 oz	110	1	21	1
Mini	1 oz	120	0	25	tr
Mini Unsalted	1 oz	110	0	25	tr
Nibblers	1 oz	120	0	25	tr
Nibblers Honey Mustard & Onions	1 oz	130	3	23	tr
Nibblers Oat Bran	1 oz	130	3	23	1
Nibblers Unsalted	1 oz	120	0	25	tr
Oat Bran	1 oz	100	3	22	tr
Old Fashioned Dipping Stix	1 oz	100	0	22	tr

FOOD	PORTION	CAL	FAT	CARB	SUG
Olde Tyme	1 oz	120	1	24	tr
Olde Tyme Stix	1 oz	120	1	23	tr
Olde Tyme Unsalted	1 oz	120	1	24	tr
Pieces Buttermilk Ranch	1 oz	130	5	19	tr
Pieces Cheddar Cheese	1 oz	190	6	18	tr
Pieces Honey Mustard & Onions	1 oz	140	7	18	3
Pieces Peppered Pizza	1 oz	150	8	16	1
Rods	1 oz	120	2	24	tr
Snaps	24 (1 oz)	120	1	25	tr
Thin	1 oz	130	0	23	1
Whole Wheat Honey	1 oz	120	1	24	4
Utz					
Country Store Stix	5 (1 oz)	110	1	22	tr
Fat Free Hard	1 (0.8 oz)	90	0	18	tr
Fat Free Hard No Salt Added	1 (0.8 oz)	90	0	19	tr
Fat Free Sour Dough Nuggets	10 (1 oz)	100	0	22	tr
Fat Free Stix	14 (1 oz)	100	0	23	1
Fat Free Thin	10 (1 oz)	100	0	22	1
Honey Mustard & Onion	⅓ cup (1 oz)	130	6	18	1
Rods	3 (1 oz)	120	1	24	1
Specials	5 (1 oz)	110	1	21	tr
Specials Extra Dark	5 (1 oz)	110	1	21	tr
Specials Unsalted	5 (1 oz)	110	1	21	tr
Wheels	20 (1 oz)	100	0	22	1
Weight Watchers					
Oat Bran Nuggets	1 pkg (1.5 oz)	170	3	33	0

FOOD	PORTION	CAL	FAT	CARB	SUG
PRUNES					
Sonoma					
Pitted	¼ cup (1.4 oz)	120	0	29	15
PUDDING					
mix					
Betty Crocker					
Rice as prep	1 serv	200	3	33	21
Jell-O					
Americana Rice as prep w/ skim milk	½ cup (5.2 oz)	140	0	29	19
Americana Tapioca as prep w/ skim milk	½ cup (5.1 oz)	130	0	28	21
Banana Cream as prep w/ 2% milk	½ cup (5.1 oz)	140	3	26	21
Butterscotch as prep w/ 2% milk	½ cup (5.2 oz)	160	3	30	25
Chocolate as prep w/ 2% milk	½ cup (5.2 oz)	150	3	28	21
Chocolate Fudge as prep w/ 2% milk	½ cup (5.2 oz)	150	3	28	21
Coconut Cream as prep w/ 2% milk	½ cup (5.1 oz)	150	5	24	19
Fat Free Chocolate as prep w/ skim milk	½ cup (5.2 oz)	130	0	29	21
Fat Free Vanilla as prep w/ skim milk	½ cup (5.1 oz)	130	0	28	22
Instant Banana Cream as prep w/ 2% milk	½ cup (5.2 oz)	150	3	29	24
Instant Butterscotch as prep w/ 2% milk	½ cup (5.2 oz)	150	3	29	24

FOOD	PORTION	CAL	FAT	CARB	SUG
Instant Chocolate as prep w/ 2% milk	½ cup (5.2 oz)	160	3	31	25
Instant Chocolate Fudge as prep w/ 2% milk	½ cup (4.2 oz)	160	3	31	23
Instant Coconut Cream as prep w/ 2% milk	½ cup (4.2 oz)	160	5	27	22
Instant French Vanilla as prep w/ 2% milk	½ cup (4.2 oz)	150	3	29	24
Instant Lemon as prep w/ 2% milk	½ cup (4.2 oz)	150	3	29	25
Instant Pistachio as prep w/ 2% milk	½ cup (4.2 oz)	160	3	29	24
Instant Vanilla as prep w/ 2% milk	½ cup (4.2 oz)	150	3	29	25
Instant Fat Free Chocolate as prep w/ skim milk	½ cup (5.3 oz)	140	0	31	25
Instant Fat Free Devil's Food as prep w/ skim milk	½ cup (5.3 oz)	140	0	31	25
Instant Fat Free Sugar Free Banana as prep w/ skim milk	½ cup (4.6 oz)	70	0	12	6
Instant Fat Free Sugar Free Butterscotch as prep w/ skim milk	½ cup (4.6 oz)	70	0	12	6
Instant Fat Free Sugar Free Chocolate Fudge as prep w/ skim milk	½ cup (4.7 oz)	80	0	14	6
Instant Fat Free Sugar Free Chocolate as prep w/ skim milk	½ cup (4.6 oz)	80	0	14	6

FOOD	PORTION	CAL	FAT	CARB	SUG
Instant Fat Free Sugar Free Vanilla as prep w/ skim milk	½ cup (4.6 oz)	70	0	12	6
Instant Fat Free Sugar Free White Chocolate as prep w/ skim milk	½ cup (4.6 oz)	70	0	12	6
Instant Fat Free Vanilla as prep w/ skim milk	½ cup (5.2 oz)	140	0	29	25
Instant Fat Free White Chocolate as prep w/ skim milk	½ cup (5.2 oz)	140	0	29	25
Lemon as prep	½ cup (4.4 oz)	140	2	29	23
Milk Chocolate as prep w/ 2% milk	½ cup (5.2 oz)	150	3	28	22
Sugar Free Chocolate as prep w/ 2% milk	½ cup (4.6 oz)	90	3	13	6
Sugar Free Vanilla as prep w/ 2% milk	½ cup (4.5 oz)	80	3	11	6
Vanilla as prep w/ 2% milk	½ cup (5.1 oz)	150	3	30	19
Louisiana Purchase					
Bread	1 serv (1.3 oz)	150	3	28	16
Lundberg					
Elegant Rice Cinnamon Raisin	½ cup (3.9 oz)	70	0	16	7
Elegant Rice Coconut	½ cup (3.9 oz)	70	2	13	5
Elegant Rice Honey Almond	½ cup (3.9 oz)	70	1	15	5
Uncle Ben's					
Rice Pudding Cinnamon & Raisins as prep	½ cup (1.5 oz)	160	1	37	16

FOOD	PORTION	CAL	FAT	CARB	SUG
ready-to-eat					
banana	1 pkg (5 oz)	180	5	30	23
chocolate	1 pkg (5 oz)	189	6	32	23
Handi-Snacks					
Banana	1 serv (3.5 oz)	120	4	22	16
Butterscotch	1 serv (3.5 oz)	120	4	22	17
Chocolate	1 serv (3.5 oz)	130	4	23	18
Chocolate Fudge	1 serv (3.5 oz)	130	4	23	18
Fat Free Chocolate	1 serv (3.5 oz)	90	0	21	16
Fat Free Vanilla	1 serv (3.5 oz)	90	0	21	16
Tapioca	1 serv (3.5 oz)	120	4	21	14
Vanilla	1 serv (3.5 oz)	120	4	21	17
Healthy Choice					
Low Fat Chocolate Raspberry	½ cup (3.5 oz)	102	2	19	15
Low Fat Chocolate Almond	½ cup (3.5 oz)	109	2	21	15
Low Fat Double Chocolate Fudge	½ cup (3.5 oz)	101	1	20	14
Low Fat French Vanilla	½ cup (3.5 oz)	98	1	20	16
Low Fat Tapioca	½ cup (3.5 oz)	101	1	21	14
Hunt's					
Snack Pack Banana	1 serv (3.5 oz)	119	4	18	14
Snack Pack Butterscotch	1 serv (3.5 oz)	130	4	21	14
Snack Pack Chocolate	1 serv (3.5 oz)	143	5	22	17
Snack Pack Chocolate Fudge	1 serv (3.5 oz)	147	5	23	17
Snack Pack Chocolate Marshmallow	1 serv (3.5 oz)	134	5	21	16
Snack Pack Fat Free Chocolate	1 serv (3.5 oz)	86	tr	19	14

FOOD	PORTION	CAL	FAT	CARB	SUG
Snack Pack Fat Free Tapioca	1 serv (3.5 oz)	82	tr	18	14
Snack Pack Fat Free Vanilla	1 serv (3.5 oz)	81	tr	18	13
Snack Pack Lemon	1 serv (3.5 oz)	124	3	24	21
Snack Pack Milk Chocolate Variety	1 serv (3.5 oz)	143	5	22	18
Snack Pack Swirl Chocolate Caramel	1 serv (3.5 oz)	143	5	23	17
Snack Pack Swirl Chocolate Peanut Butter	1 serv (3.5 oz)	146	6	21	15
Snack Pack Swirl Smores	1 serv (3.5 oz)	136	5	21	18
Snack Pack Tapioca	1 serv (3.5 oz)	125	4	21	15
Snack Pack Toppers Chocolate Fudge w/ Rainbow Sprinkles	1 serv (4 oz)	164	6	25	16
Snack Pack Toppers Chocolate w/ Dinosaurs	1 serv (4 oz)	161	6	25	18
Snack Pack Toppers Chocolate w/ Fun Chips	1 serv (4 oz)	176	6	28	21
Snack Pack Toppers Vanilla w/ Chocolate Sprinkles	1 serv (4 oz)	164	6	26	16
Snack Pack Vanilla	1 serv (3.5 oz)	135	5	21	17
Imagine					
Banana	1 pkg (4 oz)	150	3	30	19
Butterscotch	1 pkg (4 oz)	150	3	31	17
Chocolate	1 pkg (4 oz)	170	3	38	22
Lemon	1 pkg (4 oz)	150	3	33	19

FOOD	PORTION	CAL	FAT	CARB	SUG
Jell-O					
Chocolate	1 serv (4 oz)	160	5	28	23
Chocolate Marshmallow	1 serv (4 oz)	160	5	27	22
Chocolate Vanilla Swirls	1 serv (4 oz)	160	5	27	22
Free Chocolate	1 serv (4 oz)	100	0	23	17
Free Chocolate Vanilla Swirl	1 serv (4 oz)	100	0	23	17
Free Devil's Food	1 serv (4 oz)	100	0	23	18
Free Rocky Road	1 serv (4 oz)	100	0	23	17
Free Vanilla	1 serv (4 oz)	100	0	23	18
Tapioca	1 serv (4 oz)	140	4	26	21
Tapioca	1 serv (4 oz)	100	0	23	17
Vanilla	1 serv (4 oz)	160	5	25	21
Swiss Miss					
Butterscotch	1 pkg (4 oz)	156	6	24	19
Chocolate	1 pkg (4 oz)	166	6	26	23
Chocolate Fudge	1 pkg (4 oz)	175	6	28	22
Fat Free Chocolate	1 pkg (4 oz)	98	tr	22	16
Fat Free Chocolate Fudge	1 pkg (4 oz)	101	tr	23	17
Fat Free Tapioca	1 pkg (4 oz)	98	tr	22	14
Fat Free Vanilla	1 pkg (4 oz)	93	tr	21	14
Fat Free Parfait Vanilla Chocolate	1 pkg (4 oz)	96	tr	21	16
Milk Chocolate	1 pkg (4 oz)	166	6	26	20
Parfait Vanilla Chocolate	1 pkg (4 oz)	164	6	25	22
Swirl Chocolate Caramel	1 pkg (4 oz)	169	6	26	20
Swirl Chocolate Vanilla	1 pkg (4 oz)	169	6	26	21
Swirl Chocolate Vanilla Chocolate	1 pkg (4 oz)	169	6	26	22

FOOD	PORTION	CAL	FAT	CARB	SUG
Tapioca	1 pkg (4 oz)	138	4	24	20
Vanilla	1 pkg (4 oz)	156	6	24	19
take-out					
blancmange	1 serv (4.7 oz)	154	5	25	—
bread pudding	1 serv (6.7 oz)	564	18	94	—
chocolate	½ cup (5.5 oz)	206	4	41	—
queen of puddings	1 serv (4.4 oz)	266	10	41	—
rice pudding	1 serv (3 oz)	110	4	17	—
tapioca	½ cup (5.3 oz)	189	7	26	—
vanilla	½ cup (4.3 oz)	130	4	20	—
yorkshire	1 serv (3 oz)	177	8	22	—
PUDDING POPS					
chocolate	1 (1.6 oz)	72	2	12	10
vanilla	1 (1.6 oz)	75	2	13	11
PUFFERFISH					
raw	3 oz	72	0	0	0
PUMMELO					
fresh	1	228	tr	59	—
PUMPKIN					
canned					
Libby					
Solid Pack	½ cup	40	1	9	4
fresh					
cooked mashed	½ cup	24	tr	6	—
flowers cooked	½ cup	10	tr	2	—
PURSLANE					
cooked	1 cup	21	tr	4	—
QUAHOGS					
(*see* CLAM)					

FOOD	PORTION	CAL	FAT	CARB	SUG
QUICHE					
take-out					
cheese	1 slice (3 oz)	283	20	16	—
lorraine	⅛ of 8 in pie	600	48	29	—
mushroom	1 slice (3 oz)	256	18	17	—
QUINCE					
fresh	1	53	tr	14	—
QUINOA					
quinoa not prep	1 cup (6 oz)	636	10	117	—
RABBIT					
domestic w/o bone roasted	3 oz	167	7	0	0
wild w/o bone stewed	3 oz	147	3	0	0
RACCOON					
roasted	3 oz	217	12	0	0
RADISHES					
fresh					
red raw	10	7	tr	2	—
take-out					
korean kimchee	½ cup	31	1	6	—
moo namul saengche korean salad	1 serv (3.7 oz)	34	tr	8	6
RAISINS					
seedless	1 tbsp	27	tr	7	—
sultanas	1 oz	88	0	23	—
Dole					
CinnaRaisins	1 pkg (1 oz)	95	0	22	20
Estee					
Chocolate Covered	¼ cup	180	6	27	16

FOOD	PORTION	CAL	FAT	CARB	SUG
Mariana					
Fruitn Yogurt Milk Chocolate Covered Raisins	32 pieces (1 oz)	130	5	20	17
Nestle					
Chocolate Covered	1⅛ tbsp	70	3	11	9
Sonoma					
Monukka Thompson	¼ cup (1.4 oz)	130	0	31	29
RASPBERRIES					
fresh	1 cup	61	1	14	—
Birds Eye					
Red	5 oz	90	0	22	22
RASPBERRY JUICE					
Crystal Light					
Raspberry Ice Drink	1 serv (8 oz)	5	0	0	0
Raspberry Ice Drink Mix as prep	1 serv (8 oz)	5	0	0	0
Kool-Aid					
Drink Mix as prep	1 serv (8 oz)	60	0	17	17
Raspberry Drink as prep w/ sugar	1 serv (8 oz)	100	0	25	25
Splash Blue Raspberry Drink	1 serv (8 oz)	120	0	30	30
RED BEANS canned					
Green Giant					
Red Beans	½ cup (4.5 oz)	100	1	19	2
Hunt's					
Small	½ cup (4.5 oz)	89	1	19	4
Van Camp					
Red Beans	½ cup (4.6 oz)	90	0	20	3

FOOD	PORTION	CAL	FAT	CARB	SUG
dried					
Hurst					
HamBeens w/ Ham	1 serv	120	1	20	1
mix					
Bean Cuisine					
Pasta & Beans Barcelona Red With Radiatore	1 serv	210	1	29	2
RELISH					
Claussen					
Sweet Pickle	1 tbsp (0.5 oz)	15	0	3	2
Green Giant					
Corn	1 tbsp (0.6 oz)	20	0	5	2
Vlasic					
Fancy Sweet	1 tbsp	15	0	4	4
RHUBARB					
fresh	½ cup	13	tr	3	—
RICE					
Birds Eye					
Rice & Broccoli In Cheese Sauce	1 pkg	290	9	15	4
White & Wild w/ Green Beans	1 cup (6.6 oz)	180	4	31	2
Carolina					
Red Beans & Rice as prep	¼ pkg	190	1	40	1
Chun King					
Fried Rice Mix	½ cup (1.4 oz)	126	tr	29	5
Goya					
Arroz Amarillo	¼ cup (1.6 oz)	170	0	37	0

FOOD	PORTION	CAL	FAT	CARB	SUG
Green Giant					
Rice & Broccoli	1 pkg (10 oz)	320	12	44	1
Rice Medley	1 pkg (10 oz)	240	3	46	3
Rice Pilaf	1 pkg (10 oz)	230	3	44	3
White & Wild	1 pkg (10 oz)	250	5	45	3
La Choy					
Fried Rice	1 cup (4.9 oz)	236	1	53	6
Lipton					
Oriental Stir Fry as prep	1 cup	270	8	47	2
Rice & Sauce Alfredo Broccoli as prep	1 cup	320	12	46	4
Rice & Sauce Beef as prep	1 cup	270	8	47	1
Rice & Sauce Cajun Style as prep	1 cup	270	7	46	1
Rice & Sauce Cajun Style w/ Beans as prep	1 cup	310	8	52	1
Rice & Sauce Cheddar Broccoli as prep	1 cup	280	9	46	1
Rice & Sauce Chicken & Parmesan Risotto as prep	1 cup	270	9	43	0
Rice & Sauce Chicken Broccoli as prep	1 cup	280	9	46	1
Rice & Sauce Chicken Flavor as prep	1 cup	280	9	45	1

FOOD	PORTION	CAL	FAT	CARB	SUG
Rice & Sauce Creamy Chicken as prep	1 cup	290	11	45	2
Rice & Sauce Herb & Butter as prep	1 cup	280	11	43	0
Rice & Sauce Medley as prep	1 cup	270	9	44	1
Rice & Sauce Mushroom as prep	1 cup	270	8	45	1
Rice & Sauce Mushroom & Herb as prep	1 cup	290	8	49	0
Rice & Sauce Oriental as prep	1 cup	280	8	48	2
Rice & Sauce Pilaf as prep	1 cup	260	11	44	1
Rice & Sauce Scampi Style as prep	1 cup	270	9	44	1
Rice & Sauce Spanish as prep	1 cup	270	8	47	2
Rice & Sauce Teriyaki as prep	1 cup	270	8	45	2
Roasted Chicken as prep	1 cup	260	8	46	1
Salsa Style as prep	1 cup	220	7	37	1
Southwestern Chicken Flavor as prep	1 cup	260	11	47	1
Lundberg					
One-Step Curry	1 cup (7.4 oz)	160	1	38	0
Quick Brown Rice Savory Vegetarian Chicken	1 cup (2.5 oz)	260	3	53	1

FOOD	PORTION	CAL	FAT	CARB	SUG
Risotto Tomato Basil	1 serv	140	1	30	2
Melting Pot					
Risotto Melanese w/ Saffron	1 cup	210	0	48	1
Risotto Primavera	1 cup	200	1	44	3
Risotto Sun-Dried Tomatoes & Peas	1 cup	200	1	45	2
Risotto Three Cheese	1 cup	200	2	44	1
Risotto Wild Mushroom	1 cup	200	1	44	3
Minute					
Boil-In-Bag White as prep	1 cup (5.7 oz)	190	0	42	0
Instant White as prep	1 cup (5.7 oz)	160	0	36	0
Long Grain & Wild Seasoned w/ Herbs as prep	1 cup (7.8 oz)	230	1	50	2
Success					
Brown & Wild Mix as prep	½ cup	120	3	21	1
Van Camp					
Spanish	½ cup (4.5 oz)	90	2	19	5
Zatarain's					
Dirty Rice Mix as prep w/o meat and oil	½ cup	130	0	29	0
Red Beans & Rice as prep w/o oil	½ cup	100	0	21	1
take-out					
nasi goreng indonesian rice & vegetables	1 cup (4.9 oz)	130	0	28	1
paella	1 serv (7 oz)	308	16	17	—
pilaf	½ cup	84	3	11	—

FOOD	PORTION	CAL	FAT	CARB	SUG
risotto	6.6 oz	426	18	65	—
spanish	¾ cup	363	27	19	—
RICE CAKES					
Estee					
Banana Nut	5	60	1	14	0
Cinnamon Spice	5	60	0	14	0
Granny Smith Apple	5	60	0	13	0
Mixed Berry	5	60	0	14	0
Peanut Butter Crunch	5	60	0	13	0
Lundberg					
Organic Koku Sesame	1 (0.7 oz)	80	0	17	tr
Weight Watchers					
Apple Cinnamon	1 oz	110	1	25	8
Butter	1 oz	110	2	21	0
Caramel	1 oz	110	1	24	8
White Cheddar	1 oz	100	1	22	0
ROCKFISH					
pacific cooked	3 oz	103	2	0	0
ROE					
fish	1 oz	11	tr	tr	—
fresh baked	1 oz	58	2	1	—
ROLL					
frozen					
New York					
Garlic	1 (2 oz)	210	10	26	1
Sara Lee					
Deluxe Cinnamon Rolls w/o Icing	1 (2.7 oz)	370	15	41	21
ready-to-eat					
bialy	1 (2.2 oz)	138	0	32	—

FOOD	PORTION	CAL	FAT	CARB	SUG
brioche sweet roll	1 (3.5 oz)	410	23	41	5
hamburger multi-grain	1 (1½ oz)	113	2	19	—
hot cross bun	1	202	4	38	—
hotdog whole wheat	1 (1.5 oz)	110	2	19	2
rye	1 (1 oz)	81	1	15	—
whole wheat	1 (1 oz)	75	1	15	—
Bread Du Jour					
Cracked Wheat	1 (1.2 oz)	100	1	17	2
Italian	1 (1.2 oz)	90	1	16	2
Sourdough	1 (1.2 oz)	90	1	17	1
Freihofer's					
Brown 'N Serve	1 (1 oz)	80	2	13	1
Pepperidge Farm					
Brown & Serve Club	1 (1.6 oz)	120	1	22	1
Dinner Rolls Finger Poppy	1 (0.9 oz)	80	2	12	2
Parker House	1 (0.9 oz)	80	2	13	2
Stroehmann					
Hamburger	1 (1.4 oz)	100	2	21	3
Hamburger Potato	1 (1.9 oz)	140	2	28	5
Hot Dog	1 (1.4 oz)	100	2	21	3
Hot Dog Potato	1 (1.9 oz)	140	2	28	5
Wonder					
Brown & Serve	1 (1 oz)	80	2	13	1
Brown & Serve Sourdough	1 (1 oz)	70	2	13	1
Brown & Serve Wheat	1 (1 oz)	80	2	13	1
Bun	1 (3 oz)	220	3	42	6
Club French	1 (1.6 oz)	120	2	23	2
Club Grain	1 (1.6 oz)	120	2	23	2
Club Sourdough	1 (1.6 oz)	120	2	23	1

FOOD	PORTION	CAL	FAT	CARB	SUG
Dinner	2 (1.6 oz)	130	1	25	3
Dinner Honey Rich	1 (1.3 oz)	100	2	17	3
Dinner Wheat	2 (1.6 oz)	140	3	24	4
Hamburger	1 (2.5 oz)	190	3	36	8
Hamburger	1 (2 oz)	150	2	28	4
Hamburger	1 (2.5 oz)	180	3	32	2
Hamburger	1 (1.5 oz)	110	2	21	3
Hamburger Wheat	1 (1.9 oz)	140	2	24	1
Hamburger Wheat	1 (1.5 oz)	120	2	21	1
Hoagie French	1 (3 oz)	220	3	41	3
Hoagie Grain	1 (3 oz)	220	3	41	4
Hoagie Sourdough	1 (3 oz)	220	3	41	2
Hot Dog	1 (2 oz)	160	3	29	6
Kaiser	1 (2.2 oz)	180	3	33	2
Kaiser Hoagie	1 (3 oz)	220	3	41	3
Multigrain	1 (1.8 oz)	140	2	25	4
Potato Bun	1 (1.5 oz)	110	1	22	3
Steak	1 (2.5 oz)	190	3	36	1
refrigerated					
Pillsbury					
Apple Cinnamon	1 (1.5 oz)	150	6	23	11
Caramel	1 (1.7 oz)	170	7	24	10
Cinnamon w/ Icing	1 (1.5 oz)	150	6	23	10
Cinnamon w/ Icing Reduced Fat	1 (1.5 oz)	140	4	24	10
Cinnamon Raisin w/ Icing	1 (1.7 oz)	170	6	26	11
Cornbread Twists	1 (1.4 oz)	140	6	18	4
Crecents Reduced Fat	1 (1 oz)	100	5	12	3
Crescent	1 (1 oz)	110	6	11	2
Dinner	1 (1.4 oz)	110	2	18	3

FOOD	PORTION	CAL	FAT	CARB	SUG
Dinner Wheat	1 (1.4 oz)	110	2	18	3
Orange Sweet Roll w/ Icing	1 (1.7 oz)	150	7	25	10
ROSE APPLE					
fresh	3.5 oz	32	tr	7	—
ROSE HIP					
fresh	1 oz	26	0	5	—
ROSELLE					
fresh	1 cup	28	tr	6	—
ROSEMARY					
dried	1 tsp	4	tr	1	—
ROUGHY					
orange baked	3 oz	75	1	0	0
RUTABAGA					
cooked mashed	½ cup	41	tr	9	—
SABLEFISH					
baked	3 oz	213	17	0	0
smoked	1 oz	72	6	0	0
SAFFLOWER					
seeds dried	1 oz	147	11	10	—
SAFFRON					
saffron	1 tsp	2	tr	tr	—
SAGE					
ground	1 tsp	2	tr	tr	—
SALAD mix					
Dole					
All American Toss	2 cups (3.5 oz)	50	1	7	4
American Blend	1½ cups (3 oz)	15	0	3	2

FOOD	PORTION	CAL	FAT	CARB	SUG
Classic	1½ cups (3 oz)	15	0	4	2
Classic Romaine Blend	1½ cups (3 oz)	15	0	3	2
Coleslaw	1½ cups (3 oz)	25	0	5	3
European Special Blend	2 cups (3 oz)	15	0	3	2
Garlic Caesar Complete w/ Dressing	1½ cups (3.5 oz)	180	15	8	7
Greek Marinade	1½ cups (3.5 oz)	100	8	5	3
Greener Selection	1½ cups (3 oz)	15	0	3	2
Light Caesar Complete w/ Dressing	1½ cups (3.5 oz)	60	1	10	5
Light Herb Ranch Complete w/ Dressing	1½ cups (3.5 oz)	50	1	10	5
Light Roasted Garlic Caesar Complete w/ Dressing	1½ cups (3.5 oz)	60	1	11	4
Light Zesty Italian Complete w/ Dressing	1½ cups (3.5 oz)	50	1	11	5
Mediterranean Marinade	2 cups (3.5 oz)	90	8	5	3
Oriental Complete w/ Dressing	1½ cups (3.5 oz)	120	6	13	5
Romano Complete w/ Dressing	1½ cups (3.5 oz)	150	12	9	2
Sunflower Ranch Complete w/ Dressing	1½ cups (3.5 oz)	160	16	5	3
Tomato & Mozzarella Medley	2 cups (3.5 oz)	60	2	7	4
Triple Cheese Toss	2 cups (3.5 oz)	80	5	4	2

FOOD	PORTION	CAL	FAT	CARB	SUG
Earthbound Farm					
Baby Caesar Mix	1 pkg (5 oz)	25	0	3	3
Baby Greens w/ Low Fat Honey Dijon Vinaigrette & Tomato Croutons	1 serv (3.5 oz)	90	3	15	6
Caesar w/ Garlic Croutons	1 serv (3.5 oz)	170	15	7	1
Italian Salad Organic	1⅔ cups (2.9 oz)	15	0	3	2
Mixed Baby Greens Organic	1 pkg (4 oz)	30	0	4	0
Organic Baby Greens w/ Vinaigrette & Garlic Croutons	1 serv (3.5 oz)	230	20	11	0
Organic Baby Spinach w/ Sesame Soy Vinaigrette & Peanuts	1 serv (3.5 oz)	150	11	8	4
Organic Italian Salad w/ Blue Cheese Dressing & Walnuts	1 serv (3.5 oz)	190	17	4	2
Romaine Blend Organic	1⅔ cups (2.9 oz)	15	0	3	2
Fresh Express					
Fancy Field Greens	1½ cups (3 oz)	15	0	3	1
Original Iceberg Garden w/ Zip	1½ cups (3 oz)	15	0	3	2
Veggie Lover's	1½ cups (3 oz)	20	0	4	2
Suddenly Salad					
Caesar	¾ cup	220	9	30	3
Caesar Low Fat Recipe	¾ cup	170	3	30	3
Italian Pepperoni	1 cup	190	4	35	7
Italian Pepperoni Low Fat Recipe	1 cup	180	2	35	7

FOOD	PORTION	CAL	FAT	CARB	SUG
Ranch & Bacon	¾ cup	330	20	30	3
Ranch & Bacon Low Fat Recipe	¾ cup	180	2	30	3
Weight Watchers					
Caesar Salad	1 serv (3.5 oz)	60	0	11	1
Caesar Salad w/ Cookies	1 pkg (4.3 oz)	160	3	29	12
European Salad	1 serv (3.5 oz)	60	0	13	9
European Salad w/ Cookies	1 pkg (4.3 oz)	160	3	31	11
Garden Salad	1 serv (3.5 oz)	60	0	12	4
Garden Salad w/ Cookies	1 pkg (4 oz)	120	2	24	10
take-out					
caesar	2 cups (5 oz)	235	20	11	3
chef w/o dressing	1½ cups	386	28	9	—
tossed w/o dressing	1½ cups	32	tr	7	—
tossed w/o dressing w/ cheese & egg	1½ cups	102	6	5	—
tossed w/o dressing w/ chicken	1½ cups	105	2	4	—
tossed w/o dressing w/ pasta & seafood	1½ cups (14.6 oz)	380	21	32	—
tossed w/o dressing w/ shrimp	1½ cups	107	2	7	—
waldorf	½ cup	79	6	6	—

SALAD DRESSING
mix

Et Tu

Caesar Salad Kit	1 serv	140	12	6	0
Good Seasons					
Cheese Garlic as prep	2 tbsp (1 oz)	140	16	1	1

FOOD	PORTION	CAL	FAT	CARB	SUG
Fat Free Honey Mustard as prep	2 tbsp (1.2 oz)	20	0	5	4
Fat Free Italian as prep	2 tbsp (1.1 oz)	10	0	2	3
Fat Free Ranch as prep	2 tbsp (1.2 oz)	20	0	5	4
Fat Free Zesty Herb as prep	2 tbsp (1.1 oz)	10	0	2	1
Garlic & Herbs as prep	2 tbsp (1 oz)	140	15	1	1
Gourmet Caesar as prep	2 tbsp (1.1 oz)	150	16	3	2
Gourmet Parmesan Italian as prep	2 tbsp (1.1 oz)	150	16	2	1
Honey French as prep	2 tbsp (1.2 oz)	160	15	5	4
Honey Mustard as prep	2 tbsp (1.1 oz)	150	15	3	2
Italian as prep	2 tbsp (1 oz)	140	15	1	1
Mexican Spice as prep	2 tbsp (1.1 oz)	140	15	2	1
Mild Italian as prep	2 tbsp (1.1 oz)	150	15	2	2
Oriental Sesame as prep	2 tbsp (1.1 oz)	150	16	3	2
Reduced Calorie Italian as prep	2 tbsp (1 oz)	50	5	2	1
Reduced Calorie Zesty Italian as prep	2 tbsp (1 oz)	50	5	2	1
Roasted Garlic as prep	2 tbsp (1.1 oz)	150	15	2	1
Zesty Italian as prep	2 tbsp (1 oz)	140	15	1	1

FOOD	PORTION	CAL	FAT	CARB	SUG
McCormick					
Mediterrenean Potato Salad	1 tbsp	25	0	4	3
Pasta Salad Vinagarette	1 tsp (5 g)	15	0	2	1
ready-to-eat					
Benecol					
Creamy Italian	2 tbsp	100	10	10	2
French	2 tbsp (0.8 oz)	130	11	6	6
Ranch	2 tbsp	130	13	3	2
Thousand Island	2 tbsp	130	12	5	4
Estee					
Creamy French	2 tbsp (1 oz)	10	0	2	2
Italian	2 tbsp	5	0	1	1
Hellmann's					
Citrus Splash Ruby Red Ginger	2 tbsp (1 oz)	90	7	8	7
Kraft					
⅓ Less Fat Catalina	2 tbsp (1.2 oz)	80	5	9	8
⅓ Less Fat Cucumber Ranch	2 tbsp (1.1 oz)	60	5	2	2
⅓ Less Fat Italian	2 tbsp (1.1 oz)	70	7	3	2
⅓ Less Fat Ranch	2 tbsp (1.1 oz)	110	11	1	1
⅓ Less Fat Thousand Island	2 tbsp (1.2 oz)	70	5	7	5
Bacon & Tomato	2 tbsp (1.1 oz)	140	14	2	2
Buttermilk Ranch	2 tbsp (1.1 oz)	150	16	1	tr
Caesar Italian	2 tbsp (1.1 oz)	100	10	2	1
Caesar Ranch	2 tbsp (1.1 oz)	110	11	1	0
Catalina	2 tbsp (1.1 oz)	120	10	7	7
Catalina With Honey	2 tbsp (1.1 oz)	130	11	7	6
Classic Caesar	2 tbsp (1.1 oz)	110	11	1	0

FOOD	PORTION	CAL	FAT	CARB	SUG
Coleslaw	2 tbsp (1.1 oz)	130	11	7	7
Creamy French	2 tbsp (1.1 oz)	160	15	5	5
Creamy Garlic	2 tbsp (1.1 oz)	110	11	2	2
Creamy Italian	2 tbsp (1.1 oz)	110	11	2	2
Cucumber Ranch	2 tbsp (1.1 oz)	140	15	2	2
Free Blue Cheese	2 tbsp (1.2 oz)	45	0	11	2
Free Caesar Italian	2 tbsp (1.2 oz)	25	0	4	3
Free Catalina	2 tbsp (1.2 oz)	35	0	8	7
Free Classic Caesar	2 tbsp (1.2 oz)	45	0	11	2
Free Creamy Italian	2 tbsp (1.2 oz)	50	0	12	4
Free French	2 tbsp (1.2 oz)	45	0	11	5
Free Garlic Ranch	2 tbsp (1.2 oz)	45	0	11	2
Free Honey Dijon	2 tbsp (1.2 oz)	45	0	10	4
Free Italian	2 tbsp (1.2 oz)	20	0	4	2
Free Peppercorn Ranch	2 tbsp (1.2 oz)	45	0	11	2
Free Ranch	1 tbsp (1.2 oz)	50	0	11	2
Free Red Wine Vinegar	2 tbsp (1.1 oz)	15	0	3	3
Free Thousand Island	2 tbsp (1.2 oz)	40	0	9	5
Garlic Ranch	2 tbsp (1.1 oz)	180	19	1	tr
Herb Vinaigrette	2 tbsp (1.1 oz)	140	15	tr	0
Honey Dijon	2 tbsp (1.1 oz)	110	10	6	4
Honey Mustard	2 tbsp (1.1 oz)	110	10	6	4
House Italian w/ Olive Oil Blend	2 tbsp (1.1 oz)	120	12	2	2
Peppercorn Ranch	2 tbsp (1 oz)	170	18	1	1
Pesto Italian	2 tbsp (1.1 oz)	90	9	2	1
Ranch	2 tbsp (1 oz)	170	18	1	1
Roka Blue Cheese	2 tbsp (1.1 oz)	130	13	2	tr

FOOD	PORTION	CAL	FAT	CARB	SUG
Russian	2 tbsp (1.2 oz)	130	10	10	10
Sour Cream & Onion Ranch	2 tbsp (1 oz)	170	18	1	1
Thousand Island	2 tbsp (1.1 oz)	110	10	5	4
Thousand Island With Bacon	2 tbsp (1.1 oz)	130	12	5	5
Tomato & Herb Italian	2 tbsp (1.1 oz)	100	9	3	3
Zesty Italian	2 tbsp (1.1 oz)	110	11	2	1
LaMartinique					
Blue Cheese Vinaigrette	2 tbsp	160	17	0	0
Poppy Seed	2 tbsp	170	15	8	7
Newman's Own					
Balsamic Vinaigrette	2 tbsp (1.1 oz)	90	9	3	1
Caesar	2 tbsp (1.1 oz)	150	16	1	1
Light Italian	2 tbsp (1.1 oz)	20	1	3	2
Olive Oil & Vinegar	2 tbsp (1 oz)	150	16	1	1
Ranch	2 tbsp (1 oz)	180	19	2	1
Old Dutch					
Sweet & Sour	2 tbsp	50	0	13	13
Seven Seas					
⅓ Less Fat Creamy Italian	2 tbsp (1.1 oz)	60	5	2	2
⅓ Less Fat Italian w/ Olive Oil Blend	2 tbsp (1.1 oz)	45	4	2	2
⅓ Less Fat Ranch	2 tbsp (1.1 oz)	100	9	5	2
⅓ Less Fat Red Wine Vinegar & Oil	2 tbsp (1.1 oz)	45	4	3	2
⅓ Less Fat Viva Italian	2 tbsp (1.1 oz)	45	4	2	1
2 Cheese Italian	2 tbsp (1.1 oz)	70	7	3	2
Chunky Blue Cheese	2 tbsp (1.1 oz)	130	13	2	tr

FOOD	PORTION	CAL	FAT	CARB	SUG
Classic Caesar	2 tbsp (1.1 oz)	100	10	2	1
Creamy Italian	2 tbsp (1.1 oz)	120	12	1	1
Free Ranch	2 tbsp (1.2 oz)	45	0	11	2
Free Red Wine Vinegar	2 tbsp (1.1 oz)	15	0	3	3
Free Sour Cream & Onion Ranch	2 tbsp (1.2 oz)	50	0	11	3
Free Viva Italian	2 tbsp (1.1 oz)	10	0	2	1
Green Goddess	2 tbsp (1.1 oz)	130	13	1	tr
Herbs & Spices	2 tbsp (1.1 oz)	90	9	1	1
Ranch	2 tbsp (1.1 oz)	160	17	2	1
Red Wine Vinegar & Oil	2 tbsp (1.1 oz)	90	9	2	2
Viva Italian	2 tbsp (1.1 oz)	90	9	2	1
Viva Russian	2 tbsp (1.1 oz)	150	16	3	2
Weight Watchers					
Fat Free Caesar	1 pkg (0.75 oz)	5	0	1	1
Fat Free Caesar	2 tbsp	10	0	1	1
Fat Free Creamy Italian	2 tbsp	30	0	7	2
Fat Free French Style	2 tbsp	40	0	9	6
Fat Free Honey Dijon	2 tbsp	45	0	11	6
Fat Free Italian	2 tbsp	10	0	2	1
Fat Free Ranch	1 pkg (0.75 oz)	25	0	6	2
Fat Free Ranch	2 tbsp	35	0	7	3
Wishbone					
Caesar	2 tbsp (1 oz)	90	10	2	2
Chunky Blue Cheese	2 tbsp (1 oz)	150	17	3	1
Classic House Italian	2 tbsp (1 oz)	140	14	2	1
Classic Olive Oil Italian	2 tbsp (1 oz)	60	5	4	3
Creamy Caesar	2 tbsp (1 oz)	180	18	1	1
Creamy Italian	2 tbsp (1 oz)	110	10	4	1
Creamy Roasted Garlic	2 tbsp (1 oz)	110	10	3	3

FOOD	PORTION	CAL	FAT	CARB	SUG
Deluxe French	2 tbsp (1 oz)	120	11	5	4
Fat Free Chunky Blue Cheese	2 tbsp (1 oz)	35	0	7	1
Fat Free Creamy Italian	2 tbsp (1 oz)	35	0	9	3
Fat Free Creamy Roasted Garlic	2 tbsp (1 oz)	40	0	9	3
Fat Free Deluxe French	2 tbsp (1 oz)	30	0	7	6
Fat Free Honey Dijon	2 tbsp (1 oz)	45	0	10	9
Fat Free Italian	2 tbsp (1 oz)	10	0	2	1
Fat Free Parmesan & Onion	2 tbsp (1 oz)	45	0	9	2
Fat Free Ranch	2 tbsp (1 oz)	40	0	9	2
Fat Free Red Wine Vinaigrette	2 tbsp (1 oz)	35	0	7	6
Fat Free Sweet N' Spicy French	2 tbsp (1 oz)	30	0	7	6
Fat Free Thousand Island	2 tbsp (1 oz)	35	0	9	6
Italian	2 tbsp (1 oz)	80	8	3	2
Lite French	2 tbsp (1 oz)	50	2	8	7
Lite Italian	2 tbsp (1 oz)	15	1	2	1
Lite Ranch	2 tbsp (1 oz)	100	8	5	1
Olive Oil Vinaigrette	2 tbsp (1 oz)	60	5	4	3
Oriental	2 tbsp (1 oz)	70	5	5	3
Parmesan & Onion	2 tbsp (1 oz)	110	10	5	1
Ranch	2 tbsp (1 oz)	160	17	1	1
Red Wine Vinaigrette	2 tbsp (1 oz)	80	5	9	8
Robusto Italian	2 tbsp (1 oz)	90	8	4	3
Russian	2 tbsp (1 oz)	110	6	15	7
Sweet N' Spicy French	2 tbsp (1 oz)	140	12	6	5

FOOD	PORTION	CAL	FAT	CARB	SUG
SALMON					
canned					
Bumble Bee					
Keta	½ cup (3.5 oz)	160	8	0	0
Red	½ cup (3.5 oz)	180	10	0	0
fresh					
atlantic baked	3 oz	155	7	0	0
coho cooked	3 oz	157	6	0	0
roe raw	1 oz	59	3	tr	—
smoked					
Lascco					
Nova Sliced	2 oz	60	1	3	0
take-out					
roulette w/ spinach stuffing	1 serv (4 oz)	160	6	10	0
salmon cake	1 (3 oz)	241	15	6	—
SALSA					
black bean & corn	2 tbsp (1 oz)	15	0	3	1
citrus	2 tbsp (1 oz)	10	0	2	2
Chi-Chi's					
Con Queso	2 tbsp (1.1 oz)	90	7	4	3
Hot	2 tbsp (1 oz)	10	0	2	1
Medium	2 tbsp (1 oz)	10	0	2	1
Mild	2 tbsp (1 oz)	10	0	1	1
Picante Hot	2 tbsp (1 oz)	10	0	2	2
Picante Medium	2 tbsp (1 oz)	10	0	2	2
Picante Mild	2 tbsp (1 oz)	10	0	2	2
Verde Medium	2 tbsp (1.2 oz)	15	0	3	2
Verde Mild	2 tbsp (1.2 oz)	15	0	3	2

FOOD	PORTION	CAL	FAT	CARB	SUG
Guiltless Gourmet					
Roasted Red Pepper	2 tbsp (1 oz)	10	0	2	1
Southwestern Grill	2 tbsp (1 oz)	10	0	2	1
Hunt's					
Alfresco All Varieties	2 tbsp (1.1 oz)	10	tr	2	2
Hot	2 tbsp (1.1 oz)	27	tr	6	1
Medium	2 tbsp (1.1 oz)	27	tr	6	1
Mild	2 tbsp (1.1 oz)	27	tr	6	1
Picante All Varieties	2 tbsp (1.1 oz)	11	tr	2	1
Squeeze Mild & Medium	2 tbsp (1.1 oz)	27	tr	6	2
Muir Glen					
Black Bean & Corn Medium	2 tbsp (1.1 oz)	15	0	3	1
Chipotle Medium	2 tbsp (1.1 oz)	10	0	2	1
Fire Roasted Tomato Medium	2 tbsp (1.1 oz)	10	0	2	1
Garlic Cilantro Medium	2 tbsp (1.1 oz)	10	0	2	1
Habanero Hot	2 tbsp (1.1 oz)	10	0	2	1
Organic Medium	2 tbsp (1.1 oz)	10	0	2	1
Organic Mild	2 tbsp (1.1 oz)	10	0	2	1
Roasted Garlic Medium	2 tbsp (1.1 oz)	10	0	2	1
Newman's Own					
Bandito Hot	2 tbsp (1.1 oz)	10	0	2	1
Bandito Medium	2 tbsp (1.1 oz)	10	0	2	1
Bandito Mild	2 tbsp (1.1 oz)	10	0	2	1
Peach	2 tbsp (1.1 oz)	25	0	6	5
Pineapple	2 tbsp (1.1 oz)	15	0	3	3
Roasted Garlic	2 tbsp (1.1 oz)	10	0	2	1

FOOD	PORTION	CAL	FAT	CARB	SUG
Pace					
Picante Mild or Medium	2 tbsp	10	0	2	1
Thick & Chunky Mild or Medium	2 tbsp	10	0	2	1
Rosarita					
Extra Chunky Medium	2 tbsp (1 oz)	7	tr	1	1
Green Tomatillo Medium	2 tbsp (1 oz)	8	tr	2	2
Picante Zesty Jalapeno Hot	2 tbsp (1 oz)	8	tr	2	1
Picante Zesty Jalapeno Medium	2 tbsp (1 oz)	9	tr	2	1
Picante Zesty Jalapeno Mild	2 tbsp (1 oz)	8	tr	2	1
Roasted Mild	2 tbsp (1 oz)	10	tr	2	1
Traditional Medium	2 tbsp (1 oz)	7	tr	2	1
Traditional Mild	2 tbsp (1 oz)	7	tr	1	1
Snyder's Of Hanover					
Mild	2 tbsp	10	0	2	2
Taco Bell					
Smooth 'N Zesty Picante Medium	2 tbsp (1.1 oz)	15	0	3	2
Smooth 'N Zesty Picante Mild	2 tbsp (1.1 oz)	15	0	3	2
Thick 'N Chunky Salsa Hot	2 tbsp (1.1 oz)	15	0	2	2
Thick 'N Chunky Salsa Medium	2 tbsp (1.1 oz)	15	0	2	2
Thick 'N Chunky Salsa Mild	2 tbsp (1.1 oz)	15	0	3	2
Tostitos					
Con Queso	2.3 oz	80	5	10	tr
Hot	2.3 oz	30	0	6	2

FOOD	PORTION	CAL	FAT	CARB	SUG
Low Fat Con Queso	2.5 oz	80	3	8	tr
Medium	2.3 oz	30	0	6	2
Mild	2.3 oz	30	0	6	2
Restaurant Style	2.2 oz	30	0	6	2
Ultimate Garden	2.4 oz	30	0	6	2
Utz					
Chunky	2 tbsp (1 fl oz)	60	0	14	4

SALSIFY

fresh sliced cooked	½ cup	46	tr	10	—

SALT SUBSTITUTES

Estee					
Salt-It	¼ tsp	0	0	0	0
Halsosalt					
All Flavors	¼ tsp (7 g)	1	0	0	0
Morton					
Salt Substitute	¼ tsp (1.2 g)	tr	0	tr	—
NoSalt					
Salt Alternative	1 pkg (0.75 g)	0	0	0	0

SALT/SEASONED SALT

salt	1 tsp (6 g)	0	0	0	0
Morton					
Lite	¼ tsp (1.4 g)	tr	0	tr	—

SANDWICHES
frozen

Healthy Choice					
Bread Stuffs Chicken & Broccoli	1 (6.1 oz)	310	4	50	11
Bread Stuffs Ham & Cheese w/ Broccoli	1 (6.1 oz)	320	5	46	10
Bread Stuffs Italian Style Meatball	1 (6.1 oz)	330	5	52	12

FOOD	PORTION	CAL	FAT	CARB	SUG
Bread Stuffs Philly Beef Steak	1 (6.1 oz)	310	5	50	10
take-out					
chicken fillet plain	1	515	29	39	—
chicken fillet w/ cheese lettuce mayonnaise & tomato	1	632	39	42	—
croque monsieur	1 (12.4 oz)	765	46	43	9
fish fillet w/ tartar sauce	1	431	55	41	—
fish fillet w/ tartar sauce & cheese	1	524	29	48	—
fried egg w/ cheese	1	340	19	26	—
fried egg w/ cheese & ham	1	348	16	31	—
ham w/ cheese	1	353	15	33	—
roast beef submarine sandwich w/ tomato lettuce & mayonnaise	1	411	13	44	—
roast beef w/ cheese	1	402	18	27	—
roast beef plain	1	346	14	33	—
steak w/ tomato lettuce salt & mayonnaise	1	459	14	52	—
submarine w/ salami ham cheese lettuce tomato onion & oil	1	456	19	51	—
tuna salad submarine sandwich w/ lettuce & oil	1	584	28	55	—
SAPODILLA					
fresh	1	140	2	34	—

FOOD	PORTION	CAL	FAT	CARB	SUG
SAPOTES					
fresh	1	301	1	76	—
SARDINES					
canned					
Bumble Bee					
In Hot Sauce	½ can (2 oz)	109	8	tr	tr
In Mustard	½ can (2 oz)	88	5	1	tr
In Oil	½ can (2 oz)	125	7	0	0
In Water	½ can (2 oz)	83	3	0	0
SAUCE					
jarred					
fish sauce chinese	1 tbsp	9	0	tr	—
fish sauce vietnamese nuoc mam	1 tbsp	6	0	1	—
hoisin	1 tbsp	35	1	7	—
oyster	1 tbsp	8	0	2	—
Armour					
Chili Hot Dog	¼ cup (2.2 oz)	120	9	5	2
Meatless Sloppy Joe Sauce	¼ cup (2.2 oz)	30	0	7	6
Boar's Head					
Ham Glaze Brown Sugar & Spice	2 tbsp (1.4 oz)	120	0	30	29
Cheez Whiz					
Cheese	2 tbsp (1.2 oz)	90	7	3	tr
Cheese Jalapeno Pepper	2 tbsp (1.2 oz)	90	7	3	2
Cheese Mild Salsa	2 tbsp (1.2 oz)	100	7	3	2
Chi-Chi's					
Enchilada	¼ cup (2.1 oz)	30	2	3	0
Taco	1 tbsp (0.5 oz)	10	0	1	1

FOOD	PORTION	CAL	FAT	CARB	SUG
Chun King					
Sweet And Sour	2 tbsp (1.2 oz)	58	tr	14	14
Teriyaki	1 tbsp (0.6 oz)	17	tr	3	2
Teriyaki Hot	1 tbsp (0.6 oz)	17	tr	3	2
Fritos					
Texas-Style Chili Hearty Topping	2.3 oz	50	2	8	2
Utimate Taco Hearty Topping	2.3 oz	50	2	8	2
Gebhardt					
Enchilada Sauce	¼ cup (2.2 oz)	35	2	4	0
Hot Dog Chili Sauce	¼ cup (2.2 oz)	60	3	6	0
Hot Sauce	1 tsp (5 g)	1	tr	tr	0
Green Giant					
Sloppy Joe	¼ cup (2.6 oz)	50	0	11	8
Sloppy Joe as prep w/ meat	1 serv (4.4 oz)	200	11	11	8
Hormel					
Not-So-Sloppy-Joe Sauce	¼ cup (2.2 oz)	70	0	15	3
House Of Tsang					
Bangkok Padang	1 tbsp (0.6 oz)	45	3	4	3
Hoisin	1 tsp (6 g)	15	0	4	3
Mandarin Marinade	1 tbsp (0.6 oz)	25	0	6	5
Saigon Sizzle	1 tbsp (0.6 oz)	40	1	8	6
Spicy Brown Bean	1 tsp (6 g)	15	0	3	3
Stir Fry Classic	1 tbsp (0.6 oz)	25	1	4	3
Stir Fry Sweet & Sour	1 tbsp (0.6 oz)	30	0	7	6
Stir Fry Szechuan Spicy	1 tbsp (0.6 oz)	20	1	4	3
Sweet & Sour Concentrate	1 tsp (6 g)	10	0	3	2
Teriyaki Korean	1 tbsp (0.6 oz)	30	1	6	4

FOOD	PORTION	CAL	FAT	CARB	SUG
Hunt's					
Light w/ Mushrooms	½ cup (4.4 oz)	42	tr	8	5
Steak	1 tbsp (0.6 oz)	10	tr	2	2
Just Rite					
Hot Dog	¼ cup (2.2 oz)	50	3	5	0
Kraft					
Cocktail	¼ cup (2.3 oz)	60	1	13	9
Fat Free Tartar Sauce	2 tbsp (1.1 oz)	25	0	5	4
Lemon & Herb Tartar Sauce	2 tbsp (1 oz)	150	16	tr	tr
Reduced Fat Sandwich Spread	1 tbsp (0.5 oz)	35	3	3	3
Sandwich Spread	1 tbsp (0.5 oz)	50	4	3	2
Sweet'n Sour	2 tbsp (1.2 oz)	60	0	14	12
Tartar	2 tbsp (1.1 oz)	90	9	4	0
La Choy					
Duck Sauce Sweet & Sour	2 tbsp (1.3 oz)	61	tr	15	15
Sweet & Sour	2 tbsp (1.2 oz)	58	tr	14	14
Teriyaki	1 tbsp (0.6 oz)	17	tr	3	2
Manwich					
BBQ Sloppy Joe	¼ cup (2.2 oz)	57	tr	14	10
Bold	¼ cup (2.2 oz)	62	1	13	11
Mexican	¼ cup (2.2 oz)	27	tr	5	5
Original	¼ cup (2.2 oz)	32	tr	6	5
Taco Season	¼ cup (2.2 oz)	27	tr	6	4
Thick & Chunky	¼ cup (2.3 oz)	44	tr	9	7
McCormick					
Flavor Medleys Garlic & Herb	2 tbsp	50	5	5	4
Flavor Medleys Italian Herb	2 tbsp	50	4	4	3

FOOD	PORTION	CAL	FAT	CARB	SUG
Flavor Medleys Lemon Pepper	2 tbsp	50	4	4	3
Flavor Medleys Tomato & Basil	2 tbsp	50	3	4	3
Newman's Own					
Spicy Simmer Sauce Diavolo	½ cup (4.4 oz)	70	3	10	4
Open Range					
Hot Dog Chili	¼ cup (2.2 oz)	61	3	6	1
Pace					
Enchilada Sauce	¼ cup	36	0	6	4
Taco Sauce	¼ cup	32	2	4	2
Progresso					
Alfredo	½ cup (4.4 oz)	200	15	7	2
Sauce Arturo					
Original	¼ cup (2.2 fl oz)	50	1	8	4
Tabasco					
Caribbean Steak Sauce	1 tbsp (0.6 oz)	15	0	4	3
Garlic Basting Sauce	1 tbsp (0.6 oz)	20	0	4	4
Habanero Sauce	1 tsp (0.2 oz)	5	0	1	tr
Hot Sauce w/ Garlic	1 tsp (0.2 oz)	0	0	0	0
Jalapeno Pepper Sauce	1 tbsp	15	0	3	0
New Orleans Steak Sauce	1 tbsp (0.6 oz)	15	0	4	3
Pepper Sauce	1 tsp (0.2 oz)	0	0	0	0
Taco Bell					
Taco Sauce Medium	2 tbsp (1.1 oz)	15	0	3	1
Taco Sauce Mild	2 tbsp (1.1 oz)	15	0	3	1
The Restaurant Hot Sauce	1 tsp (5 g)	0	0	0	0

FOOD	PORTION	CAL	FAT	CARB	SUG
Tostitos					
Beef Fiesta Nacho	2.4 oz	120	8	6	2
Chicken Quesadilla Topping	2.5 oz	90	6	6	2
mix					
Durkee					
A La King as prep	1 cup	60	4	8	2
Cheese as prep	¼ cup	25	2	4	0
Hollandaise as prep	2 tbsp	10	0	2	0
White as prep	¼ cup	20	1	5	0
French's					
Cheese as prep	¼ cup	25	1	4	0
Hollandaise as prep	2 tbsp	10	0	2	0
Manwich					
Mix	¼ oz	22	tr	5	0
McCormick					
Chicken Dijon Blend	1⅔ tbsp (10 g)	40	2	5	1
Green Peppercorn Blend as prep	¼ cup	20	0	3	1
Grill Mates Mesquite Marinade as prep	1 tbsp	15	0	2	2
Hunter Blend as prep	¼ cup	25	0	4	1
Meat Marinade	1 tsp (4 g)	15	0	2	tr
Pepper Medley Blend as prep	¼ cup	30	2	3	tr
shelf-stable					
Cheez Whiz					
Cheese Sqeezable	2 tbsp (1.2 oz)	100	8	4	1
take-out					
bearnaise	1 oz	177	19	1	—

FOOD	PORTION	CAL	FAT	CARB	SUG
SAUERKRAUT					
B&G					
Sauerkraut	2 tbsp (1 oz)	6	0	1	0
Boar's Head					
Sauerkraut	2 tbsp (1 oz)	5	0	1	0
Claussen					
Sauerkraut	¼ cup (1.1 oz)	5	0	1	0
SAUSAGE					
chipolata	3.5 oz	342	32	1	1
chorizo	3.5 oz	499	45	4	4
Armour					
Vienna Sausage 25% Less Fat	3 (1.9 oz)	130	11	1	0
Vienna Sausage 50% Less Fat	3 (1.9 oz)	90	7	1	1
Vienna Sausage Chicken & Beef	3 (1.9 oz)	120	10	1	1
Vienna Sausage Hot'n Spicy	3 (2.1 oz)	150	13	2	0
Vienna Sausage In BBQ Sauce	3 (2.1 oz)	150	13	3	3
Vienna Sausage In Beef Stock	3 (1.9 oz)	150	14	0	0
Vienna Sausage Jalapeno In Beef Stock	3 (1.9 oz)	170	16	1	0
Banner					
Sausage Stomachs	2 oz	90	5	0	0
Sausage Tripe	2 oz	90	5	2	0
Boar's Head					
Bratwurst	1 (4 oz)	300	25	0	0
Hot Smoked	1 (3.2 oz)	280	25	1	0

FOOD	PORTION	CAL	FAT	CARB	SUG
Kielbasa	2 oz	120	10	0	0
Knockwurst	1 (4 oz)	310	27	1	0
Brown'N Serve					
Turkey	3 (2.1 oz)	120	8	2	1
Hormel					
Light & Lean 97 Dinner Smoked	2 oz	60	2	2	2
Pickled Hot	6 (2 oz)	140	11	1	1
Pickled Smoked	6 (2 oz)	140	11	1	1
Smoked Summer	2 oz	200	18	2	2
Vienna	2 oz	140	14	0	0
Vienna Chicken	2 oz	110	9	1	0
Little Sizzlers					
Brown & Serve	3 links (2.1 oz)	190	22	1	1
Brown & Serve	2 patties (1.8 oz)	190	18	1	1
Cooked	2 patties (1.8 oz)	230	22	0	0
Cooked	3 links (1.8 oz)	230	22	0	0
Heat & Serve Pork cooked	3 links (1.8 oz)	230	22	0	0
Louis Rich					
Polska Kielbasa	2 oz	90	5	2	tr
Turkey Hot	2.5 oz	120	8	1	0
Turkey Original	2.5 oz	120	8	1	0
Turkey Smoked	2 oz	90	5	2	1
Old Smokehouse					
Summer Sausage	2 oz	200	18	2	2
Oscar Mayer					
Pork cooked	2 links (1.7 oz)	170	15	1	0
Smokies Beef	1 (1.5 oz)	120	11	1	tr
Smokies Cheese	1 (1.5 oz)	130	12	1	tr
Smokies Link	1 (1.5 oz)	130	12	1	tr

FOOD	PORTION	CAL	FAT	CARB	SUG
Smokies Little	6 (2 oz)	170	15	1	tr
Smokies Little Cheese	6 (2 oz)	180	16	1	0
Wampler					
Breakfast Turkey	2 (2.4 oz)	110	6	1	1
Italian Turkey	1 (2.7 oz)	120	6	1	1

SAUSAGE DISHES
take-out

FOOD	PORTION	CAL	FAT	CARB	SUG
italian sausage w/ peppers & onions	1 cup	210	11	14	—
sausage roll	1 (2.3 oz)	311	24	22	—

SAUSAGE SUBSTITUTES

FOOD	PORTION	CAL	FAT	CARB	SUG
Boca Burgers					
Breakfast Patties	1 (1.3 oz)	70	3	4	1
GardenSausage					
Patty	1 (2.5 oz)	140	3	20	2
Lightlife					
Gimme Lean	2 oz	70	0	8	1
Lean Links Breakfast	1 (1.2 oz)	60	3	4	1
Lean Links Italian	1 (1.4 oz)	60	2	5	1
Light	2 patties (2.3 oz)	80	0	10	1
Loma Linda					
Linketts	1 (1.2 oz)	70	5	1	0
Little Links	2 (1.6 oz)	90	6	2	0
Morningstar Farms					
Breakfast Links	2 (1.6 oz)	60	2	2	0
Breakfast Patties	1 (1.3 oz)	80	3	3	tr
Grillers	1 patty (2.2 oz)	140	7	5	tr
Sausage Style Recipe Crumbles	⅔ cup (1.9 oz)	90	3	5	tr
Natural Touch					
Vegan Sausage Crumbles	½ cup (1.9 oz)	60	0	4	0

FOOD	PORTION	CAL	FAT	CARB	SUG
Worthington					
Leanies	1 link (1.4 oz)	100	7	2	tr
Prosage Links	2 (1.6 oz)	60	3	2	0
Saucettes	1 link (1.3 oz)	90	6	1	0
Super Links	1 (1.7 oz)	110	8	2	0
Veja Links	1 (1.1 oz)	50	3	1	0
Yves					
Veggie Breakfast Links	1 (1.6 oz)	60	0	3	1
Veggie Breakfast Patties	1 (2 oz)	70	2	4	1
SAVORY					
ground	1 tsp	4	tr	1	—
SCALLOP					
take-out					
breaded & fried	2 lg	67	3	3	—
SCONE					
Finnegan's					
Cranberry	1 (2.7 oz)	90	2	20	1
Health Valley					
Apple Kiwi	1	180	0	43	18
Cinnamon Raisin	1	180	0	43	18
Cranberry Orange	1	180	0	43	18
Mountain Blueberry	1	180	0	43	18
Pineapple Banana	1	180	0	43	18
take-out					
cheese	1 (1.75 oz)	182	9	22	—
fruit	1 (1.75 oz)	158	5	27	—
orange poppy	1 (3 oz)	260	6	47	12
plain	1 (1.75 oz)	181	7	27	—
raisin	1 (3 oz)	270	6	50	15

FOOD	PORTION	CAL	FAT	CARB	SUG
SCUP					
fresh baked	3 oz	115	3	0	0
SEA BASS					
(see BASS)					
SEA CUCUMBER					
dried	1 oz	74	1	1	—
fresh	1 oz	20	tr	tr	—
SEA TROUT					
(see TROUT)					
SEA URCHIN					
canned	1 oz	39	1	3	—
fresh	1 oz	36	1	3	—
roe paste	1 tbsp	19	tr	3	—
SEAWEED					
agar dried	1 oz	87	tr	23	—
agar fresh	1 oz	tr	tr	2	—
hijiki dried	1 tbsp	9	0	2	—
irishmoss fresh	1 oz	14	tr	4	—
kelp fresh	1 oz	12	tr	3	—
kombu fresh	1 oz	12	tr	3	—
laver fresh	1 oz	10	tr	1	—
nori fresh	1 oz	10	tr	1	—
nori sheet dried	1 (8 x 8 in)	5	0	1	—
seahair dried	1 tbsp	13	0	3	—
spirulina dried	1 oz	83	2	7	—
spirulina fresh	1 oz	7	tr	1	—
tangle fresh	1 oz	12	tr	3	—
wakame fresh	1 oz	13	tr	3	—

FOOD	PORTION	CAL	FAT	CARB	SUG
SEITAN					
(see WHEAT)					
SESAME					
seeds	1 tsp	16	2	tr	—
SESBANIA					
flowers cooked	1 cup	23	tr	5	—
SHAD					
american baked	3 oz	214	15	0	0
roe baked w/ butter & lemon	1 oz	36	1	tr	—
SHARK					
batter-dipped & fried	3 oz	194	12	5	—
SHEEPSHEAD FISH					
cooked	3 oz	107	1	0	0
SHELLFISH					
(see individual names and SHELLFISH SUBSTITUTES)					
SHELLFISH SUBSTITUTES					
Louis Kemp					
Crab Delights	½ cup (3 oz)	90	0	12	8
Lobster Delights	½ cup (3 oz)	80	0	12	4
Scallop Delights	13 pieces (3 oz)	80	0	12	3
SHELLIE BEANS					
canned	½ cup	37	tr	8	—
SHERBET					
Breyers					
Fat Free Orange	½ cup (3 oz)	110	0	27	21
Fat Free Rainbow	½ cup (3 oz)	110	0	28	21
Fat Free Raspberry	½ cup (3 oz)	120	0	28	22

FOOD	PORTION	CAL	FAT	CARB	SUG
Fat Free Tropical	½ cup (3 oz)	110	0	27	21
Orange	½ cup (3 oz)	120	1	26	19
Rainbow	½ cup (3 oz)	120	2	27	21
Raspberry	½ cup (3 oz)	120	2	28	21
Tropical	½ cup (3 oz)	120	1	27	21
SHRIMP					
canned	1 cup	154	3	1	—
chinese shrimp pasta	1 tbsp	15	tr	1	—
cooked	4 large	22	tr	0	0
Bumble Bee					
Medium	⅛ can (2 oz)	45	tr	0	1
Orleans Tiny Cocktail	½ can (3 oz)	44	0	0	1
Gorton's					
Popcorn Garlic & Herb	22 pieces (3.6 oz)	270	14	24	3
Popcorn Original	20 pieces (3.2 oz)	240	13	22	1
take-out					
breaded & fried	3 oz	206	10	10	—
jambalaya	¾ cup	188	5	26	—
SMELT					
rainbow cooked	3 oz	106	3	0	0
SNACKS					
Baken-ets					
BBQ	9 (0.5 oz)	70	5	tr	0
Hot N'Spicy	7 (0.5 oz)	70	5	tr	0
Hot N'Spicy Cracklins	8 (0.5 oz)	80	5	tr	0
Regular	9 (0.5 oz)	80	5	tr	0
Regular Cracklins	8 (0.5 oz)	40	6	tr	0

FOOD	PORTION	CAL	FAT	CARB	SUG
Barbara's Bakery					
Cheese Puffs Bakes	1½ cups (1 oz)	160	11	13	1
Cheese Puffs Jalapeno	¾ cup (1 oz)	150	10	16	0
Cheese Puffs Original	¾ cup (1 oz)	150	10	16	0
Bugles					
Baked Cheddar Cheese	1½ cups (1 oz)	130	4	23	2
Baked Original	1½ cups (1 oz)	130	4	23	2
Baked Original	1 pkg (1.4 oz)	170	5	30	3
Nacho	1⅓ cups (1 oz)	160	9	18	1
Nacho	1 pkg (0.9 oz)	130	7	15	1
Original	1 pkg (1.5 oz)	230	13	25	1
Original	1⅓ cups (1 oz)	160	9	18	1
Ranch	1⅓ cups (1 oz)	160	9	18	2
Smokin BBQ	1⅓ cups (1 oz)	150	8	19	2
Sour Cream & Onion	1⅓ cups (1 oz)	160	9	18	1
Cheetos					
Crunchy	21 pieces (1 oz)	160	10	15	1
Curls	15 pieces (1 oz)	150	10	15	1
Flamin' Hot	21 pieces (1 oz)	160	10	15	1
Nacho Cheese	23 pieces (1 oz)	160	10	15	0
Puffed Balls	38 pieces (1 oz)	150	10	15	1
Puffs	29 pieces (1 oz)	160	10	15	tr
Zig Zags	17 pieces (1 oz)	170	11	17	tr
Chex Mix					
Bold'n Zesty	1 pkg (1.7 oz)	230	9	33	3
Cheddar Cheese	1 pkg (1.7 oz)	220	9	33	4
Hot'n Spicy	1 pkg (1.7 oz)	210	7	35	3
Traditional	1 pkg (1.7 oz)	210	7	35	3
Dakota Gourmet					
Heart Smart Toasted Corn	⅓ cup (1 oz)	110	2	22	0

FOOD	PORTION	CAL	FAT	CARB	SUG
Toasted Corn Heart Smart	1 pkg (1.75 oz)	177	3	39	0
Trail Mix Heart Smart	1 pkg (1.75 oz)	172	0	39	25
Frito Lay					
Funyuns	13 (1 oz)	140	7	18	tr
Munchos	16 (1 oz)	160	10	16	0
Munchos BBQ	14 (1 oz)	160	10	15	2
Health Valley					
Cheddar Lites Green Onion	1¾ cups	120	3	21	1
Cheddar Lites Original	1¾ cups	120	3	21	1
Corn Puffs Caramel	2 cups	120	2	25	7
Low Fat Potato Puffs Cheddar Cheese	1½ cups	110	3	21	1
Low Fat Potato Puffs Garlic w/ Cheese	1½ cups	260	3	21	1
Low Fat Potato Puffs Zesty Ranch	1½ cups	110	3	21	1
Lance					
Cheese Balls	1 pkg (1 oz)	150	8	16	1
Crunchy Cheese Twists	1 pkg (1.25 oz)	100	4	15	0
Gold-N-Chees	1 pkg (1 oz)	130	5	18	0
Onion Rings	1 pkg (0.9 oz)	100	8	7	1
Pork Skins	1 pkg (0.4 oz)	65	4	1	0
Pork Skins BBQ	1 pkg (0.4 oz)	60	4	1	0
Old Dutch Foods					
Baked Cheese Curls	2 cups (1.1 oz)	180	12	15	1
Cheese Puffcorn Curls	2 cups (1.1 oz)	170	12	15	1
Planters					
Cheez Mania Original	42 pieces (1 oz)	150	10	15	tr

FOOD	PORTION	CAL	FAT	CARB	SUG
Robert's American Gourmet					
Pirate's Booty Puffed Rice & Corn w/ Cheddar	1 oz	120	3	22	0
Rold Gold					
Snack Mix Colossal Cheddar	1 pkg (1 oz)	140	7	17	2
Snyder's Of Hanover					
Cheese Twists	1 oz	230	14	10	0
Fried Pork Skins	1 oz	80	4	1	0
Fried Pork Skins Barbecue	1 oz	80	4	1	0
Kruncheez	1.25 oz	200	10	19	tr
Onion Toasters	1 oz	188	10	21	tr
Utz					
Caramel Corn Clusters	1⅛ cups (1 oz)	120	2	24	13
Cheese Balls	50 (1 oz)	150	9	16	tr
Cheese Curls	18 (1 oz)	150	9	16	tr
Cheese Curls Crunchy	30 (1 oz)	160	10	16	tr
Cheese Curls Reduced Fat	32 (1 oz)	140	6	18	tr
Onion Rings	41 (1 oz)	140	7	18	2
Party Mix	¾ cup (1 oz)	140	6	19	tr
Pork Cracklins	0.5 oz	90	7	0	0
Pork Cracklins Hot & Spicy	0.5 oz	80	5	0	0
Pork Rinds	0.5 oz	80	5	0	0
Pork Rinds BBQ	0.5 oz	80	5	0	0
Weight Watchers					
Cheese Curls	1 pkg (0.5 oz)	70	3	10	0

FOOD	PORTION	CAL	FAT	CARB	SUG
SNAIL					
take-out					
escargot cooked	5	25	0	1	—
SNAKE					
fresh	3 oz	78	tr	3	—
SNAPPER					
cooked	3 oz	109	1	0	0
SODA					
cream	12 oz	191	0	49	—
diet cola w/ saccharin	12 oz	0	0	tr	—
orange	12 oz	177	0	46	—
7 Up					
Original	1 can	140	0	39	39
A & W					
Root Beer	1 can	180	0	46	46
Barritts					
Ginger Beer	1 bottle (12 oz)	200	0	49	49
Best Health					
Root Beer	1 bottle (12 oz)	165	0	42	42
Vanilla Cream	1 bottle (12 oz)	170	0	43	43
Canada Dry					
Ginger Ale	1 can	120	0	33	33
Tonic Water	8 fl oz	90	0	24	24
Dr Pepper					
Original	1 can	150	0	40	40
Health Valley					
Ginger Ale	1 bottle	160	0	40	40
Rootbeer Old Fashioned	1 bottle	160	0	40	40
Sarsaparilla Rootbeer	1 bottle	160	0	40	40

FOOD	PORTION	CAL	FAT	CARB	SUG
IBC					
Root Beer	1 can	160	0	43	43
Saranac					
Diet Root Beer	1 bottle (12 oz)	35	0	9	9
Ginger Beer	1 bottle (12 oz)	160	0	42	42
Root Beer	1 bottle (12 oz)	180	0	46	46
Shasta					
Black Cherry	1 can (12 oz)	170	0	41	41
Caffeine Free Cola	1 can (12 oz)	160	0	41	41
Cherry Cola	1 can (12 oz)	160	0	39	39
Club Soda	1 can (12 oz)	0	0	0	0
Cola	1 can (12 oz)	170	0	42	42
Creme	1 can (12 oz)	190	0	47	47
Diet Black Cherry	1 can (12 oz)	0	0	0	0
Diet Caffeine Free Cola	1 can (12 oz)	0	0	0	0
Diet Cherry Cola	1 can (12 oz)	0	0	0	0
Diet Cola	1 can (12 oz)	0	0	0	0
Diet Creme	1 can (12 oz)	0	0	0	0
Diet Doc Shasta	1 can (12 oz)	0	0	0	0
Diet Ginger Ale	1 can (12 oz)	0	0	0	0
Diet Grape	1 can (12 oz)	0	0	0	0
Diet Grapefruit	1 can (12 oz)	0	0	0	0
Diet Kiwi-Strawberry	1 can (12 oz)	0	0	0	0
Diet Lemon-Lime Twist	1 can (12 oz)	0	0	0	0
Diet Orange	1 can (12 oz)	0	0	0	0
Diet Pineapple-Orange	1 can (12 oz)	0	0	0	0
Diet Raspberry Creme	1 can (12 oz)	0	0	0	0
Diet Red Pop	1 can (12 oz)	0	0	0	0
Diet Root Beer	1 can (12 oz)	0	0	0	0
Diet Strawberry	1 can (12 oz)	0	0	0	0

FOOD	PORTION	CAL	FAT	CARB	SUG
Diet Strawberry-Peach	1 can (12 oz)	0	0	0	0
Doc Shasta	1 can (12 oz)	160	0	39	39
Fruit Punch	1 can (12 oz)	200	0	50	50
Ginger Ale	1 can (12 oz)	130	0	32	32
Grape	1 can (12 oz)	190	0	48	48
Kiwi-Strawberry	1 can (12 oz)	170	0	43	43
Lemon-Lime Twist	1 can (12 oz)	150	0	38	38
Moon Mist	1 can (12 oz)	180	0	46	46
Orange	1 can (12 oz)	200	0	49	49
Peach	1 can (12 oz)	170	0	43	43
Pineapple	1 can (12 oz)	200	0	51	51
Pineapple-Orange	1 can (12 oz)	180	0	46	46
Quinine/Tonic	1 can (12 oz)	130	0	32	32
Raspberry Creme	1 can (12 oz)	170	0	44	44
Red Pop	1 can (12 oz)	170	0	43	43
Root Beer	1 can (12 oz)	170	0	42	42
Strawberry	1 can (12 oz)	190	0	46	46
Strawberry-Peach	1 can (12 oz)	170	0	42	42
Sunkist					
Orange	1 can	190	0	52	52

SOLE

cooked	3 oz	99	1	0	0

take-out

battered & fried	3.2 oz	211	11	15	—
breaded & fried	3.2 oz	211	11	15	—

SORBET

(*see* ICES AND ICE POPS)

SORGHUM

sorghum	1 cup (6.7 oz)	651	6	143	—

FOOD	PORTION	CAL	FAT	CARB	SUG
SOUP					
canned					
Boston Market					
Chicken Broth Reduced Sodium	1 cup	15	1	1	0
Butterball					
Chicken Broth Reduced Sodium 99% Fat Free	1 cup	10	0	2	0
Campbell					
98% Fat Free Cream Of Chicken as prep	1 cup	80	3	10	0
Bean With Bacon as prep	1 cup	168	4	26	3
Beef Barley as prep	1 cup	81	2	11	1
Beef Noodle as prep	1 cup	73	2	8	1
Cheddar Cheese	1 cup	130	8	11	2
Cheddar Cheese as prep	1 cup	134	8	11	1
Chicken Vegetable as prep	1 cup	74	3	9	1
Chicken Gumbo as prep	1 cup	55	1	9	2
Chunky Savory Chicken w/ White & Wild Rice	1 cup	140	3	18	2
Clam Chowder New England as prep	1 cup	89	3	13	tr
Classic Chicken Noodle	1 cup	70	2	10	1
Classic Chicken Rice	1 cup (8.4 oz)	80	2	14	0
Consomme as prep	1 cup	24	tr	1	1

FOOD	PORTION	CAL	FAT	CARB	SUG
Cream Of Asparagus as prep	1 cup	72	4	9	3
Cream Of Mushroom as prep	1 cup	108	7	9	1
Cream Of Celery as prep	1 cup	107	7	9	1
Cream Of Chicken as prep	1 cup	120	8	10	1
Cream Of Potato as prep	1 cup	102	4	15	1
Fiesta Tomato as prep	1 cup	72	tr	16	8
Garden Vegetable as prep	1 cup	69	2	11	2
Green Pea as prep	1 cup	173	3	29	4
Healthy Request Chicken Noodle as prep	1 cup	60	2	8	1
Healthy Request Cream Of Mushroom as prep	1 cup	66	2	10	2
Healthy Request Cream Of Chicken & Broccoli as prep	1 cup	78	3	10	2
Healthy Request Cream Of Chicken as prep	1 cup	72	2	12	1
Healthy Request Hearty Pasta w/ Vegetables	1 cup	87	1	17	7
Healthy Request Tomato as prep	1 cup	91	2	18	9
Healthy Request Vegetable as prep	1 cup	84	1	17	5

FOOD	PORTION	CAL	FAT	CARB	SUG
Home Cookin' Chicken Vegetable	1 cup (8.4 oz)	130	4	20	6
Home Cookin' Chicken Rice	1 cup	110	1	20	3
Home Cookin' Chicken With Egg Noodles	1 cup (8.4 oz)	90	2	13	2
Home Cookin' Oriental Noodles w/ Vegetables	1 cup (8.4 oz)	100	1	18	5
Italian Tomato as prep	1 cup	105	tr	23	16
Low Sodium Chicken Broth	1 can (10.75 oz)	27	1	2	1
Low Sodium Chicken w/ Noodles	1 can (10.75 oz)	162	5	16	3
Low Sodium Chunky Vegetable Beef	1 can (10.75 oz)	159	4	17	5
Low Sodium Cream of Mushroom	1 can (10.75 oz)	200	13	18	5
Low Sodium Green Pea	1 can (10.75 oz)	235	4	38	4
Low Sodium Tomato w/ Pieces	1 can (10.75 oz)	170	5	28	17
Minestrone as prep	1 cup	81	2	12	2
Plus! Hearty Minestrone	2 cup (8.4 oz)	130	1	25	7
Plus! Roasted Vegetable w/ Barley & Wild Rice	1 cup (8.4 oz)	130	1	25	4
Ready To Serve Bean w/ Bacon 'N Ham	1 can (10.5 oz)	274	7	41	8
Ready To Serve Chicken Noodle	1 can (10.5 oz)	134	4	18	4

FOOD	PORTION	CAL	FAT	CARB	SUG
Ready To Serve Chicken w/ Rice	1 can (10.5 oz)	122	2	20	4
Ready To Serve Vegetable Beef	1 can (10.5 oz)	143	1	26	5
Savory Tomato & Dill as prep	1 cup	99	2	20	11
Select Chicken & Pasta With Roasted Garlic	1 cup (8.4 oz)	110	2	17	3
Select Chicken Rice	1 cup	110	1	18	2
Select Fiesta Vegetable	1 cup (8.4 oz)	120	1	24	7
Select Mushroom w/ White & Wild Rice	1 cup	90	1	16	2
Select Split Pea w/ Ham	1 cup (8.4 oz)	170	2	30	6
Select Tuscany-Style Minestrone	1 cup (8.4 oz)	190	9	21	5
Simply Home Chicken Noodle	1 cup (8.4 oz)	80	1	12	2
Simply Home Chicken With Rice	1 cup (8.4 oz)	100	1	19	2
Tomato as prep	1 cup	80	0	18	10
Vegetable Beef as prep	1 cup	68	2	9	1
Vegetarian Vegetable as prep	1 cup	79	2	14	3
Gold's					
Russian Borscht	8 oz	70	0	17	15
Health Valley					
5 Bean Vegetable	1 cup	250	0	32	9
Beef Broth Fat Free	1 cup	20	0	0	2

FOOD	PORTION	CAL	FAT	CARB	SUG
Beef Broth Fat Free No Salt	1 cup	20	0	0	2
Black Bean & Vegetable	1 cup	110	0	24	8
Chicken Broth	1 cup	45	2	0	0
Chicken Broth Fat Free	1 cup	30	0	0	0
Chicken Broth No Salt	1 cup	45	2	0	0
Country Corn & Vegetable	1 cup	70	0	17	8
Garden Vegetable	1 cup	80	0	17	8
Italian Plus Carotene	1 cup	80	0	19	5
Lentil & Carrot	1 cup	100	0	25	7
Organic Black Bean	1 cup	110	0	28	14
Organic Lentil No Salt	1 cup	90	0	20	7
Organic Minestrone	1 cup	100	0	23	6
Organic Mushroom Barley No Salt	1 cup	60	0	15	5
Organic Potato Leek	1 cup	70	0	15	5
Organic Potato Leek No Salt	1 cup	70	0	15	5
Organic Split Pea	1 cup	110	0	23	5
Organic Split Pea No Salt	1 cup	110	0	23	5
Organic Tomato	1 cup	90	0	22	20
Organic Vegetable No Salt	1 cup	80	0	18	10
Pasta Bolognese	1 cup	100	0	20	4
Pasta Cacciatore	1 cup	100	0	20	6
Pasta Romano	1 cup	100	0	20	6
Real Italian Minestrone	1 cup	90	0	21	6
Rotini & Vegetable	1 cup	100	0	20	4
Split Pea & Carrots	1 cup	110	0	17	7
Super Broccoli Carotene	1 cup	70	0	16	12

FOOD	PORTION	CAL	FAT	CARB	SUG
Tomato Vegetable	1 cup	80	0	17	9
Vegetable Barley	1 cup	90	0	19	4
Vegetable Power Carotene	1 cup	70	0	17	7
Healthy Choice					
Bean & Ham	1 cup (8.7 oz)	166	1	31	3
Beef & Potato	1 cup (8.5 oz)	116	1	16	3
Broccoli Cheddar	1 cup (8.4 oz)	116	2	22	1
Chicken Corn Chowder	1 cup (8.8 oz)	176	3	30	2
Chicken Pasta	1 cup (8.6 oz)	119	3	18	0
Chicken Rice	1 cup (8.4 oz)	119	2	19	3
Chili Beef	1 cup (9.1 oz)	189	2	32	5
Clam Chowder	1 cup (8.8 oz)	123	1	23	3
Classic Italian Bean and Pasta	1 cup (8 oz)	100	2	17	0
Country Vegetable	1 cup (8.6 oz)	112	1	24	5
Cream Of Mushroom	1 cup (8.8 oz)	77	1	14	0
Cream Of Celery as prep	1 cup	73	2	14	2
Cream Of Chicken Vegetable	1 cup (8.9 oz)	127	2	21	0
Cream Of Roasted Chicken as prep	1 cup	80	3	13	1
Cream Of Roasted Garlic as prep	1 cup	57	1	13	0
Garden Tomato Herbs as prep	1 cup	80	1	18	11
Garden Vegetable	1 cup (8.6 oz)	108	1	22	0
Hearty Chicken	1 cup (8.7 oz)	136	3	20	1
Lentil	1 cup (8.7 oz)	135	1	28	2
Minestrone	1 cup (8.6 oz)	107	1	24	4

FOOD	PORTION	CAL	FAT	CARB	SUG
Old Fashion Chicken Noodle	1 cup (8.8 oz)	137	3	19	0
Split Pea & Ham	1 cup (8.8 oz)	164	2	26	6
Tomato Garden	1 cup (8.6 oz)	101	1	19	8
Turkey Wild Rice	1 cup (8.4 oz)	72	1	9	5
Vegetable Beef	1 cup (8.8 oz)	96	1	14	3
Herb-Ox					
Beef Liquid	2 tsp (0.4 oz)	20	0	2	1
Chicken Liquid	2 tsp (0.4 oz)	15	0	1	0
Imagine					
Creamy Broccoli	1 serv (8 oz)	70	2	10	4
Creamy Butternut Squash	1 serv (8 oz)	120	2	23	14
Creamy Mushroom	1 serv (8 oz)	80	3	10	1
Creamy Potato Leek	1 serv (8 oz)	90	3	14	tr
Creamy Sweet Corn	1 serv (8 oz)	100	3	15	6
Creamy Tomato	1 serv (8 oz)	90	2	17	10
Vegetable Broth	1 serv (8 oz)	45	1	7	5
Zesty Gazpacho	1 serv (8 oz)	80	0	8	5
Natural Choice					
Orangic Vegan Classic Tomato	1 cup	100	1	22	8
Organic Vegan Classic Mushroom	1 cup	50	2	9	3
Organic Vegan Country Corn	1 cup	100	1	24	6
Organic Vegan Kabocha Squash	1 cup	60	1	14	8
Organic Vegan Southern Greens	1 cup	80	3	13	5
Organic Vegan Split Pea	1 cup	120	1	21	4

FOOD	PORTION	CAL	FAT	CARB	SUG
Organic Vegan Vegetable Curry	1 cup	110	4	17	4
Progresso					
99% Fat Free Beef Barley	1 cup (8.5 oz)	140	2	20	4
99% Fat Free Beef Vegetable	1 cup (8.5 oz)	160	2	24	4
99% Fat Free Chicken Noodle	1 cup (8.3 oz)	90	2	13	2
99% Fat Free Chicken Rice w/ Vegetables	1 cup (8.4 oz)	110	2	16	2
99% Fat Free Creamy Mushroom Chicken	1 cup (8.3 oz)	90	2	12	2
99% Fat Free Lentil	1 cup (8.5 oz)	130	2	20	1
99% Fat Free Minestrone	1 cup (8.5 oz)	130	2	23	3
99% Fat Free Roasted Chicken w/ Italian Style Vegetable	1 cup (8 oz)	90	2	12	2
99% Fat Free Split Pea	1 cup (8.9 oz)	170	2	29	5
99% Fat Free Tomato Garden Vegetable	1 cup (8.6 oz)	100	2	19	7
99% Fat Free Vegetable	1 cup (8.4 oz)	70	1	13	3
99% Fat Free White Cheddar Potato	1 cup (8.6 oz)	140	3	26	2
Basil Rotini Tomato	1 cup (8.9 oz)	120	2	22	6
Bean & Ham	1 cup (8.4 oz)	160	2	25	3
Beef Barley	1 cup (8.5 oz)	130	4	13	4

FOOD	PORTION	CAL	FAT	CARB	SUG
Beef Minestrone	1 cup (8.5 oz)	140	3	18	3
Beef Noodle	1 cup (8.5 oz)	140	4	15	2
Beef Vegetable & Rotini	1 cup (8.4 oz)	130	3	14	3
Cheese & Herb Tortellini Tomato	1 cup (8.6 oz)	140	3	23	9
Chickarina	1 cup (8.3 oz)	130	5	12	tr
Chicken Minestrone	1 cup (8.4 oz)	110	2	15	2
Chicken Vegetable	1 cup (8.4 oz)	90	2	13	2
Chicken & Wild Rice	1 cup (8.4 oz)	100	2	15	1
Chicken Barley	1 cup (8.5 oz)	110	2	16	2
Chicken Broth	1 cup (8.2 oz)	20	2	1	0
Chicken Noodle	1 cup (8.4 oz)	90	2	9	1
Chicken Rice w/ Vegetable	1 cup (8.4 oz)	90	2	13	1
Clam & Rotini Chowder	1 cup (8.8 oz)	190	9	21	3
Escarole In Chicken Broth	1 cup (8.1 oz)	25	1	3	tr
Green Split Pea	1 cup (8.6 oz)	170	3	25	4
Hearty Black Bean	1 cup (8.5 oz)	170	2	30	2
Hearty Penne In Chicken Broth	1 cup (8.4 oz)	80	1	14	1
Hearty Tomato	1 cup (8.7 oz)	100	2	19	11
Herb Rotini Vegetable	1 cup (9.1 oz)	120	2	21	5
Homestyle Chicken w/ Vegetable	1 cup (8.4 oz)	90	2	11	1
Italian Herb Shells Minestrone	1 cup (9.1 oz)	120	2	22	4
Lentil	1 cup (8.5 oz)	140	2	22	2
Macaroni & Bean	1 cup (8.6 oz)	160	4	23	1
Manhattan Clam Chowder	1 cup (8.4 oz)	110	2	11	3
Meatballs & Pasta Pearls	1 cup (8.3 oz)	140	7	13	0

FOOD	PORTION	CAL	FAT	CARB	SUG
Minestrone	1 cup (8.4 oz)	120	2	21	4
Minestrone Parmesan	1 cup (8.3 oz)	100	3	16	3
New England Clam Chowder	1 cup (8.4 oz)	190	10	20	3
Oregano Penne Italian Style Vegetable	1 cup (8.7 oz)	90	2	15	2
Peppercorn Penne Vegetable	1 cup (9.1 oz)	100	1	20	3
Potato Broccoli & Cheese	1 cup (8.8 oz)	160	6	21	4
Potato Ham & Cheese	1 cup (8.6 oz)	170	7	21	3
Roasted Garlic Pasta Lentil	1 cup (9.3 oz)	120	2	20	2
Rotisserie Seasoned Chicken	1 cup (8.5 oz)	100	2	15	2
Spicy Chicken & Penne	1 cup (8.5 oz)	110	2	14	2
Split Pea w/ Ham	1 cup (8.4 oz)	150	4	20	3
Tomato	1 cup (8.5 oz)	100	2	19	10
Tomato Basil	1 cup (8.8 oz)	100	2	19	10
Tomato Vegetable	1 cup (8.5 oz)	90	2	15	8
Tortellini In Chicken Broth	1 cup (0.0 oz)	70	0	10	1
Turkey Noodle	1 cup (8.4 oz)	90	2	11	2
Turkey Rice w/ Vegetables	1 cup (8.5 oz)	110	1	18	2
Vegetable	1 cup (8.4 oz)	90	2	15	3
White Meat Roasted Chicken Rotini	1 cup (8.1 oz)	80	2	11	1
Swanson					
Beef Broth	1 cup	19	1	1	1
Beef Broth Onion Seasoned	1 cup (8.4 oz)	20	0	2	1

FOOD	PORTION	CAL	FAT	CARB	SUG
Chicken Broth	1 cup	19	1	1	1
Chicken Broth Seasoned Italian Herbs	1 cup (8.4 oz)	20	1	3	0
Chicken Broth Seasoned w/ Italian Herbs	1 cup (8 oz)	25	1	4	2
Vegetable Broth	1 cup	19	1	3	3
Ultra Slim-Fast					
Chicken Alfredo Pasta	1 cup (8.3 oz)	132	2	17	3
Walnut Acres					
Organic Country Corn Chowder	1 cup (8.8 oz)	150	3	28	8
Weight Watchers					
Chicken & Rice	1 can (10.5 oz)	110	2	17	11
Chicken Noodle	1 can (10.5 oz)	150	2	25	15
Minestrone	1 can (10.5 oz)	130	2	23	7
Vegetable	1 can (10.5 oz)	130	1	27	11
frozen					
Nature's Entree					
Chowder	1 pkg (12 oz)	230	6	26	5
Tortellini Minestone	1 pkg (12 oz)	360	9	48	6
mix					
asparagus cream of as prep w/ water	1 cup	59	2	9	—
Armour					
Bouillon Cubes Beef	1 (4 g)	5	0	1	0
Bouillon Cubes Chicken	1 (4 g)	5	0	1	0
Bean Cuisine					
13 Bean Bouillabisse	1 cup	220	0	17	1

FOOD	PORTION	CAL	FAT	CARB	SUG
Island Black Bean	1 cup	210	0	17	1
Lots of Lentil	1 cup	230	0	17	1
Mesa Maize	1 cup	160	0	18	2
White Bean Provencal	1 cup	250	1	32	4
Cup-a-Soup					
Broccoli & Cheese as prep	1 serv (6 oz)	70	3	9	2
Chicken Vegetable as prep	1 serv (6 oz)	50	1	10	1
Chicken Broth as prep	1 serv (6 oz)	20	0	3	0
Chicken Broth w/ Pasta Fat Free as prep	1 serv (6 oz)	45	0	8	0
Chicken Noodle as prep	1 serv (6 oz)	50	1	8	0
Cream Of Chicken as prep	1 serv (6 oz)	70	2	12	2
Creamy Chicken Vegetable as prep	1 serv (6 oz)	80	5	10	2
Creamy Mushroom as prep	1 serv (6 oz)	60	2	10	1
Green Pea as prep	1 serv (6 oz)	80	1	12	1
Hearty Chicken Noodle as prep	1 serv (6 oz)	60	1	10	0
Ring Noodle as prep	1 serv (6 oz)	50	1	9	0
Spring Vegetable as prep	1 serv (6 oz)	45	1	21	1
Tomato as prep	1 serv (6 oz)	100	1	20	14
Health Valley					
Chicken Noodles w/ Vegetables	1 serv	110	0	24	1
Corn Chowder w/ Tomatoes	1 serv	100	0	21	1

FOOD	PORTION	CAL	FAT	CARB	SUG
Creamy Potato w/ Broccoli	1 serv	70	0	17	2
Garden Split Pea w/ Carrots	1 serv	130	0	22	2
Lentil w/ Couscous	1 serv	130	0	28	1
Pasta Italiano	1 serv	140	0	31	1
Pasta Marinara	1 serv	100	0	20	1
Pasta Parmesan	1 serv	100	0	20	1
Spicy Black Bean w/ Couscous	1 serv	130	0	29	3
Zesty Black Bean w/ Rice	1 serv	100	0	22	2
Herb-Ox					
Beef Bouillon	1 cube (3.5 g)	5	0	tr	0
Beef Instant Bouillon Powder	1 tsp (4 g)	5	0	tr	0
Beef Instant Broth & Seasoning Pack	1 pkg (4.5 g)	5	0	tr	0
Beef Instant Broth & Seasoning Pack Low Sodium	1 pkg (4 g)	10	0	2	1
Chicken Bouillon	1 cube (4 g)	5	0	tr	0
Chicken Instant Bouillon Powder	1 tsp (4 g)	5	0	tr	0
Chicken Instant Broth & Seasoning Pack	1 pkg (4 g)	5	0	tr	0
Chicken Instant Broth & Seasoning Pack Low Sodium	1 pkg (4 g)	10	0	2	1
Vegetable Bouillon	1 cube (4 g)	5	0	tr	0

FOOD	PORTION	CAL	FAT	CARB	SUG
Hodgson Mill					
Choice Bean not prep	¼ cup (1.5 oz)	150	0	27	2
Hurst					
15 Bean Soup Beef	1 serv (6 oz)	120	1	20	1
15 Bean Soup Cajun	1 serv	120	1	20	1
15 Bean Soup Chicken	1 serv (6 oz)	120	1	20	1
15 Bean Soup Chili	1 serv (6 oz)	120	1	20	1
15 Bean Soup Ham	1 serv	120	1	20	1
HamBeens Great Northern Bean	1 serv	120	1	22	1
HamBeens Navy Bean	1 serv	120	1	21	1
Pasta Fagioli	1 serv	120	1	23	1
Spanish-American Pinto Bean	1 serv	120	1	22	1
Spanish-American Black Bean	1 serv	120	1	22	1
Lipton					
Chicken Noodle w/ White Chicken Meat as prep	1 cup	80	2	11	0
Extra Noodle w/ Chicken Broth as prep	1 cup	90	2	15	1
Giggle Noodle w/ Chicken Broth as prep	1 cup	70	2	11	1
Recipe Secrets Beefy Mushroom	1½ tbsp (0.4 oz)	35	0	7	2
Recipe Secrets Beefy Onion	1 tbsp (0.3 oz)	25	1	5	0
Recipe Secrets Fiesta Herb w/ Red Pepper as prep	1 cup	30	0	6	tr

FOOD	PORTION	CAL	FAT	CARB	SUG
Recipe Secrets Golden Herb w/ Lemon as prep	1 cup	35	1	7	0
Recipe Secrets Golden Onion	1⅔ tbsp (0.5 oz)	50	1	9	2
Recipe Secrets Italian Herb w/ Tomato as prep	1 cup	40	1	9	3
Recipe Secrets Onion as prep	1 cup	20	0	4	0
Recipe Secrets Onion Mushroom as prep	1 cup	30	1	5	0
Recipe Secrets Savory Herb w/Garlic as prep	1 cup	30	0	6	0
Recipe Secrets Vegetable as prep	1 cup	30	0	7	2
Ring-O-Noodle w/ Chicken Broth as prep	1 cup	70	2	10	1
Soup Secrets Chicken 'N Onion as prep	1 cup	120	2	24	1
Soup Secrets Chicken w/ Pasta & Beans as prep	1 cup	110	2	19	1
Soup Secrets Country Chicken w/ Pasta & Herbs as prep	1 cup	100	2	18	1
Soup Secrets Homestyle Lentil w/ Bow Tie Pasta as prep	1 cup	130	1	22	1

FOOD	PORTION	CAL	FAT	CARB	SUG
Soup Secrets Minestrone as prep	1 cup	110	1	21	4
Spiral Pasta w/ Chicken Broth as prep	1 cup	60	1	11	1
Ramen Noodle					
Beef Low Fat as prep	1 pkg (2.2 oz)	216	1	45	3
Beef as prep	1 pkg (2.2 oz)	280	11	40	3
Chicken Low Fat as prep	1 pkg (2.2 oz)	216	1	44	3
Chicken as prep	1 pkg (2.2 oz)	279	11	40	3
Oriental Low Fat as prep	1 pkg (2.2 oz)	217	1	45	3
Shrimp Low Fat as prep	1 pkg (2.2 oz)	218	1	45	3
Shrimp as prep	1 pkg (2.2 oz)	294	13	39	3
Tomato as prep	1 pkg (2.2 oz)	295	13	39	4
Weight Watchers					
Instant Beef Broth	1 pkg (0.16 oz)	10	0	2	2
Instant Chicken Broth	1 pkg (0.16 oz)	10	0	2	2
Wyler's					
Beef Bouillon Cube Reduced Sodium	1 (3.5 g)	5	0	1	—
shelf-stable					
Hormel					
Micro Cup Bean & Ham	1 cup (7.5 oz)	190	4	29	2
Micro Cup Beef Vegetable	1 cup (7.5 oz)	90	1	15	3
Micro Cup Broccoli Cheese w/ Ham	1 cup (7.5 oz)	170	13	10	3

FOOD	PORTION	CAL	FAT	CARB	SUG
Micro Cup Chicken & Rice	1 cup (7.5 oz)	110	3	17	3
Micro Cup Chicken Noodle	1 cup (7.5 oz)	110	3	13	0
Micro Cup New England Clam Chowder	1 cup (7.5 oz)	130	5	17	0
Micro Cup Potato Cheese w/ Ham	1 cup (7.5 oz)	190	13	15	2
Lunch Bucket					
Chicken Noodle	1 pkg (7.25 oz)	80	2	13	0
Country Vegetable	1 pkg (7.25 oz)	60	1	14	1
take-out					
beef stew soup	1 cup (8.8 oz)	221	5	20	—
black bean turtle soup	1 cup	241	1	45	—
brunswick stew soup	1 cup (8.5 oz)	232	6	17	—
corn & cheese chowder	¾ cup	215	12	21	—
gazpacho	1 cup	46	tr	5	—
greek	¾ cup	63	2	7	—
hot & sour	1 serv (14 oz)	173	8	8	1
onion soup gratinee	1 serv	492	27	38	6
oxtail	5 oz	64	3	7	—
pasta e fagioll	1 cup (8.8 oz)	194	5	30	—
ratatouille	1 cup (7.5 oz)	266	25	12	—
vietnamese pho beef noodle	1 serv (7.8 oz)	480	12	78	2

SOUR CREAM
Breakstone's

Free	2 tbsp (1.1 oz)	35	0	6	2
Reduced Fat	2 tbsp (1.1 oz)	45	4	2	2
Sour Cream	2 tbsp (1 oz)	60	5	1	1

FOOD	PORTION	CAL	FAT	CARB	SUG
Knudsen					
Free	2 tbsp (1.1 oz)	35	0	6	2
Hampshire	2 tbsp (1 oz)	60	6	1	1
Light	2 tbsp (1.1 oz)	50	3	2	2
Land O Lakes					
Fat Free	2 tbsp (1.1 oz)	25	0	4	2
Light	2 tbsp (1 oz)	40	3	3	2
Sour Cream	2 tbsp (1 oz)	60	6	1	1
SOURSOP					
fresh	1	416	2	105	—
fresh cut up	1 cup	150	1	38	—
SOY					
lecithin	1 tbsp	104	14	0	0
I.M. Healthy					
SoyNut Butter Chocolate	2 tbsp (1.1 oz)	190	14	12	7
SoyNut Butter Honey Creamy	2 tbsp (1.1 oz)	170	11	12	2
SoyNut Butter Original Creamy	2 tbsp (1.1 oz)	170	11	10	3
SoyNut Butter Unsweetened Chunky	2 tbsp (1.1 oz)	160	13	5	1
SoyNut Butter Unsweetened Creamy	2 tbsp (1.1 oz)	160	13	5	1
Loma Linda					
Soyagen All Purpose	¼ cup (1 oz)	130	6	12	7
Soyagen Carob	¼ cup (1 oz)	130	6	13	7
Soyagen No Sucrose	¼ cup (1 oz)	130	6	12	7
Natural Touch					
Roasted Soy Butter	2 tbsp (1.1 oz)	170	11	10	3

FOOD	PORTION	CAL	FAT	CARB	SUG
Revival					
Chocolate Soy Nuts!	12–14 pieces (0.5 oz)	70	4	7	6
Soy Shake Plain as prep w/ water	1 pkg (1 oz)	110	2	2	1
Soy Shakes Chocolate Daydream Equal as prep w/ water	1 pkg (1.2 oz)	130	3	7	1
Soy Shakes Chocolate Daydream Unsweetened as prep w/ water	1 pkg (1.2 oz)	130	3	7	1
Soy Shakes Chocolate Daydreams as prep w/ water	1 pkg (2.2 oz)	240	3	36	32
Soy Shakes Vanilla Pleasures Equal as prep w/ water	1 pkg (1.2 oz)	120	2	6	1
Soy Shakes Vanilla Pleasures Unsweetened as prep w/ water	1 pkg (1.2 oz)	120	2	6	1
Soy Shakes Vanilla Pleasures as prep w/ water	1 pkg (2 oz)	220	2	31	28
Tree Of Life					
Soy Wonder Spread	2 tbsp (1.1 oz)	170	11	10	3
SOY SAUCE					
Chun King					
Lite	1 tbsp (0.5 oz)	15	tr	2	2
Soy Sauce	1 tbsp (0.6 oz)	11	tr	1	1

FOOD	PORTION	CAL	FAT	CARB	SUG
House Of Tsang					
Ginger Flavored	1 tbsp (0.6 oz)	20	0	4	3
Light	1 tbsp (0.6 oz)	5	0	0	0
Low Sodium	1 tbsp (0.6 oz)	5	0	0	0
Low Sodium Ginger	1 tbsp (0.6 oz)	10	0	2	1
Low Sodium Mushroom	1 tbsp (0.6 oz)	10	0	2	1
Just Rite					
Soy Sauce	1 tbsp (0.5 oz)	11	tr	1	1
Kikkoman					
Soy Sauce	1 tbsp (0.5 oz)	10	0	0	0
La Choy					
Lite	1 tbsp (0.5 oz)	15	tr	2	2
Soy Sauce	1 tbsp (0.6 oz)	11	tr	1	1
SOYBEANS					
dried cooked	1 cup	298	15	17	—
honey toasted	¼ cup (1 oz)	130	4	19	15
Seapoint Farms					
Edamame Organic	½ cup (2.6 oz)	100	3	9	1
Edamame In Pods frozen	½ cup (2.6 oz)	100	3	9	1
Edamame Rice Bowl Kung Pao Vegetable	1 pkg (12 oz)	420	6	72	14
Edamame Rice Bowl Szechwan Vegetables	1 pkg (12 oz)	420	4	80	22
Edamame Rice Bowl Teriyaki Vegetable	1 pkg (12 oz)	430	5	83	21
Edamame Rice Bowl Vegetable Fried Rice	1 pkg (11 oz)	220	6	31	6
Edamame Shelled	½ cup (2.6 oz)	100	3	9	1

FOOD	PORTION	CAL	FAT	CARB	SUG

SPAGHETTI

(*see* PASTA, PASTA DINNERS, PASTA SALAD, SPAGHETTI SAUCE)

SPAGHETTI SAUCE
jarred

Francesco Rinaldi

FOOD	PORTION	CAL	FAT	CARB	SUG
Dolce Sweet & Tasty Tomato	½ cup (4.4 oz)	110	5	15	11
Dolce Three Cheese	½ cup (4.4 oz)	90	2	15	11
Dulce Super Mushroom	½ cup (4.4 oz)	110	5	15	11
Hearty Diavolo	½ cup (4.4 oz)	70	4	7	4
Hearty Mushroom Pepper & Onion	½ cup (4.4 oz)	80	3	10	7
Hearty Tomato & Basil	½ cup (4.4 oz)	80	3	11	7
Puttanesca	½ cup (4.3 oz)	70	4	8	7
Tomato Alfredo	¼ cup (2.1 oz)	60	4	4	4
Traditional Meat Flavored	½ cup (4.4 oz)	90	4	11	7
Traditional Mushroom	1.2 cup (4.4 oz)	90	4	11	7
Traditional Original	½ cup (4.4 oz)	90	4	11	7
Traditional Original	½ cup (4.4 oz)	90	4	11	2
Vodka Sauce	¼ cup (2.1 oz)	60	4	4	4
Healthy Choice					
Chunky Italian Vegetable	½ cup (4.4 oz)	40	tr	9	7
Chunky Mushroom	½ cup (4.4 oz)	42	tr	9	8
Garlic & Herbs	½ cup (4.4 oz)	49	tr	10	7
Garlic Lovers Garlic & Mushroom	½ cup (4.4 oz)	44	tr	10	8
Garlic Lovers Roasted Garlic	½ cup (4.4 oz)	52	tr	12	8

FOOD	PORTION	CAL	FAT	CARB	SUG
Garlic Lovers Roasted Garlic & Sun Dried Tomato	½ cup (4.4 oz)	52	tr	11	8
Super Chunky Mushroom & Sweet Peppers	½ cup (4.4 oz)	43	tr	9	6
Super Chunky Tomato Mushroom & Garlic	½ cup (4.4 oz)	45	tr	10	8
Super Chunky Vegetable Primavera	½ cup (4.4 oz)	43	tr	9	7
Traditional	½ cup (4.4 oz)	48	tr	11	8
With Mushrooms	½ cup (4.4 oz)	48	tr	11	8
Hunt's					
Angela Mia Marinara	¼ cup (2.2 oz)	24	1	4	3
Chunky	½ cup (4.4 oz)	38	1	8	7
Chunky Italian Sausage	½ cup (4.5 oz)	72	3	45	8
Chunky Italian Style Vegetable	½ cup (4.4 oz)	63	1	13	5
Chunky Marinara	½ cup (4.4 oz)	61	1	12	5
Chunky Tomato Garlic & Onion	½ cup (4.4 oz)	63	1	13	5
Classic Four Cheese	½ cup (4.4 oz)	50	1	9	7
Classic Garlic & Herb	½ cup (4.4 oz)	53	2	9	6
Classic Parmesan	½ cup (4.4 oz)	49	2	8	6
Classic Tomato & Basil	½ cup (4.4 oz)	48	1	9	7
Family Favorites Seasoned Diced Tomato Sauce	½ cup (4.3 oz)	50	1	11	9
Homestyle Meat Flavored	½ cup (4.4 oz)	51	2	9	5

FOOD	PORTION	CAL	FAT	CARB	SUG
Homestyle Mushrooms	½ cup (4.4 oz)	48	1	9	7
Homestyle Traditional	½ cup (4.4 oz)	49	1	9	7
Light Meat Flavored	½ cup (4.4 oz)	45	1	8	6
Light w/ Garlic & Herb	½ cup (4.5 oz)	40	1	7	5
Original Meat Flavored	½ cup (4.4 oz)	68	2	12	9
Original Traditional	½ cup (4.4 oz)	67	2	11	9
Original w/ Mushrooms	½ cup (4.4 oz)	62	2	11	9
Original w/ Italian Cheese & Garlic	½ cup (4.5 oz)	64	2	10	7
Tomato Bits	½ cup (4.5 oz)	49	tr	11	6
Traditional Light	½ cup (4.4 oz)	40	tr	7	6
Muir Glen					
Organic Balsamic Roasted Onion	½ cup (4.4 oz)	50	1	10	5
Organic Cabernet Marinara	½ cup (4.4 oz)	50	1	10	4
Organic Chunky Herb	½ cup (4.4 oz)	50	1	10	5
Organic Garden Vegetable	½ cup (4.4 oz)	50	1	10	4
Organic Garlic & Onion	½ cup (4.4 oz)	55	1	10	5
Organic Garlic Roasted Garlic	½ cup (4.4 oz)	50	1	10	4
Organic Green Olive	½ cup (4.4 oz)	60	2	10	4
Organic Italian Herb	½ cup (4.4 oz)	55	1	10	5
Organic Mushroom Marinara	½ cup (4.4 oz)	45	0	10	4

FOOD	PORTION	CAL	FAT	CARB	SUG
Organic Portabello Mushroom	½ cup (4.4 oz)	50	0	10	4
Organic Sun Dried Tomato	½ cup (4.4 oz)	55	1	10	4
Organic Tomato Basil	½ cup (4.4 oz)	50	1	12	4
Newman's Own					
Marinara Ventian	½ cup (4.4 oz)	60	2	9	7
Marinara Ventian w/ Mushrooms	½ cup (4.4 oz)	60	2	9	7
Pasta Sauce Bambolina	½ cup (4.5 oz)	100	5	15	9
Pasta Sauce Roasted Garlic & Red & Green Peppers	½ cup (4.7 oz)	70	3	11	6
Pasta Sauce Say Cheese	½ cup (4.4 oz)	90	3	14	8
Sockarooni	½ cup (4.4 oz)	60	2	9	7
Prego					
Pasta Bake Sauce Tomato Garlic & Basil	1 serv (3.4 oz)	80	4	11	10
Traditional	½ cup (4.2 oz)	140	5	23	15
Progresso					
Marinara	½ cup (4.3 oz)	80	5	8	5
Meat Flavored	½ cup (4.4 oz)	100	5	12	9
Sauce	½ cup (4.4 oz)	100	5	12	8
Ragu					
Chunky Garden Style Tomato Garlic & Onion	½ cup (4.5 oz)	110	3	18	13

FOOD	PORTION	CAL	FAT	CARB	SUG
Sara Lee					
Chunky Garden Mushroom & Peppers	½ cup (4.4 oz)	80	2	12	6
mix					
Durkee					
Spaghetti Sauce as prep	½ cup	15	0	5	1
With Mushrooms as prep	½ cup	15	0	4	2
French's					
Italian as prep	½ cup	16	0	5	1
Mushroom as prep	½ cup	20	1	4	1
Thick as prep	½ cup	10	0	4	1
McCormick					
Alfredo Pasta Blend as prep	½ cup	60	2	4	2
Pasta Rosa Blend	1 tbsp (10 g)	40	2	4	2
Primavera Pasta Blend	1 tbsp (7 g)	30	1	4	tr
Spaghetti Sauce	1 tbsp (8 g)	25	0	5	3
refrigerated					
Di Giorno					
Alfredo	¼ cup (2.2 oz)	180	18	3	2
Basil Pesto	¼ cup (2.2 oz)	320	31	2	tr
Four Cheese	¼ cup (2.2 oz)	160	15	3	2
Garlic Pesto	¼ cup (2.1 oz)	340	33	3	tr
Light Alfredo Sauce	¼ cup (2.4 oz)	140	9	9	3
Marinara	½ cup (4.5 oz)	70	0	15	10
Plum Tomato Cream Sauce	½ cup (4.4 oz)	160	13	8	6
Plum Tomato & Mushroom	½ cup (4.4 oz)	60	0	13	10

FOOD	PORTION	CAL	FAT	CARB	SUG
Roasted Red Bell Pepper Cream Sauce	¼ cup (2.3 oz)	140	10	8	3
take-out					
bolognese	5 oz	195	15	4	—

SPANISH FOOD
canned

Chi-Chi's

Pico De Gallo	2 tbsp (1.2 oz)	10	0	2	2

Derby

Tamales	3 (6.5 oz)	253	17	21	0

Gebhardt

Enchiladas	2 (5.7 oz)	258	19	20	0
Tamales	2 (5.7 oz)	268	21	19	1
Tamales Jumbo	2 (6.9 oz)	332	25	24	0

Hormel

Tamales Beef	3 (7.5 oz)	280	21	20	1
Tamales Chicken	3 (7.5 oz)	210	11	22	2
Tamales Hot Spicy Beef	3 (7.5 oz)	280	21	20	1
Tamales Jumbo Beef	2 (6.9 oz)	270	20	18	1

Rosarita

Enchilada Sauce Mild	¼ cup (2.1 oz)	23	1	3	3

Van Camp

Tamales	2 (5 oz)	210	13	20	1

frozen

Amy's Organic

Black Bean Vegetable Enchilada	1 (4.75 oz)	130	4	20	1
Burritos Bean & Cheese	1 (6 oz)	280	8	43	1
Burritos Bean & Rice Non-Dairy	1 (6 oz)	250	5	44	1

FOOD	PORTION	CAL	FAT	CARB	SUG
Burritos Black Bean Vegetable	1 (6 oz)	320	8	54	4
Burritos Breakfast	1 (6 oz)	230	5	38	4
Cheese Enchilada	1 (4.7 oz)	210	9	16	0
Mexican Tamale Pie	1 (8 oz)	220	3	41	4
Pocket Sandwich Tamale	1 (4.5 oz)	250	7	39	4
Whole Meals Cheese Enchilada	1 pkg (9 oz)	330	14	38	6
Whole Meals Enchilada	1 pkg (10 oz)	250	8	41	4
Banquet					
Chimichanga Meal	1 meal (9.5 oz)	500	24	56	9
Enchilada Beef	1 pkg (11 oz)	370	12	54	7
Enchilada Cheese	1 pkg (11 oz)	360	10	56	7
Enchilada Chicken	1 pkg (11 oz)	350	10	54	7
Enchilada Beef & Tamale Combo	1 pkg (11 oz)	450	20	50	7
Mexican Style Enchilada Combo	1 meal (11 oz)	360	11	55	7
Chi-Chi's					
Burro Beef	1 pkg (15.9 oz)	590	19	76	7
Burro Chicken	1 pkg (15.9 oz)	540	14	77	8
Chimichanga Beef	1 pkg (15.9 oz)	630	24	75	8
Chimichanga Chicken	1 pkg (15.9 oz)	580	19	78	8
Enchilada Chicken Suprema	1 pkg (15.9 oz)	600	20	80	9
Enchilida Baja	1 pkg (15.9 oz)	590	20	75	7
Health Is Wealth					
Burrito Munchees	10 (5 oz)	310	7	53	2
Mexican Munchees	2 (1 oz)	49	1	8	0
Healthy Choice					
Chicken Enchilada Suprema	1 meal (11.3 oz)	300	7	46	8

FOOD	PORTION	CAL	FAT	CARB	SUG
Chicken Enchiladas Suiz	1 meal (10 oz)	280	6	43	4
Chicken Breast Con Queso Burrito	1 meal (10.55 oz)	350	6	60	11
Lean Cuisine					
Everyday Favorites Chicken Enchilada Suiza	1 pkg (9 oz)	280	5	48	7
Patio					
Beef & Cheese Enchiladas Chili 'N Beans	1 meal (15.5 oz)	670	30	80	6
Burrito Bean & Cheese	1 (5 oz)	300	9	45	4
Burrito Beef & Bean Hot	1 (5 oz)	320	12	43	4
Burrito Beef & Bean Mild	1 (5 oz)	330	12	45	3
Burrito Chicken	1 (5 oz)	290	6	44	6
Burritos Beef & Bean Medium	1 (5 oz)	310	10	45	5
Burritos Beef & Bean Red Chili Pepper Red Hot	1 (5 oz)	320	12	42	4
Enchilada Beef	1 meal (12 oz)	320	12	52	4
Enchilada Cheese	1 meal (12 oz)	370	12	54	7
Enchilada Chicken	1 meal (12 oz)	400	12	60	6
Fiesta	1 meal (12 oz)	350	11	53	5
Mexican Style	1 meal (13.25 oz)	470	19	59	5
Stouffer's					
Chicken Enchilada	1 serv (4.8 oz)	230	11	25	4
Tyson					
Beef Fajita	3½ pieces (12.5 oz)	550	16	75	8
Chicken Fajita	3½ pieces (13.1 oz)	460	11	61	10

FOOD	PORTION	CAL	FAT	CARB	SUG
Weight Watchers					
Smart Ones Chicken Enchiladas Suiza	1 pkg (9 oz)	270	9	33	8
Smart Ones Santa Fe Style Rice & Beans	1 pkg (10 oz)	290	8	43	6
mix					
Gebhardt					
Menudo Mix	¼ tsp (0.4 g)	1	tr	tr	tr
McCormick					
Burrito Seasoning	1 tbsp (8 g)	25	1	5	1
Taco Seasoning Hot	2 tsp (6 g)	20	0	3	1
Taco Seasoning Mild	2 tsp (7 g)	20	0	4	1
Taco Bell					
Home Originals Chicken Fajita Dinner as prep	2 (6.9 oz)	340	9	45	7
Home Originals Chicken Fajita Seasoning Mix	1 tbsp (8 g)	25	0	5	1
Home Originals Soft Taco Dinner as prep	2 (6.3 oz)	410	18	41	5
Home Originals Taco Dinner as prep	2 (4.4 oz)	280	15	19	2
Home Originals Taco Seasoning Mix	2 tsp (6 g)	20	0	3	0
Home Originals Ultimate Bean Burrito Dinner as prep	1 (4.4 oz)	200	5	34	4

FOOD	PORTION	CAL	FAT	CARB	SUG
Home Originals Ultimate Nachos as prep	12 pieces (4.6 oz)	240	11	31	2
ready-to-eat					
Chi-Chi's					
Taco Shells White Corn	2 (1.2 oz)	170	8	22	0
Taco Shells Yellow Corn	2 shells (1.2 oz)	170	8	22	0
Gebhardt					
Taco Shells	3 (1.1 oz)	155	8	19	0
La Mexicana					
Flour Burritos	1 (1.6 oz)	160	5	26	2
Rosarita					
Taco Shells	3 (1.1 oz)	155	8	19	0
Tostada Shells	2 (1 oz)	125	5	17	tr
Taco Bell					
Home Originals Taco Shells	3 (1.1 oz)	150	6	21	0
take-out					
burrito w/ beans	2 (7.6 oz)	448	14	71	—
burrito w/ beans & cheese	2 (6.5 oz)	377	12	55	—
burrito w/ beans & chili peppers	2 (7.2 oz)	413	15	58	—
burrito w/ beans & meat	2 (8.1 oz)	508	18	66	—
burrito w/ beans cheese & beef	2 (7.1 oz)	331	13	40	—
burrito w/ beans cheese & chili peppers	2 (11.8 oz)	663	23	85	—
burrito w/ beef	2 (7.7 oz)	523	21	59	—
burrito w/ beef & chili peppers	2 (7.1 oz)	426	17	49	—

FOOD	PORTION	CAL	FAT	CARB	SUG
burrito w/ beef cheese & chili peppers	2 (10.7 oz)	634	25	64	—
chimichanga w/ beef	1 (6.1 oz)	425	20	43	—
chimichanga w/ beef & cheese	1 (6.4 oz)	443	23	39	—
enchilada w/ cheese	1 (5.7 oz)	320	19	29	—
enchilada w/ cheese & beef	1 (6.7 oz)	324	18	30	—
enchirito w/ cheese beef & beans	1 (6.8 oz)	344	16	34	—
frijoles w/ cheese	1 cup (5.9 oz)	226	8	29	—
nachos w/ cheese	6 to 8 (4 oz)	345	19	36	—
nachos w/ cheese beans ground beef & peppers	6 to 8 (8.9 oz)	568	31	56	—
taco	1 sm (6 oz)	370	21	27	—
taco salad	1½ cups	279	15	24	—
taco salad w/ chili con carne	1½ cups	288	13	27	—
tostada w/ beans & cheese	1 (5.1 oz)	223	10	27	—
tostada w/ beans beef & cheese	1 (7.9 oz)	334	17	30	—
tostada w/ beef & cheese	1 (5.7 oz)	315	16	23	—
tostada w/ guacamole	2 (9.2 oz)	360	23	32	—

SPARE RIBS

(*see* PORK)

SPICES

(*see individual names and* HERBS/SPICES)

FOOD	PORTION	CAL	FAT	CARB	SUG
SPINACH					
fresh					
cooked	½ cup	21	tr	3	—
Dole					
Baby Spinach	3½ cups (3 oz)	35	0	9	0
frozen					
Amy's Organic					
Pocket Sandwich Spinach Feta	1 (4.5 oz)	200	7	27	4
Birds Eye					
Creamed	½ cup (4.3 oz)	100	7	7	3
Cut Leaf	1 cup (2.8 oz)	20	0	2	1
Green Giant					
Butter Sauce	½ cup (3.4 oz)	40	2	5	tr
Creamed	½ cup (3.8 oz)	80	3	10	4
Cut Leaf	¾ cup (2.6 oz)	25	0	3	0
Harvest Fresh	½ cup (3.5 oz)	25	0	3	0
Health Is Wealth					
Spinach Munchees	2 (1 oz)	60	3	9	0
Spinach Feta Munchees	2 (1 oz)	70	3	9	0
Stouffer's					
Creamed	1 serv (4.5 oz)	160	12	8	2
Souffle	1 serv (4 oz)	150	10	9	4
take-out					
indian saag	1 serv	28	2	2	—
spanakopita spinach pie	1 cup (6 oz)	196	3	35	4
SPINACH JUICE					
juice	7 oz	14	0	2	—

FOOD	PORTION	CAL	FAT	CARB	SUG

SPORTS DRINKS

(*see also* ENERGY DRINKS)

Powerade

FOOD	PORTION	CAL	FAT	CARB	SUG
Fruit Punch	8 fl oz	70	0	19	15
Lemon Lime	8 fl oz	70	0	19	15
Mountain Blast	8 fl oz	70	0	19	15

SPOT

baked	3 oz	134	5	0	0

SPROUTS

Chun King

Bean Sprouts	1 cup (3 oz)	11	tr	1	0

Fresh Alternatives

BroccoSprouts	½ cup (1 oz)	10	0	1	0
Deli Blend	½ cup (1 oz)	10	0	1	0
Salad Blend	½ cup (1 oz)	10	0	2	0
Sandwich Blend	½ cup (1 oz)	5	0	1	0

La Choy

Bean Sprouts	1 cup (2.9 oz)	11	tr	1	0

take-out

mung bean stir fried	½ cup	31	tr	7	—

SQUAB

boneless baked	3.5 oz	175	3	0	0

SQUASH

(*see also* ZUCCHINI)

fresh

acorn cooked mashed	½ cup	41	tr	11	—
butternut baked	½ cup	41	tr	11	—
crookneck sliced cooked	½ cup	18	tr	4	—
hubbard baked	½ cup	51	tr	11	—

FOOD	PORTION	CAL	FAT	CARB	SUG
scallop sliced cooked	½ cup	14	tr	3	—
spaghetti cooked	½ cup	23	tr	5	—
frozen					
Birds Eye					
Sliced Yellow	⅔ cup (2.7 oz)	15	0	2	1
SQUID					
fried	3 oz	149	6	7	—
SQUIRREL					
roasted	3 oz	147	4	0	0
STARFRUIT					
fresh	1	42	tr	10	—
STRAWBERRIES					
fresh					
strawberries	1 cup	45	1	10	—
frozen					
Birds Eye					
In Syrup	½ cup (4.7 oz)	120	0	31	28
Lite Syrup	1 pkg (10 oz)	120	0	31	28
Whole	½ cup (4.5 oz)	100	0	25	23
STRAWBERRY JUICE					
Capri Sun					
Strawberry Cooler Drink	1 pkg (7 oz)	90	0	25	25
Kool-Aid					
Drink as prep w/ sugar	1 serv (8 oz)	100	0	25	25
Drink Mix as prep	1 serv (8 oz)	60	0	16	16
Veryfine					
Juice-Ups	8 fl oz	140	0	36	36

FOOD	PORTION	CAL	FAT	CARB	SUG

STUFFING/DRESSING

Kellogg's

FOOD	PORTION	CAL	FAT	CARB	SUG
Croutettes Mix	1 cup (1.2 oz)	120	0	25	0
Pepperidge Farm					
Corn Bread	¾ cup (1.5 oz)	170	2	33	2
Herb Seasoned	¾ cup (1.5 oz)	170	2	33	2
Herb Seasoned Cubed	¾ cup (1.3 oz)	140	2	28	2
One Step Chicken	½ cup (1.2 oz)	140	4	23	tr
One Step Southwestern Corn Bread	½ cup (1.2 oz)	150	5	23	2
One Step Turkey	½ cup (1.2 oz)	150	5	22	3
Stove Top					
Chicken as prep w/ margarine	½ cup (3.6 oz)	170	9	20	3
Cornbread as prep w/ margarine	½ cup (3.6 oz)	170	8	21	3
Flexible Serve Chicken as prep w/ margarine	½ cup (3.3 oz)	170	8	19	3
Flexible Serve Cornbread as prep w/ margarine	½ cup (3.3 oz)	160	8	19	3
Flexible Serve Homestyle Herb as prep w/ margarine	½ cup (3.3 oz)	170	8	19	3
For Beef as prep w/ margarine	½ cup (3.7 oz)	180	9	22	4
For Pork as prep w/ margarine	½ cup (3.6 oz)	170	9	20	3
For Turkey as prep w/ margarine	½ cup (3.6 oz)	170	9	20	3

FOOD	PORTION	CAL	FAT	CARB	SUG
Long Grain & Wild Rice as prep w/ margarine	½ cup (3.7 oz)	180	9	22	3
Lower Sodium Chicken as prep w/ margarine	½ cup (3.6 oz)	180	9	21	3
Microwave Chicken as prep w/ margarine	½ cup (3.5 oz)	160	7	20	3
Microwave Homestyle Cornbread as prep w/ margarine	½ cup (3 oz)	160	7	20	3
Mushroom & Onion as prep w/ margarine	½ cup (3.6 oz)	180	9	20	3
San Francisco Style as prep w/ margarine	½ cup (3.6 oz)	170	9	20	3
Savory Herb as prep w/ margarine	½ cup (3.6 oz)	170	9	20	3
Traditional Sage as prep w/ margarine	½ cup (3.6 oz)	180	9	21	3
take-out					
bread	½ cup (3½ oz)	195	8	26	—
sausage	½ cup	292	11	40	—
STURGEON					
cooked	3 oz	115	4	0	0
smoked	1 oz	48	1	0	0
SUCKER					
white baked	3 oz	101	3	0	0
SUGAR					
brown packed	1 cup (7.7 oz)	828	0	214	214
maple	1 piece (1 oz)	100	tr	26	—
powdered	1 tbsp (0.3 oz)	31	0	8	8
white	1 cup (7 oz)	773	0	200	200
white	1 tsp (4 g)	15	0	4	4

FOOD	PORTION	CAL	FAT	CARB	SUG
Domino					
Dark Brown	1 tsp	15	0	4	4
Maui Brand					
Raw Sugar	1 tsp	15	0	4	4

SUGAR SUBSTITUTES
Weight Watchers

Sweetener	1 serv (1 g)	5	0	1	1

SUGAR-APPLE

fresh	1	146	tr	37	—

SUNDAE TOPPINGS

(*see* ICE CREAM TOPPINGS)

SUNFISH

pumpkinseed baked	3 oz	97	1	0	0

SUNFLOWER
Dakota Gourmet

Honey Roasted Kernels	1 pkg (1 oz)	158	12	8	4
Lightly Salted Kernels	1 pkg (1 oz)	168	14	5	1
Frito Lay					
Seeds	1 oz	180	15	5	tr
Lance					
Seeds In Shell	⅔ cup (1.8 oz)	160	13	5	1
Seeds Roasted & Shelled	1 pkg (1⅛ oz)	190	16	6	1

SUSHI
take-out

california roll	1 piece (0.8 oz)	28	1	4	tr
sashimi	1 serv (6 oz)	198	7	4	1
tuna roll	1 piece (0.7 oz)	23	tr	3	tr
vegetable roll	1 piece (1.2 oz)	27	1	5	tr
vinegared ginger	⅛ cup (1.6 oz)	48	tr	12	4

FOOD	PORTION	CAL	FAT	CARB	SUG
wasabi	2 tsp (0.3 oz)	5	tr	1	—
yellowtail roll	1 piece (0.6 oz)	25	1	3	tr
SWAMP CABBAGE					
chopped cooked	½ cup	10	tr	2	—
SWEET POTATO					
fresh					
baked w/ skin	1 (3½ oz)	118	tr	28	—
mashed	½ cup	172	tr	40	—
take-out					
candied	3½ oz	144	3	29	—
SWEETBREADS					
beef braised	3 oz	230	15	0	0
lamb braised	3 oz	199	13	0	0
veal braised	3 oz	218	12	0	0
SWISS CHARD					
cooked	½ cup	18	tr	4	—
SWORDFISH					
cooked	3 oz	132	4	0	0
SYRUP					
corn light	1 tbsp (0.7 oz)	56	0	15	10
maple	1 tbsp (0.8 oz)	52	0	13	12
rose hip	1 oz	9	0	2	2
sorghum	1 tbsp (0.7 oz)	61	0	16	16
Estee					
Blueberry	¼ cup	80	0	20	20
Karo					
Corn Syrup Light	2 tbsp (1 oz)	120	0	31	12
Quik					
Strawberry	2 tbsp (1.5 oz)	110	0	27	26

FOOD	PORTION	CAL	FAT	CARB	SUG
Smucker's					
Apricot	¼ cup	210	0	52	52
Blackberry	¼ cup	210	0	52	52
Plate Scapers Kiwi Lime	2 tbsp (1.3 oz)	100	0	25	13
Plate Scapers Mango Orange	2 tbsp	100	0	24	13
Plate Scapers Raspberry	2 tbsp (1.3 oz)	100	0	25	13

TACO

(*see* SPANISH FOOD)

TAMARIND

fresh	1	5	tr	1	—

TANGERINE
fresh
Chiquita

Tangerine	1 med (3.5 oz)	50	1	15	12

TAPIOCA
Minute

Minute Tapioca	1½ tsp (6 g)	20	0	5	0

TARO

sliced cooked	½ cup (2.3 oz)	94	tr	23	—

TARPON

fresh	3 oz	87	2	0	0

TARRAGON

ground	1 tsp	5	tr	1	—

TEA/HERBAL TEA

(*see also* ICED TEA)
herbal
Celestial Seasonings

Mandarin Orange Spice	1 tea bag	0	0	tr	0

FOOD	PORTION	CAL	FAT	CARB	SUG
Lipton					
Bedtime Story	1 tea bag	0	0	1	0
Cinnamon Apple	1 tea bag	0	0	1	0
Gentle Orange	1 tea bag	0	0	1	0
Lemon Soother	1 tea bag	0	0	1	0
Peppermint	1 tea bag	0	0	1	0
Quietly Chamomile	1 tea bag	0	0	1	0
regular					
brewed tea	6 oz	2	0	tr	—
Activitea					
Green Tea	1 cup	36	0	3	tr
General Foods					
International Instant Tea Decaffeinated English Breakfast Creme	1 serv (8 oz)	70	2	13	10
International Instant Tea Decaffeinated Viennese Cinnamon Creme	1 serv (8 oz)	70	2	13	10
International Instant Tea English Breakfast Creme as prep	1 serv (8 oz)	70	2	13	10
International Instant Tea English Raspberry Creme as prep	1 serv (8 oz)	70	2	13	11
International Instant Tea Island Orange Creme as prep	1 serv (8 oz)	70	2	13	11
International Instant Tea Viennese Cinnamon Creme as prep	1 serv (8 oz)	70	2	13	11

FOOD	PORTION	CAL	FAT	CARB	SUG
Lipton					
Brisk Tea as prep	1 serv	0	0	0	0
Decaffeinated Brisk Tea as prep	1 serv	0	0	0	0
English Blend as prep	1 cup	0	0	0	0
Flavored Decaffeinated Orange & Spice	1 tea bag	0	0	0	0
Green Tea	1 tea bag	0	0	0	0
Loose Tea	1 tsp (2 g)	0	0	0	0
Paradise					
Tropical Tea	8 fl oz	1	0	tr	0
Tropical Tea Decafe	8 fl oz	1	0	tr	0
Tropical Tea Passion Fruit	8 fl oz	1	0	tr	0
Salada					
Green Tea	1 cup	0	0	0	0
Tetley					
British Blend Round Teabags	1 cup	0	0	0	0
Tea Bag as prep	1	0	0	0	0

TEMPEH

FOOD	PORTION	CAL	FAT	CARB	SUG
Lightlife					
Garden Vege	4 oz	200	8	12	3
Quinoa Sesame	4 oz	220	8	15	3
Smokey Strips	3 slices (2 oz)	80	3	6	0
Soy	4 oz	210	8	11	3
Three Grain	4 oz	200	7	13	3
Wild Rice	4 oz	190	7	13	3
Turtle Island					
Five Grain	3 oz	190	6	20	0
Low Fat Millet	3 oz	130	2	20	0

FOOD	PORTION	CAL	FAT	CARB	SUG
Soy	3 oz	160	4	20	0
Wild Rice Rhapsody	3 oz	160	4	20	0
THYME					
ground	1 tsp	4	tr	1	—
TILEFISH					
cooked	3 oz	125	4	0	0
TOFU					
Galaxy					
Slices Hickory Smoked	1 slice (1 oz)	50	2	5	2
Slices Italian Garlic Herb	1 slice (1 oz)	50	2	5	2
Slices Original	1 slice (1 oz)	50	2	5	2
Slices Savory	1 slice (1 oz)	50	2	5	2
Hinoichi					
Firm	1 inch slice (3 oz)	60	3	2	0
Long Life					
Tofu	3 oz	60	3	2	0
Tree Of Life					
30% Reduced Fat Firm	⅕ block (3.2 oz)	90	4	4	0
Easymeal Pasta Primavera as prep	1 serv	460	16	54	4
Easymeal Southwest Medley as prep	1 serv	380	14	44	4
Easymeal Teriyaki Stir Fry as prep	1 serv	270	14	24	8
Easymeal Thai Stir Fry	1 serv	270	14	21	8
Organic Firm	⅕ block (3.2 oz)	100	5	2	0
Raw Firm	⅕ block (3.2 oz)	100	5	2	0
TOMATILLO					
fresh	1 (1.2 oz)	11	tr	2	—

FOOD	PORTION	CAL	FAT	CARB	SUG
TOMATO					
canned					
Amore					
Sun-Dried Tomato Paste	1 tsp (6 g)	15	1	tr	0
Big R					
Cajun Stewed	½ cup (4.2 oz)	25	0	4	4
Diced w/ Chilies	½ cup (4.2 oz)	25	0	4	3
Mexican Stewed	½ cup (4.2 oz)	25	0	5	3
Stewed	½ cup (4.2 oz)	25	0	5	3
Whole	½ cup (4.2 oz)	25	0	5	3
Contadina					
Paste	2 tbsp (1.2 oz)	30	0	6	3
Puree	¼ cup (2.2 oz)	20	0	4	1
Recipe Ready Diced Roasted Garlic	½ cup (4.3 oz)	45	0	10	7
Del Monte					
Zesty Diced w/ Mild Green Chilies	½ cup (4.4 oz)	30	0	6	3
Hunt's					
Angela Mia Puree	¼ cup (2.2 oz)	16	tr	3	3
Choice Cut	½ cup (4.2 oz)	23	tr	5	5
Choice Cut Diced Tomatoes & Italian Herb	½ cup (4.2 oz)	24	0	5	5
Choice Cut Diced Tomatoes & Roasted Garlic	½ cup (4.2 oz)	24	0	5	5
Choice Cut Diced Tomatoes w/ Red Pepper & Basil	¼ cup (4.2 oz)	27	tr	6	5
Crushed Pear Tomatoes	½ cup (4.2 oz)	29	tr	7	6
Diced In Juice	½ cup (4.2 oz)	20	tr	4	5

FOOD	PORTION	CAL	FAT	CARB	SUG
Diced In Puree	½ cup (4.3 oz)	23	tr	5	5
Diced w/ Green Chilies	2 tbsp (0.4 oz)	1	tr	tr	tr
Paste	2 tbsp (1.2 oz)	30	tr	6	4
Paste Italian	2 tbsp (1.2 oz)	27	tr	6	4
Paste No Salt Added	2 tbsp (1.2 oz)	30	tr	6	4
Paste With Garlic	2 tbsp (1.2 oz)	28	tr	6	4
Puree	¼ cup (2.2 oz)	24	tr	5	3
Ready Sauce Chunky Chili	¼ cup (2.2 oz)	22	tr	4	3
Ready Sauce Chunky Italian	¼ cup (2.2 oz)	30	1	4	4
Ready Sauce Chunky Mexican	¼ cup (2.2 oz)	21	tr	4	3
Ready Sauce Chunky Salsa	¼ cup (2.2 oz)	18	tr	3	3
Ready Sauce Chunky Tomato	¼ cup (2.2 oz)	15	tr	3	2
Ready Sauce Garlic & Herb	¼ cup (2.2 oz)	26	tr	5	4
Sauce	¼ cup (2.2 oz)	16	tr	3	3
Sauce Herb	¼ cup (2.2 oz)	32	1	5	5
Sauce Italian	¼ cup (2.2 oz)	32	1	5	5
Sauce Meatloaf Fixins	¼ cup (2.2 oz)	23	tr	4	5
Sauce No Salt Added	¼ cup (2.2 oz)	16	tr	3	3
Sauce Special	¼ cup (2.2 oz)	21	1	4	3
Stewed	½ cup (4.2 oz)	33	tr	7	6
Stewed No Salt Added	½ cup (4.2 oz)	33	tr	7	6
Whole Peeled	2 (5.2 oz)	24	tr	5	5
Whole Peeled No Salt Added	2 (4.8 oz)	21	tr	4	4
Muir Glen					
Diced Fire Roasted	¼ cup	30	0	6	4

FOOD	PORTION	CAL	FAT	CARB	SUG
Diced w/ Green Chilies	½ cup (4.5 oz)	25	0	4	4
Organic Chunky Sauce	¼ cup (2.3 oz)	20	0	4	2
Organic Crushed Fire Roasted	¼ cup	20	0	5	4
Organic Diced	½ cup (4.5 oz)	25	0	4	4
Organic Diced No Salt Added	½ cup (4.5 oz)	25	0	4	4
Organic Diced w/ Basil & Garlic	½ cup (4.5 oz)	25	0	4	4
Organic Diced w/ Italian Herbs	½ cup (4.4 oz)	25	0	4	4
Organic Ground Peeled	¼ cup (2.3 oz)	10	0	2	2
Organic Paste	2 tbsp (1.2 oz)	30	0	6	3
Organic Puree	¼ cup (2.2 oz)	20	0	5	3
Organic Sauce	¼ cup (2.2 oz)	20	0	5	3
Organic Sauce No Salt Added	¼ cup (2.2 oz)	20	0	5	3
Organic Stewed	½ cup (4.5 oz)	30	0	7	3
Organic Whole Peeled	½ cup (4.6 oz)	30	0	5	4
Whole Peeled w/ Basil	½ cup (4.6 oz)	30	0	5	4
Progresso					
Crushed	¼ cup (2.1 oz)	20	0	4	2
Italian Style Peeled	½ cup (4.2 oz)	20	0	4	3
Paste	2 tbsp (1.2 oz)	30	0	6	3
Puree	¼ cup (2.2 oz)	25	0	5	3
Puree Thick Style	¼ cup (2.2 oz)	20	0	5	3
Sauce	¼ cup (2.1 oz)	20	0	4	2
Whole Peeled	½ cup (4.2 oz)	25	0	5	3
Red Pack					
Puree	¼ cup (2.2 oz)	25	0	5	3

FOOD	PORTION	CAL	FAT	CARB	SUG
Sonoma					
Pesto	¼ cup (2 oz)	110	9	6	2
Tapenade	1 tbsp (0.7 oz)	70	6	4	1
dried					
Sonoma					
Dried	2–3 halves (5 g)	15	0	3	1
fresh					
green	1	30	tr	6	—
red	1 (4.5 oz)	26	tr	6	—
Chiquita					
Tomato	1 med (5.2 oz)	35	1	7	4
take-out					
stewed	1 cup	80	3	13	—
TOMATO JUICE					
Campbell					
Juice	8 oz	51	1	10	8
Hunt's					
Juice	1 can (6 oz)	22	tr	5	4
No Salt Added	8 fl oz	34	tr	8	7
Muir Glen					
Organic	5.5 oz	40	0	8	3
TONGUE					
beef simmered	3 oz	241	18	tr	—
lamb braised	3 oz	234	17	0	0
pork braised	3 oz	230	16	0	0
TOPPINGS					
(*see* ICE CREAM TOPPINGS)					
TORTILLA					
La Mexicana					
Corn	1 (0.8 oz)	50	1	10	0

FOOD	PORTION	CAL	FAT	CARB	SUG
Flour	1 (0.8 oz)	80	3	13	1
Tortillas de Trigo	1 (1 oz)	140	7	18	0
Old El Paso					
Flour	1 (1.4 oz)	130	4	21	0
Tyson					
Flour	1 (1.7 oz)	150	4	24	1
Flour Heat Pressed	2 (2 oz)	170	4	30	1
White Corn	2 (1.8 oz)	100	1	21	0
Whole Wheat Heat Pressed	1 (1.4 oz)	120	3	20	2
Yellow Corn	3 (1.9 oz)	140	2	27	0

TORTILLA CHIPS

(*see* CHIPS)

TREE FERN

chopped cooked	½ cup	28	tr	8	—

TRITICALE

dry	1 cup (6.7 oz)	645	4	138	—

TROUT

baked	3 oz	162	7	0	0

TRUFFLES

fresh	0.5 oz	4	tr	9	—

TUMERIC

ground	1 tsp	8	tr	1	—

TUNA
canned

Bumble Bee					
Albacore In Water	2 oz	60	1	0	0
Chunk Light In Water	2 oz	60	1	0	0
Chunk Light In Water Pouch	2 oz	60	1	0	0
Solid White In Water	2 oz	70	1	0	0

FOOD	PORTION	CAL	FAT	CARB	SUG
Progresso					
In Olive Oil drained	¼ cup (2 oz)	160	12	0	0
StarKist					
Chunk Light No Drain Package	¼ cup (2 oz)	60	1	0	0
Solid White Albacore In Spring Water	¼ cup (2 oz)	70	1	0	0
Tuna Fillet In Spring Water	¼ cup (2 oz)	60	1	0	0
Low Sodium Chunk White In Water	2 oz	60	1	0	0
fresh					
bluefin cooked	3 oz	157	5	0	0
yellowfin baked	3 oz	118	1	0	0

TUNA DISHES
mix

Tuna Helper

FOOD	PORTION	CAL	FAT	CARB	SUG
AuGratin 50% Less Fat Recipe as prep	1 cup	240	6	37	5
AuGratin as prep	1 cup	300	11	37	5
Cheesy Broccoli 50% Less Fat Recipe as prep	1 cup	240	5	00	0
Cheesy Broccoli as prep	1 cup	290	9	38	6
Cheesy Pasta 50% Less Fat Recipe as prep	1 cup	230	5	32	5
Cheesy Pasta as prep	1 cup	280	11	32	5
Creamy Broccoli 50% Less Fat Recipe as prep	1 cup	240	5	35	6

FOOD	PORTION	CAL	FAT	CARB	SUG
Creamy Broccoli as prep	1 cup	310	12	35	6
Creamy Pasta 50% Less Fat Recipe as prep	1 cup	230	6	31	4
Creamy Pasta as prep	1 cup	300	13	31	4
Fettuccine Alfredo 50% Less Fat Recipe as prep	1 cup	240	6	32	6
Fettuccine Alfredo as prep	1 cup	310	14	32	6
Garden Cheddar 50% Less Fat Recipe as prep	1 cup	240	5	36	7
Garden Cheddar as prep	1 cup	290	11	36	7
Pasta Salad Low Fat Recipe as prep	⅔ cup	230	2	26	4
Pasta Salad as prep	⅔ cup	380	27	26	4
Tetrazzini 50% Less Fat Recipe as prep	1 cup	230	5	34	3
Tetrazzini as prep	1 cup	300	12	34	3
Tuna Melt Reduced Fat Recipe as prep	1 cup	240	6	34	9
Tuna Melt as prep	1 cup	300	12	34	9
Tuna Pot Pie as prep	1 cup	440	24	40	9
Tuna Romanoff 50% Less Fat Recipe as prep	1 cup	240	3	38	3
Tuna Romanoff as prep	1 cup	280	8	38	3

FOOD	PORTION	CAL	FAT	CARB	SUG
ready-to-eat					
Bumble Bee					
Tuna Salad Fat Free	1 pkg (3.5 oz)	190	2	25	7
Tuna Salad Kit	1 pkg (3.8 oz)	250	13	15	2
StarKist					
Lunch To-Go	1 pkg	310	13	26	11
Ready-Mixed Tuna Salad Kit	1 pkg (3.5 oz)	190	6	25	11
Tuna Salad Lunch Kit	1 pkg (4.3 oz)	230	9	17	4
take-out					
tuna salad	1 cup	383	19	19	—
TURBOT					
european baked	3 oz	104	3	0	0
TURKEY					
fresh					
breast w/ skin roasted	4 oz	212	8	0	0
ground cooked	3 oz	188	11	0	0
leg w/ skin roasted	1 (1.2 lbs)	1133	54	0	0
neck simmered	1 (5.3 oz)	274	11	0	0
skin roasted	1 oz	141	13	0	0
w/o skin roasted	1 cup (5 oz)	238	7	0	0
wing w/ skin roasted	1 (6.5 oz)	426	23	0	0
Louis Rich					
Ground	4 oz	190	12	0	0
Patties White	1 (4 oz)	170	10	0	0
Perdue					
Burger Cooked	1 (4 oz)	160	9	0	0
Drumsticks Cooked	1 (2.2 oz)	110	6	0	0
Ground Cooked	3 oz	160	9	0	0
Thighs Cooked	1 (3.2 oz)	240	19	0	0

FOOD	PORTION	CAL	FAT	CARB	SUG
Shady Brook					
Ground Breast	4 oz	120	1	0	0
Wampler					
Boneless Breast Roast	4 oz	160	6	0	0
Breast Half	4 oz	160	6	0	0
Breast Steaks	4 oz	120	1	0	0
Drumsticks	4 oz	180	10	0	0
Ground	4 oz	210	15	0	0
Ground Breast	4 oz	130	1	0	0
Ground Lean	4 oz	160	8	0	0
Thighs	4 oz	170	10	0	0
Wings	4 oz	220	14	0	0
frozen					
Wampler					
Burgers Cracked Peppercorn & Garlic	1 (3 oz)	170	9	0	0
Seasoned Burgers Cracked Peppercorn & Garlic	1 (3 oz)	170	9	0	0
ready-to-eat					
patties battered & fried	1 (3.3 oz)	266	17	15	—
Alpine Lace					
Breast Fat Free	2 oz	45	0	0	0
Boar's Head					
Breast Cracked Pepper Smoked	2 oz	60	1	1	0
Breast Golden Skin on	2 oz	60	2	0	0
Breast Golden Skinless	2 oz	60	1	tr	0
Breast Hickory Smoked	2 oz	70	2	tr	0
Breast Low Sodium Skinless	2 oz	60	1	tr	0

FOOD	PORTION	CAL	FAT	CARB	SUG
Breast Lower Sodium Skin On	2 oz	60	2	tr	0
Breast Maple Glazed Honey Coat	2 oz	70	1	2	2
Breast Ovengold Skin On	2 oz	60	2	1	0
Breast Ovengold Skinless	2 oz	60	1	0	0
Breast Roasted Mesquite Smoked Skinless	2 oz	60	1	0	0
Breast Roasted Salsalito	2 oz	60	1	1	0
Pastrami Seasoned	2 oz	60	1	1	0
Carl Buddig					
Honey Roasted Turkey Breast	1 pkg (2.5 oz)	120	7	3	3
Lean Slices Honey Roasted Breast	1 pkg (2.5 oz)	70	1	4	4
Lean Slices Oven Roasted Breast	1 pkg (2.5 oz)	70	1	1	1
Lean Slices Smoked Breast	1 pkg (2.5 oz)	70	1	1	1
Oven Roasted Breast	1 pkg (2.5 oz)	110	7	1	1
Smoked Breast	1 pkg (2.5 oz)	110	7	1	1
Turkey Ham	1 pkg (2.5 oz)	100	5	1	1
Hormel					
Light & Lean 97 Breast Sliced	1 slice (1 oz)	30	1	0	0
Light & Lean 97 Mesquite Smoked Breast	1 slice (1 oz)	30	1	0	0
turkey pepperoni	17 slices (1 oz)	80	4	0	0

FOOD	PORTION	CAL	FAT	CARB	SUG
Louis Rich					
Bologna	1 slice (28 g)	50	4	1	0
Breaded Nuggets	4 (3.2 oz)	260	16	15	0
Breaded Patties	1 (3 oz)	220	13	13	0
Breaded Sticks	3 (3 oz)	230	15	12	0
Breast Skinless Hickory Smoked	2 oz	50	0	1	0
Breast Skinless Honey Roasted	2 oz	60	0	3	2
Breast Skinless Oven Roasted	2 oz	50	0	1	0
Breast Skinless Rotisserie	2 oz	50	0	1	1
Breast Slices Hickory Smoked	1 slice (2 oz)	50	0	1	0
Breast Slices Honey Roasted	1 slice (2 oz)	60	0	3	2
Breast Slices Oven Roasted	1 slice (2 oz)	50	0	1	0
Breast Slices Rotisserie	1 slice (2 oz)	50	0	1	1
Carving Board Hickory Smoked	2 slices (1.6 oz)	40	1	0	0
Carving Board Oven Roasted Thin	6 slices (2.1 oz)	60	1	1	0
Carving Board Oven Roasted Traditional	2 slices (1.6 oz)	40	1	0	0
Carving Board Rotisserie	2 slices (1.6 oz)	40	1	0	0
Cotto Salami	1 slice (28 g)	40	3	0	0
Deli-Thin Oven Roasted	4 slices (1.8 oz)	50	1	2	0
Deli-Thin Smoked	4 slices (1.8 oz)	50	2	1	tr

FOOD	PORTION	CAL	FAT	CARB	SUG
Fat Free Hickory Smoked Breast	1 slice (1 oz)	25	0	1	0
Fat Free Oven Roasted Breast	1 slice (1 oz)	25	0	1	tr
Fat Free Oven Roasted Deli-Thin Breast	4 slices (1.8 oz)	45	0	2	tr
Fat Free Turkey Ham Honey	2 slices (1.7 oz)	35	0	2	1
Fat Free Turkey Ham Smoked	2 slices (1.7 oz)	35	0	1	tr
Hickory Smoked	1 slice (1 oz)	30	1	1	0
Oven Roasted	1 slice (1 oz)	30	1	1	0
Pastrami	1 slice (1 oz)	30	1	1	0
Smoked	1 slice (1 oz)	30	1	0	0
Turkey Ham	1 slice (1 oz)	30	1	1	0
Turkey Ham Chopped	1 slice (1 oz)	45	3	1	0
Turkey Ham Honey Cured	1 slice (1 oz)	30	1	1	tr
Oscar Mayer					
Free Oven Roasted Breast	4 slices (1.8 oz)	40	0	2	tr
Free Smoked Breast	4 slices (1.8 oz)	40	0	2	tr
Oven Roasted White	1 slice (1 oz)	30	1	1	tr
Smoked White	1 slice (1 oz)	30	1	1	0
Perdue					
Breast Sliced Honey Smoked	2 oz	50	0	2	2
Breast Sliced Pan Roasted	2 oz	70	2	0	0
Healthsense Breast Sliced Oven Roasted	2 oz	60	0	3	1

FOOD	PORTION	CAL	FAT	CARB	SUG
Shady Brook					
Meatballs Italian Style	3 (3 oz)	130	7	5	1
Wampler					
Deli Roast Breast	2 oz	50	1	0	0
Turkey Ham	2 oz	60	3	0	0

TURKEY DISHES
canned
Dinty Moore

Stew	1 cup (8.5 oz)	140	3	19	3

frozen
Banquet

Sandwich Toppers Gravy & Sliced Turkey	1 pkg (5 oz)	160	11	6	1

shelf-stable
Dinty Moore

Microwave Cup Stew	1 pkg (7.5 oz)	130	3	16	3

TURKEY SUBSTITUTES
Lightlife

Smart Deli Turkey	3 slices (1.5 oz)	40	0	1	0
Tofurkey					
Deli Slices Hickory	1.5 oz	120	2	14	0
Deli Slices Original	1.5 oz	120	2	14	0
Deli Slices Peppered	1.5 oz	120	2	14	0
Drummettes	1 (3 oz)	105	2	11	2
Giblet Gravy	1 serv (3.5 oz)	42	2	5	2
Stuffed Tofu Roast	1 serv (4 oz)	193	5	10	1
Worthington					
Smoked Turkey Meatless	3 slices (2 oz)	140	10	3	tr
Turkee Slices	3 slices (3.3 oz)	130	14	3	tr

FOOD	PORTION	CAL	FAT	CARB	SUG
Yves					
Veggie Turkey Deli Slices	1 serv (2.2 oz)	85	0	4	2
TURNIPS					
fresh					
cooked mashed	½ cup (4.2 oz)	47	tr	10	—
greens chopped cooked	½ cup	15	tr	3	—
frozen					
Birds Eye					
Greens w/ Diced Turnip	1 cup (3 oz)	25	0	2	1
TURTLE					
raw	3.5 oz	85	1	0	0
TUSK FISH					
raw	3.5 oz	79	tr	0	0
VEAL					
cutlet lean only braised	3 oz	172	4	0	0
cutlet lean only fried	3 oz	156	4	0	0
ground broiled	3 oz	146	6	0	0
loin chop w/ bone lean & fat braised	1 chop (2.8 oz)	227	14	0	0
sirloin w/ bone lean & fat roasted	3 oz	171	9	0	0
VEAL DISHES					
take-out					
parmigiana	4.2 oz	279	18	6	—
VEGETABLE JUICE					
Hunt's					
Cocktail	1 can (6 oz)	20	0	7	3

FOOD	PORTION	CAL	FAT	CARB	SUG
Muir Glen					
Organic	5.5 oz	50	0	10	7
V8					
Lightly Tangy	8 oz	58	1	11	9
Low Sodium	8 oz	53	tr	11	8
Original	8 oz	51	1	10	8
Picante Vegetable	8 oz	51	tr	10	7
Spicy Hot	8 oz	49	tr	10	7
Splash Tropical Blend	8 fl oz	120	0	30	27

VEGETABLES MIXED
canned

FOOD	PORTION	CAL	FAT	CARB	SUG
Chi-Chi's					
Diced Tomatoes & Green Chilies	¼ cup (2.5 oz)	20	0	4	3
Chun King					
Chow Mein Vegetables	⅔ cup (3 oz)	14	tr	3	0
Green Giant					
Garden Medley	½ cup (4.2 oz)	40	0	9	3
Mixed	½ cup (4.3 oz)	60	0	12	4
Sweet Peas & Carrots	½ cup (4.3 oz)	50	0	11	4
Sweet Peas & Tiny Pearl Onion	½ cup (4.4 oz)	60	0	11	3
House Of Tsang					
Vegetables & Sauce Cantonese Classic	½ cup (4.2 oz)	70	1	14	8
Vegetables & Sauce Hong Kong Sweet & Sour	½ cup (4.5 oz)	160	0	40	35
Vegetables & Sauce Szechuan Hot & Spicy	½ cup (4.2 oz)	70	1	14	8
Vegetables & Sauce Tokyo Teriyaki	½ cup (4.4 oz)	100	0	23	19

FOOD	PORTION	CAL	FAT	CARB	SUG
La Choy					
Chop Suey Vegetables	½ cup (2.2 oz)	10	tr	2	0
LeSueur					
Early Peas w/ Mushrooms & Pearl Onions	½ cup (4.3 oz)	60	0	11	4
frozen					
Amy's Organic					
Pocket Sandwich Mediterranean Vegetables	1 (4.5 oz)	220	7	33	5
Pocket Sandwich Roasted Vegetables	1 (4.5 oz)	220	8	35	5
Pocket Sandwich Vegetable Pie	1 (5 oz)	230	6	37	2
Birds Eye					
Baby Sweet Peas & Pearl Onions	⅔ cup (3.2 oz)	60	1	12	6
Bavarian Vegetables	1 cup (5.5 oz)	150	8	15	3
Broccoli Cauliflower Carrots w/ Cheese	½ cup (3.9 oz)	70	4	7	3
Broccoli Cauliflower & Red Peppers	½ cup	20	0	5	3
Broccoli & Cauliflower	½ cup	20	0	4	2
Broccoli Carrots & Water Chestnuts	½ cup (3.3 oz)	30	0	7	3
Broccoli Corn & Red Peppers	½ cup	50	0	12	3
Broccoli Red Peppers Onions & Mushrooms	½ cup	25	0	5	3
Broccoli & Cauliflower & Carrots	½ cup	25	0	5	3

FOOD	PORTION	CAL	FAT	CARB	SUG
Brussels Sprouts Cauliflower & Carrots	½ cup	30	0	7	3
California Style Vegetables	½ cup (3 oz)	100	5	9	4
Cauliflower Nuggets Corn Carrots & Snow Peas Pods	½ cup (3.2 oz)	30	0	6	3
Chicken Voila! Italian Pesto Chicken	2 cups (6.6 oz)	240	9	24	5
Chicken Voila! Three Cheese Chicken	1¾ cups (5.6 oz)	220	8	24	6
French Style	⅔ cup (4.4 oz)	110	6	10	2
Gumbo Blend	¾ cup (3 oz)	40	0	10	3
Italian Style Vegetables & Bow Tie Pasta	1 cup (5.8 oz)	150	9	13	3
New England Style Vegetables & Pasta Shells	1 pkg (7.9 oz)	260	14	29	6
Peas & Pearl Onions	⅔ cup (4.2 oz)	90	1	18	9
Peas & Potatoes In Cream Sauce	½ cup (4.4 oz)	90	3	13	5
Radiatore Pasta & Vegetables	1 cup (4.6 oz)	200	8	27	5
Roasted Potatoes & Broccoli	⅔ cup (3.9 oz)	100	4	15	2
Roletti Pasta & Vegetables	1 cup (4.4 oz)	190	8	11	5
Stir Fry Asparagus	2 cups (5.8 oz)	90	1	16	4
Stir Fry Broccoli	1 cup (3.4 oz)	30	0	5	3
Stir Fry Pepper	1 cup (3 oz)	25	0	5	4

FOOD	PORTION	CAL	FAT	CARB	SUG
Stir Fry Sugar Snap	¾ cup	35	0	5	3
Stir Fry Whole Green Bean	1¾ cup (5.3 oz)	100	1	19	4
Stir Fry Style Vegetables	½ cup (3.6 oz)	60	4	5	4
Vegetables For Stew	⅔ cup (2.9 oz)	40	0	9	2
Green Giant					
Alfredo Vegetables	¾ cup	70	3	9	4
American Mixtures Broccoli Carrots Cauliflower	¾ cup (2.6 oz)	25	0	5	2
American Mixtures Broccoli Carrots Waterchestnuts	¾ cup (3 oz)	30	0	6	2
American Mixtures Carrots Green Beans Cauliflower	¾ cup (2.7 oz)	25	0	5	2
American Mixtures Cauliflower Broccoli Sugar Snap & Sweet Peas	¾ cup (2.8 oz)	35	0	7	2
American Mixtures Corn Broccoli Red Peppers	¾ cup (3.1 oz)	60	0	13	3
American Mixtures Green Beans Potatoes Onions Red Peppers	¾ cup (2.8 oz)	45	1	8	2
American Mixtures Sweet Peas Potatoes Carrots	⅔ cup (3 oz)	70	2	12	2
Butter Sauce Broccoli Cauliflower Carrots Corn Sweet Peas	¾ cup (3.6 oz)	60	2	8	3

FOOD	PORTION	CAL	FAT	CARB	SUG
Butter Sauce Broccoli Pasta Sweet Peas Corn Red Peppers	¾ cup (3.5 oz)	70	2	11	3
Butter Sauce Mixed	¾ cup (3.6 oz)	70	2	11	3
Cheese Sauce Broccoli Cauliflower Carrots	⅔ cup (4.3 oz)	80	3	11	5
Harvest Fresh Broccoli Cauliflower Carrots	1 cup (3.4 oz)	30	0	5	2
Harvest Fresh Mixed Vegetables	⅔ cup (3.1 oz)	50	0	10	3
Harvest Fresh Sweet Peas & Pearl Onions	½ cup (2.7 oz)	55	0	10	2
Mixed	¾ cup (2.9 oz)	50	0	11	1
Select Sweet Peas & Pearl Onions	⅔ cup (3.1 oz)	60	0	12	2
Health Is Wealth					
Veggie Munchees	2 (1 oz)	50	1	9	0
La Choy					
Fancy Chinese Mixed Vegetables	½ cup (2.9 oz)	9	tr	1	0
take-out					
buddha's delight	1 serv (16 oz)	174	5	17	8
curry	1 serv (7.7 oz)	398	33	22	—
gyoza potstickers vegetable	8 (4.9 oz)	210	4	34	7
pakoras	1 (2 oz)	108	5	12	—
ratatouille	1 serv (3.5 oz)	96	7	7	7
samosa	2 (4 oz)	519	46	25	—
succotash	½ cup	111	1	23	—

FOOD	PORTION	CAL	FAT	CARB	SUG
VENISON					
roasted	3 oz	134	3	0	0
VINEGAR					
cider	1 tbsp	tr	0	1	—
Progresso					
Balsamic	2 tbsp (0.5 oz)	10	0	2	2
Victoria					
Balsamic	1 tbsp (0.5 oz)	5	0	2	2
White House					
Apple Cider	1 tbsp (0.5 oz)	0	0	0	0
White	1 tbsp (0.5 oz)	0	0	0	0
WAFFLES					
frozen					
Eggo					
Apple Cinnamon	2 (2.7 oz)	220	8	33	5
Banana Bread	2 (2.7 oz)	200	7	32	5
Blueberry	2 (2.7 oz)	220	9	32	6
Buttermilk	2 (2.7 oz)	220	8	31	3
Golden Oat	2 (2.7 oz)	150	3	29	3
Homestyle	2 (2.7 oz)	220	8	32	3
Minis Cinnamon Toast	12 (3.2 oz)	290	10	45	17
Minis Homestyle	12 (3.3 oz)	260	9	38	3
Nut & Honey	2 (2.7 oz)	240	10	31	5
Nutri-Grain	2 (2.7 oz)	190	6	30	4
Nutri-Grain Multi-Bran	2 (2.7 oz)	180	6	32	4
Nutri-Grain Raisin & Bran	2 (2.9 oz)	210	6	36	10
Special K	2 (2 oz)	120	0	26	4
Strawberry	2 (2.7 oz)	220	8	32	5
Kellogg's					
Homestyle Low Fat	2 (2.7 oz)	180	3	34	5

FOOD	PORTION	CAL	FAT	CARB	SUG
Nutri-Grain Low Fat	2 (2.7 oz)	160	3	31	4
Nutri-Grain Low Fat Blueberry	2 (2.7 oz)	160	2	33	7
Kid Cuisine					
Wave Rider Waffle Sticks	1 meal (6.6 oz)	380	8	75	38
ready-to-eat					
Thomas'					
Buttermilk	1 (1.6 oz)	130	5	18	7
WALNUTS					
Planters					
Halves	⅛ cup (1.2 oz)	220	22	5	tr
WATER					
Absopure					
Natural Spring	8 fl oz	0	0	0	0
Aquess					
Purified Water w/ Soluble Fiber	1 bottle (18 oz)	30	0	8	2
Crystal Geyser					
Spring Water	8 fl oz	0	0	0	0
Dasani					
Purfied Water	8 oz	0	0	0	0
Diamond Spring					
Water	1 qt	0	0	0	0
Gerolsteiner					
Sparkling Mineral	8 fl oz	0	0	0	0
Glaceau					
Vitamin Water Tropical Citrus	1 cup (8 oz)	40	0	9	8
Glacier Springs					
Drinking Water	8 fl oz	0	0	0	0

FOOD	PORTION	CAL	FAT	CARB	SUG
LaCroix					
Spring	1 bottle (12 oz)	0	0	0	0
Meridian					
Clear All Flavors	8 oz	100	0	25	25
Mountain Valley					
Mineral Water	1 qt	0	0	0	0
Mt Shasta					
Natural Spring	1 bottle (20 oz)	0	0	0	0
Reebok					
Fitness Water Berry	1 bottle (24 oz)	30	0	0	0
Fitness Water Natural	1 bottle (24 oz)	0	0	0	0
San Pellegrino					
Acqua Panna	8 fl oz	0	0	0	0
Saratoga					
Spring	8 oz	0	0	0	0
Snapple					
Natural Spring	8 fl oz	0	0	0	0
Veryfine					
Fruit 2 O Lemon	8 oz	0	0	0	0
Fruit 2 O Lemon Lime	8 fl oz	0	0	0	0
Fruit 2 O Orange	8 fl oz	0	0	0	0
Fruit 2 O Raspberry	8 fl oz	0	0	0	0
WATER CHESTNUTS					
Chun King					
Sliced	2 tbsp (0.8 oz)	11	tr	3	tr
Whole	2 (0.7 oz)	10	tr	2	tr
La Choy					
Chopped	2 tbsp (0.6 oz)	9	tr	2	tr
Sliced	2 tbsp (0.8 oz)	11	tr	3	tr
Whole	2 (0.7 oz)	10	tr	2	tr

FOOD	PORTION	CAL	FAT	CARB	SUG
WATERCRESS					
raw chopped	½ cup	2	tr	tr	—
WATERMELON					
cut up	1 cup	50	1	11	—
wedge	1/16	152	2	35	—
WATERMELON JUICE					
Kool-Aid					
Splash Drink	1 serv (8 oz)	110	0	30	30
WHEAT					
Lightlife					
Savory Seitan Barbecue	4 oz	160	2	12	3
Savory Seitan Teriyaki	4 oz	160	2	10	2
WHEAT GERM					
Kretschmer					
Original Toasted	2 tbsp (0.5 oz)	50	1	6	1
WHEY					
whey cheese	1 oz	126	8	9	0
WHIPPED TOPPINGS					
Cool Whip					
Extra Creamy	2 tbsp (0.3 oz)	25	2	2	2
Free	2 tbsp (0.3 oz)	15	0	3	1
Lite	2 tbsp (0.3 oz)	20	1	2	1
Original	2 tbsp (0.3 oz)	25	2	2	1
Dream Whip					
Mix as prep	2 tbsp (0.3 oz)	20	1	2	2
Estee					
Whipped Topping	1 serv	10	1	1	0
Kraft					
Dairy Whip Light Cream	2 tbsp (0.2 oz)	10	1	tr	tr
Fat Free	1 tbsp (0.3 oz)	15	0	2	2

FOOD	PORTION	CAL	FAT	CARB	SUG
WHITE BEANS					
canned					
Progresso					
Cannellini	½ cup (4.6 oz)	100	1	18	0
dried					
regular cooked	1 cup	249	1	45	—
WHITEFISH					
baked	3 oz	146	6	0	0
smoked	1 oz	39	tr	0	0
WHITING					
cooked	3 oz	98	1	0	0
WILD RICE					
Haddon House					
Extra Fancy	¼ cup (1.6 oz)	170	1	35	0
WINE					
japanese plum	3 oz	139	tr	16	—
japanese sake	1 oz	33	0	2	—
madeira	3.5 oz	169	0	10	10
port	3.5 oz	156	0	11	11
red	3½ oz	74	0	2	—
rose	3½ oz	73	0	2	—
sherry	2 oz	84	0	5	—
sweet dessert	2 oz	90	0	7	—
vermouth dry	3½ oz	105	0	1	—
vermouth sweet	3½ oz	167	0	12	—
white	3½ oz	70	0	1	—
WOLFFISH					
atlantic baked	3 oz	105	3	0	0
WRAPS					
(*see* BREAD)					

FOOD	PORTION	CAL	FAT	CARB	SUG
YEAST					
brewer's dry	1 tbsp	25	tr	3	—
Hodgson Mill					
Fast Rise	1 tsp (9 g)	25	0	4	0
YELLOW BEANS					
fresh cooked	½ cup	22	tr	5	—
YELLOWTAIL					
baked	3 oz	159	6	0	0
YOGURT					
Colombo					
99% Fat Free Peach	4 oz	110	1	22	19
99% Fat Free Strawberry	4 oz	110	1	22	19
Dannon					
Chunky Fruit Nonfat Apple Cinnamon	6 oz	160	0	33	29
Chunky Fruit Nonfat Blueberry	6 oz	160	0	32	29
Chunky Fruit Nonfat Cherry Vanilla	6 oz	160	0	31	28
Chunky Fruit Nonfat Peach	6 oz	160	0	33	29
Chunky Fruit Nonfat Strawberry	6 oz	160	0	32	28
Chunky Fruit Nonfat Strawberry Banana	6 oz	160	0	32	28
Danimals Lowfat Blueberry	4.4 oz	130	1	24	21
Danimals Lowfat Grape Lemonade	4.4 oz	120	1	22	20
Danimals Lowfat Lemon Ice	4.4 oz	120	1	22	19

FOOD	PORTION	CAL	FAT	CARB	SUG
Danimals Lowfat Orange Banana	4.4 oz	130	1	24	21
Danimals Lowfat Strawberry	4.4 oz	130	1	24	21
Danimals Lowfat Tropical Punch	4.4 oz	130	1	25	22
Danimals Lowfat Vanilla	4.4 oz	120	1	23	21
Danimals Lowfat Wild Raspberry	4.4 oz	120	1	22	19
Double Delights Banana Creme Strawberry	6 oz	160	1	32	28
Double Delights Bavarian Creme Raspberry	6 oz	170	1	34	31
Double Delights Cheesecake Cherry	6 oz	170	1	34	30
Double Delights Cheesecake Strawberry	6 oz	170	1	33	39
Double Delights Chocolate Cheesecake	6 oz	220	1	45	42
Double Delights Chocolate Dipped Strawberry	6 oz	210	1	45	41
Double Delights Chocolate Eclair	6 oz	220	1	45	42
Double Delights Vanilla Strawberry	6 oz	170	1	33	29
Double Delights Vanilla Peach & Apricot	6 oz	170	1	33	29

FOOD	PORTION	CAL	FAT	CARB	SUG
Fruit On The Bottom Lowfat Apple Cinnamon	8 oz	240	3	46	45
Fruit On The Bottom Lowfat Blueberry	8 oz	240	3	46	44
Fruit On The Bottom Lowfat Boysenberry	8 oz	240	3	45	42
Fruit On The Bottom Lowfat Cherry	8 oz	240	3	46	44
Fruit On The Bottom Lowfat Minipack Mixed Berry	4.4 oz	130	2	25	24
Fruit On The Bottom Lowfat Minipack Strawberry	4.4 oz	130	2	25	24
Fruit On The Bottom Lowfat Mixed Berries	8 oz	240	3	45	43
Fruit On The Bottom Lowfat Orange	8 oz	240	3	45	44
Fruit On The Bottom Lowfat Peach	8 oz	240	3	45	44
Fruit On The Bottom Lowfat Raspberry	8 oz	240	3	45	43
Fruit On The Bottom Lowfat Strawberry	8 oz	240	3	46	44
Fruit On The Bottom Lowfat Strawberry Banana	8 oz	240	3	43	40
LaCreme Vanilla	1 pkg (4.4 oz)	140	5	20	18
Light 'N Crunchy Mint Chocolate Chip	8 oz	140	0	27	14
Light 'N Crunchy Nonfat Caramel Apple Crunch	8 oz	140	0	26	14

FOOD	PORTION	CAL	FAT	CARB	SUG
Light 'N Crunchy Nonfat Lemon Blueberry Cobbler	8 oz	140	0	25	17
Light 'N Crunchy Nonfat Mocha Cappuccino	8 oz	140	0	26	14
Light 'N Crunchy Nonfat Raspberry w/ Granola	8 oz	140	0	26	13
Light 'N Crunchy Nonfat Vanilla Chocolate Crunch	8 oz	130	0	23	13
Light Duets Cherry Cheesecake	6 oz	90	0	18	12
Light Duets Peaches N' Cream	6 oz	90	0	18	13
Light Duets Raspberry Royale	6 oz	90	0	17	12
Light Duets Strawberry Cheesecake	6 oz	90	0	18	12
Light Nonfat Banana Cream Pie	8 oz	100	0	15	9
Light Nonfat Blueberry	8 oz	100	0	18	12
Light Nonfat Cappuccino	8 oz	100	0	16	9
Light Nonfat Cherry Vanilla	8 oz	100	0	18	13
Light Nonfat Coconut Cream Pie	8 oz	100	0	16	9
Light Nonfat Creme Caramel	8 oz	100	0	15	9
Light Nonfat Lemon Chiffon	8 oz	100	0	15	9
Light Nonfat Mint Chocolate Cream Pie	8 oz	100	0	17	9

FOOD	PORTION	CAL	FAT	CARB	SUG
Light Nonfat Peach	8 oz	100	0	16	11
Light Nonfat Raspberry	8 oz	100	0	17	11
Light Nonfat Strawberry	8 oz	100	0	16	10
Light Nonfat Strawberry Banana	8 oz	100	0	17	11
Light Nonfat Strawberry Kiwi	8 oz	100	0	16	10
Light Nonfat Tangerine Chiffon	8 oz	100	0	15	9
Light Nonfat Vanilla	8 oz	100	0	15	9
Lowfat Coffee	8 oz	210	3	36	34
Lowfat Cranberry Raspberry	8 oz	210	3	36	35
Lowfat Lemon	8 oz	210	3	36	35
Lowfat Vanilla	8 oz	210	3	36	34
Minipack Blended Nonfat Blueberry	4.4 oz	120	0	25	22
Minipack Blended Nonfat Cherry	4.4 oz	110	0	24	20
Minipack Blended Nonfat Peach	4.4 oz	120	0	23	21
Minipack Blended Nonfat Raspberry	4.4 oz	120	0	24	21
Minipack Blended Nonfat Strawberry	4.4 oz	120	0	23	20
Minipack Blended Nonfat Strawberry Banana	4.4 oz	120	0	23	20
Sprinkl'ins Cherry Vanilla	1 (4.1 oz)	130	2	24	20

FOOD	PORTION	CAL	FAT	CARB	SUG
Sprinkl'ins Strawberry	1 (4.1 oz)	130	2	24	20
Sprinkl'ins Strawberry Banana	1 (4.1 oz)	130	2	24	20
Sprinkl'ins Vanilla w/ Cherry Crystals	1 (4.1 oz)	110	1	21	19
Sprinkl'ins Vanilla w/ Orange Crystals	1 (4.1 oz)	110	1	21	19
Oberweis					
Peach	1 pkg (8 oz)	210	3	39	35
Pascual					
Nonfat Cherries & Berries	1 pkg (4.4 oz)	100	0	19	12
Nonfat Peach	1 pkg (4.4 oz)	100	0	19	12
Stonyfield Farm					
Creamy Maple	1 pkg	160	6	19	18
Mocho-Ccino	1 pkg	170	6	23	22
Nonfat Apricot Mango	1 pkg (8 oz)	160	0	31	30
Nonfat Black Cherry	1 pkg (8 oz)	160	0	31	29
Nonfat Cappuccino	1 pkg (8 oz)	160	0	31	29
Nonfat Cherry Vanilla	1 pkg (8 oz)	190	0	43	41
Nonfat Chocolate Undorground	1 pkg (8 oz)	200	0	46	45
Nonfat French Vanilla	1 pkg (8 oz)	180	0	30	29
Nonfat Lotsa Lemon	1 pkg (8 oz)	160	0	30	29
Nonfat Peach	1 pkg (8 oz)	150	0	30	30
Nonfat Plain	1 pkg (8 oz)	100	8	15	15
Nonfat Raspberry	1 pkg (8 oz)	160	0	31	28
Nonfat Strawberry	1 pkg (8 oz)	180	0	32	30
Organic French Vanilla	1 pkg	170	6	23	22
Organic Wild Blueberry	1 pkg	160	6	22	21
Organic Lowfat Blueberry	1 pkg (6 oz)	130	2	23	22

FOOD	PORTION	CAL	FAT	CARB	SUG
Organic Lowfat Luscious Lemon	1 pkg (6 oz)	130	2	23	22
Organic Lowfat Maple Vanilla	1 pkg (6 oz)	120	2	19	19
Organic Lowfat Mocha Latte	1 pkg (6 oz)	120	2	20	19
Organic Lowfat Plain	1 cup (8 oz)	110	2	14	13
Organic Lowfat Raspberry	1 pkg (6 oz)	130	2	23	21
Organic Lowfat Strawberry	1 pkg (6 oz)	130	2	23	22
Organic Lowfat Vanilla	1 pkg (6 oz)	120	2	20	20
Strawberries & Cream	1 pkg	160	5	23	22
Vanilla Truffle	1 pkg	220	5	37	34
YoSelf Organic Chocolate	1 (4 oz)	110	1	21	19
YoSelf Organic Creme Carmel	1 (4 oz)	110	1	21	19
Yosqueeze Strawberry	1 tube (2 oz)	60	1	11	10
Yoplait					
Whips! Orange Creme	1 pkg (4 oz)	140	3	23	21
Whips! Raspberry Mousse	1 pkg (4 oz)	140	3	23	21

YOGURT FROZEN

FOOD	PORTION	CAL	FAT	CARB	SUG
vanilla soft serve	½ cup (4 fl oz)	114	4	17	16
Turkey Hill					
Chocolate Chip Cookie Dough	½ cup	140	5	23	21
Fat Free Chocolate Cherry Cordial	½ cup	100	0	24	21
Fat Free Chocolate Marshmallow	½ cup	130	0	30	21

FOOD	PORTION	CAL	FAT	CARB	SUG
Fat Free Mint Cookie 'N Cream	½ cup	110	0	24	18
Fat Free Neapolitan	½ cup	100	0	22	19
Fat Free Vanilla Fudge	½ cup	110	0	24	21
Peach Raspberry	½ cup	110	2	20	20
Tin Roof Sundae	½ cup	140	5	21	20
Vanilla & Chocolate	½ cup	110	3	19	18
Vanilla Bean	½ cup	110	3	17	17

ZUCCHINI
canned
Progresso

FOOD	PORTION	CAL	FAT	CARB	SUG
Italian Style	½ cup (4.2 oz)	50	2	7	4

fresh

baby raw	1 (0.5 oz)	3	tr	1	—
sliced cooked	½ cup	14	tr	4	—

take-out

indian paalkora	1 serv	46	2	7	—

Part 2

◆

Restaurant Chains

FOOD	PORTION	CAL	FAT	CARB	SUG
APPLEBEE'S					
desserts					
Apple Betty Cobbler Ala Mode	1 serv	598	22	94	57
Fudge Brownie Sundae	1 serv	739	40	87	39
Low Fat Bikini Banana Strawberry Shortcake	1 serv	248	2	48	27
Low Fat Brownie Sundae	1 serv	415	2	82	57
Low Fat Marble Cheesecake	1 serv	261	2	50	—
main menu selections					
Applebee's Burger w/ Fries	1 serv	1274	79	90	10
Basic Hamburger w/ Fries	1 serv	980	58	86	8
Beef Fajita Quesadilla	1 serv	1205	86	58	5
Bourbon Street Steak w/ Fried New Potatoes	1 serv	1115	94	50	3
Low Fat Asian Chicken Salad	1 med serv (2.5 oz)	370	6	64	—
Low Fat Blacked Chicken Salad	1 med serv (2.5 oz)	287	3	27	—
Low Fat Garlic Chicken Pasta	1 serv	587	8	89	7
Low Fat Lemon Chicken Pasta	1 serv	528	11	78	12
Low Fat Quesadilla Chicken Fajita	1 serv	518	11	63	6
Low Fat Quesadilla Veggie	1 serv	344	8	46	4
Mozzarella Stix	8 pieces	963	57	74	—

FOOD	PORTION	CAL	FAT	CARB	SUG
Quesadillas	1 serv	684	46	40	5
Riblet Basket w/ Fries	1 serv	1317	92	45	tr
Salad Dinner w/o Dressing	1 serv	303	18	13	4
Salad Santa Fe Chicken	1 med	724	42	56	12
Sandwich Bacon Cheese Chicken Grill w/o Fries	1	746	46	36	1
Sandwich Gyro	1	880	69	44	5
Stir Fry Chicken	1 serv	566	7	89	24

ARBY'S
beverages

FOOD	PORTION	CAL	FAT	CARB	SUG
Chocolate Shake	1 (14 oz)	480	16	84	—
Hot Chocolate	1 serv (8.6 oz)	110	1	23	—
Jamocha Shake	1 (14 oz)	470	15	82	—
Milk	1 serv (8 oz)	120	5	12	—
Orange Juice	1 serv (10 oz)	140	0	34	—
Strawberry Shake	1 (14 oz)	500	13	87	—
Vanilla Shake	1 (14 oz)	470	15	83	—

breakfast selections

FOOD	PORTION	CAL	FAT	CARB	SUG
Add Egg To Breakfast	1 serv (2 oz)	110	9	2	—
Biscuit w/ Bacon	1 (3.4 oz)	360	24	27	—
Biscuit w/ Butter	1 (2.9 oz)	280	17	27	—
Biscuit w/ Ham	1 (4.3 oz)	330	20	28	—
Biscuit w/ Sausage	1 (4.2)	460	33	28	—
Croissant w/ Bacon	1 (2.7 oz)	340	23	28	—
Croissant w/ Ham	1 (3.7 oz)	310	19	29	—
Croissant w/ Sausage	1 (3.6 oz)	440	32	29	—
Maple Syrup	1 serv (0.5 oz)	130	0	32	—
Sourdough w/ Bacon	1 (5.1 oz)	420	10	66	—

FOOD	PORTION	CAL	FAT	CARB	SUG
Sourdough w/ Ham	1 (6.1 oz)	390	6	67	—
Sourdough w/ Sausage	1 (5.9 oz)	520	19	67	—
Toastix w/o Syrup	6 pieces (4.4 oz)	370	17	48	—
desserts					
Apple Turnover Iced	1 (4.5 oz)	420	16	65	—
Cherry Turnover Iced	1 (4.5 oz)	410	16	63	—
main menu selections					
Arby's Sauce	1 serv (0.5 oz)	15	0	4	—
Au Jus Sauce	1 serv (3 oz)	5	tr	1	—
BBQ Dipping Sauce	1 serv (1 oz)	40	0	10	—
Baked Potato Broccoli'N Cheddar	1 (14 oz)	540	24	71	—
Baked Potato Deluxe	1 (13 oz)	650	34	67	—
Baked Potato w/ Butter & Sour Cream	1 (11.2 oz)	500	24	65	—
Bronco Berry Sauce	1 serv (1.5 oz)	90	0	23	—
Caesar Salad w/o Dressing	1 serv (8 oz)	90	4	8	—
Cheddar Curly Fries	1 serv (6 oz)	460	24	54	—
Chicken Finger 4-Pak	1 serv (6.77 oz)	640	38	42	—
Chicken Finger Salad w/o Dressing	1 serv (13 oz)	570	34	39	—
Chicken Finger Snack	1 serv (6.4 oz)	580	32	55	—
Curly Fries	1 sm (3.8 oz)	310	15	39	—
German Mustard	1 pkg (0.25 oz)	5	0	0	—
Grilled Chicken Caesar Salad w/o Dressing	1 serv (12 oz)	230	8	8	—
Homestyle Fries	1 sm (4 oz)	300	13	42	—
Homestyle Fries Child-Size	1 serv (3 oz)	220	10	32	—

FOOD	PORTION	CAL	FAT	CARB	SUG
Honey Mustard	1 serv (1 oz)	130	12	5	—
Horsey Sauce	1 pkg (0.5 oz)	60	5	3	—
Jalapeno Bites	1 serv (4 oz)	330	21	29	—
Ketchup	1 pkg (0.3 oz)	10	0	2	—
Light Grilled Chicken Salad	1 (16.3 oz)	210	5	14	—
Marinara Sauce	1 serv (1.5 oz)	35	1	4	—
Mayonnaise	1 pkg (0.4 oz)	90	10	0	—
Mayonnaise Light Cholesterol Free	1 pkg (0.4 oz)	20	2	1	—
Mozzarella Sticks	1 serv (4.8 oz)	470	29	34	—
Onion Petals	1 serv (4 oz)	410	24	43	—
Potato Cakes	2 (3.5 oz)	250	16	26	—
Roast Beef Sandwich Arby's Melt w/ Cheddar	1 (5.2 oz)	320	14	36	—
Roast Beef Sandwich Arby-Q	1 (6.4 oz)	360	14	40	—
Roast Beef Sandwich Beef'N Cheddar	1 (6.9 oz)	460	23	43	—
Roast Beef Sandwich Big Montana	1 (11 oz)	560	27	42	—
Roast Beef Sandwich Junior	1 (4.4 oz)	290	12	34	—
Roast Beef Sandwich Regular	1 (5.4 oz)	330	14	35	—
Sandwich Chicken Bacon'N Swiss	1 (7.4 oz)	610	33	49	—
Sandwich Chicken Breast Fillet	1 (7.2 oz)	550	30	47	—
Sandwich Chicken Cordon Bleu	1 (8.4 oz)	630	35	47	—
Sandwich Grilled Chicken Deluxe	1 (8.7 oz)	450	22	37	—

FOOD	PORTION	CAL	FAT	CARB	SUG
Sandwich Hot Ham 'N Swiss	1 (5.9 oz)	340	13	35	—
Sandwich Light Roast Chicken Deluxe	1 (7.2 oz)	260	5	33	—
Sandwich Light Roast Turkey Deluxe	1 (7.2 oz)	260	5	33	—
Sandwich Market Fresh Roast Beef & Swiss	1 (12.5 oz)	780	40	74	—
Sandwich Market Fresh Roast Chicken Caesar	1 (12.7 oz)	820	38	75	—
Sandwich Market Fresh Roast Ham & Swiss	1 (12.5 oz)	730	34	74	—
Sandwich Market Fresh Roast Turkey & Swiss	1 (12.5 oz)	760	33	75	—
Sandwich Roast Chicken Club	1 (8.4 oz)	520	28	38	—
Sub Sandwich French Dip	1 (10 oz)	410	16	43	—
Sub Sandwich Hot Ham 'N Swiss	1 (9.7 oz)	530	27	45	—
Sub Sandwich Italian	1 (11 oz)	780	53	49	—
Sub Sandwich Philly Beef 'N Swiss	1 (10.8 oz)	670	40	46	—
Sub Sandwich Roast Beef	1 (11.6 oz)	730	46	48	—
Sub Sandwich Turkey	1 (10.6 oz)	630	37	51	—
Tangy Southwest Sauce	1 serv (1.5 oz)	250	26	3	—
salad dressings					
Bleu Cheese	1 serv (2 oz)	300	31	3	—
Buttermilk Ranch	1 serv (2 oz)	360	39	2	—

FOOD	PORTION	CAL	FAT	CARB	SUG
Buttermilk Ranch Reduced Calorie	1 serv (2 oz)	60	0	13	—
Caesar	1 serv (2 oz)	310	34	1	—
Honey French	1 serv (2 oz)	290	24	18	—
Italian Reduced Calorie	1 serv (2 oz)	25	1	3	—
Thousand Island	1 serv (2 oz)	290	28	9	—
salads and salad bars					
Croutons Seasoned	1 serv (0.25 oz)	30	1	5	—
Croutons Cheese & Garlic	1 serv (0.63 oz)	100	6	10	—
Garden Salad	1 (12.3 oz)	70	1	14	—
Light Roast Chicken Salad	1 (14.8 oz)	160	3	15	—
Light Grilled Chicken Sandwich	1 (7.5 oz)	280	5	30	—
Side Salad	1 (6.1 oz)	30	0	6	—
Turkey Club Salad w/o Dressing	1 serv (12 oz)	350	21	9	—

AU BON PAIN

baked selections

FOOD	PORTION	CAL	FAT	CARB	SUG
Apple Coffee Cake	1 piece (4.6 oz)	480	24	60	42
Bagel Chocolate Chip	1 (5 oz)	380	7	69	14
Bagel Dutch Apple w/ Walnut Streussel	1 (5 oz)	360	5	77	21
Baguette Loaf	1 slice (1.8 oz)	140	5	29	1
Biscotti	1 (1.5 oz)	200	10	24	11
Biscotti Chocolate	1 (1.7 oz)	240	13	28	13
Braided Roll	1 (1.8 oz)	170	5	26	4
Cinnamon Roll	1 (7 oz)	710	26	110	56
Cookie Chocolate Chip	1 (2.1 oz)	280	13	40	26

FOOD	PORTION	CAL	FAT	CARB	SUG
Cookie Oatmeal Raisin	1 (2.1 oz)	250	10	40	26
Cookie Peanut Butter	1 (2.1 oz)	280	15	32	16
Cookie Shortbread	1 (2.4 oz)	390	25	39	13
Croissant Almond	1 (4.3 oz)	560	37	50	19
Croissant Apple	1 (3.4 oz)	280	10	46	19
Croissant Chocolate	1 (3.4 oz)	440	23	53	25
Croissant Cinnamon Raisin	1 (3.7 oz)	380	13	61	5
Croissant Plain	1 (2.1 oz)	270	15	30	20
Croissant Raspberry Cheese	1 (3.5 oz)	380	19	47	17
Croissant Sweet Cheese	1 (3.6 oz)	390	22	42	18
Danish Cheese Swirl	1 (3.8 oz)	450	28	46	21
Danish Lemon Swirl	1 (4 oz)	450	24	53	12
Danish Raspberry	1 (3.6 oz)	370	21	42	16
Danish Sweet Cheese	1 (3.6 oz)	420	26	42	—
Four Grain Loaf	1 slice (1.8 oz)	130	1	25	3
French Sandwich Roll	1 (1.8 oz)	120	5	25	1
Hazelnut Fudge Brownie	1 (4 oz)	380	18	56	34
Mochaccino Bar	1 (4 oz)	404	24	44	30
Muffin Blueberry	1 (4.5 oz)	410	15	64	34
Muffin Carrot	1 (5 oz)	480	23	61	34
Muffin Chocolate Chip	1 (4.5 oz)	490	20	70	30
Muffin Corn	1 (4.6 oz)	470	18	70	37
Muffin Pumpkin w/ Streusel Topping	1 (5.5 oz)	470	18	74	—
Muffin Low Fat Chocolate Cake	1 (4 oz)	290	3	68	43

FOOD	PORTION	CAL	FAT	CARB	SUG
Muffin Low Fat Triple Berry	1 (4.2 oz)	270	3	60	28
Multigrain Loaf	1 slice (1.8 oz)	130	1	26	3
Parisienne Loaf	1 slice (1.8 oz)	120	5	25	1
Pear Ginger Tea Cake	1 piece (4 oz)	380	20	47	30
Pecan Roll	1 (6.8 oz)	900	48	111	61
Roll 3 Seed Pecan Raisin	1 (2.7 oz)	250	6	43	9
Roll Hearth Sandwich	1 (2.8 oz)	220	2	43	5
Rolls Petit Pan	1 (2.5 oz)	200	1	41	2
Rye Loaf	1 slice (1.8 oz)	110	2	21	2
Scone Cinnamon	1 (4.1 oz)	520	28	60	16
Scone Current	1 (3.7 oz)	430	23	47	7
Scone Orange	1 (4.1 oz)	440	23	53	6
Sourdough Bagel Asiago Cheese	1 (4.2 oz)	380	6	66	5
Sourdough Bagel Cinnamon Raisin	1 (4.5 oz)	390	1	83	18
Sourdough Bagel Cranberry Walnut	1 (5 oz)	460	4	93	19
Sourdough Bagel Everything	1 (4.2 oz)	360	3	72	5
Sourdough Bagel Honey 8 Grain	1 (4.2 oz)	360	2	72	9
Sourdough Bagel Mocha Chip Swirl	1 (5 oz)	370	4	72	13
Sourdough Bagel Plain	1 (4 oz)	350	1	71	5
Sourdough Bagel Sesame	1 (4.2 oz)	380	4	71	5
Sourdough Bagel Wild Blueberry	1 (4.5 oz)	380	2	80	8

FOOD	PORTION	CAL	FAT	CARB	SUG
beverages					
Frozen Java Blast	1 serv (16 oz)	220	2	42	11
Frozen Mocha Blast	1 serv (16 oz)	320	3	64	58
Hot Apple Cider	1 sm (10 oz)	190	0	47	47
Hot Hazelnut Blast	1 serv (16 oz)	310	6	57	52
Hot Mocha Blast	1 sm (9 oz)	160	4	23	21
Hot Raspberry Mocha Blast	1 serv (10 oz)	180	4	29	27
Hot Strawberry Chocolate Blast	1 serv (16 oz)	330	6	57	52
Hot Vanilla Chocolate Blast	1 serv (16 oz)	310	6	57	52
Iced Caffe Latte	1 sm (9 oz)	130	5	12	12
Iced Cappuccino	1 sm (9 oz)	110	4	10	10
Iced Cocoa	1 sm (9 oz)	200	6	27	24
Iced Hazelnut Blast	1 serv (16 oz)	310	6	54	48
Iced Mocha Blast	1 sm (9 oz)	180	5	25	22
Iced Raspberry Mocha Blast	1 serv (24 oz)	330	7	54	—
Iced Raspberry Mocha Blast	1 serv (16 oz)	310	6	54	—
Iced Raspberry Mocha Blast	1 serv (12 oz)	160	4	27	—
Iced Strawberry Chocolate Blast	1 serv (16 oz)	310	6	54	48
Iced Vanilla Chocolate Blast	1 serv (16 oz)	310	6	54	48
Iced Tea Peach	1 sm (12 oz)	90	0	22	22
Iced Tea Raspberry	1 sm (8 oz)	80	0	19	19
Whipped Cream	1 serv (1.2 oz)	160	11	11	5
salad dressings					
Bleu Cheese	1 serv (3 oz)	370	41	8	5

FOOD	PORTION	CAL	FAT	CARB	SUG
Buttermilk Ranch	1 serv (3 oz)	310	32	4	3
Caesar	1 serv (3 oz)	380	39	3	1
Fat Free Tomato Basil	1 serv (3 oz)	70	0	17	13
Greek	1 serv (3 oz)	440	50	2	1
Lemon Basil Vinaigrette	1 serv (3 oz)	330	32	15	13
Lite Honey Mustard	1 serv (3 oz)	280	17	30	20
Lite Italian	1 serv (3 oz)	230	20	15	14
Sesame French	1 serv (3 oz)	370	30	26	1
salads and salad bars					
Caesar	1 serv (8.9 oz)	270	10	27	3
Chicken Caesar	1 serv (11.4 oz)	360	11	28	3
Garden	1 sm (7.5 oz)	100	1	20	6
Mozzarella & Roasted Pepper Salad	1 serv (13.7 oz)	340	18	25	5
Pesto Chicken Salad	1 serv (10.7 oz)	230	11	11	6
Tuna	1 serv (15 oz)	490	27	40	9
sandwiches and fillings					
Bagel Spreads Lite Strawberry	1 serv (2 oz)	150	11	6	5
Bagel Spreads Lite Vanilla Hazelnut	1 serv (2 oz)	150	11	6	5
Cheddar	½ serv (1.5 oz)	170	14	1	1
Chicken Tarragon	1 serv (4 oz)	240	17	1	1
Club Sandwich Hot Roasted Turkey	1 (14.9 oz)	950	50	80	6
Country Ham	1 serv (3.7 oz)	150	7	1	1
Cracked Pepper Chicken	1 serv (3.9 oz)	140	2	2	0
Cream Cheese Lite	1 serv (2 oz)	130	12	2	1
Cream Cheese Lite Honey Walnut	1 serv (2 oz)	260	12	8	—

FOOD	PORTION	CAL	FAT	CARB	SUG
Cream Cheese Lite Raspberry	1 serv (2 oz)	200	8	10	—
Cream Cheese Lite Sun-Dried Tomato	1 serv (2 oz)	130	11	2	2
Cream Cheese Plain	1 serv (2 oz)	190	18	2	1
Cream Cheese Veggie Lite	1 serv (2 oz)	100	10	6	—
Grilled Chicken	1 serv (3.9 oz)	140	2	2	0
Hot Croissant Ham & Cheese	1 (4.2 oz)	380	20	36	6
Hot Croissants Spinach & Cheese	1 (3.6 oz)	270	16	27	5
Provolone	½ serv (1.5 oz)	150	11	1	1
Roast Beef	1 serv (3.7 oz)	140	5	1	0
Sandwich Arizona Chicken	1 (12.7 oz)	720	33	57	7
Sandwich Buffalo Chicken	1 (13.7 oz)	640	19	76	5
Sandwich California Chicken	1 (13.2 oz)	820	44	55	9
Sandwich Fresh Mozzarella Tomato & Pesto	1 (10.5 oz)	650	30	69	7
Sandwich Honey Dijon Chicken	1 (15.3 oz)	730	18	85	12
Sandwich Parmesan Chicken	1 (11.1 oz)	740	24	91	4
Sandwich Steak & Cheese Melt	1 (11.7 oz)	750	32	79	9
Sandwich Thai Chicken	1 (8.3 oz)	420	6	72	9
Swiss	½ serv (1.5 oz)	160	12	1	1
Tuna Salad	1 serv (4.5 oz)	360	29	3	2
Turkey Breast	1 serv (3.7 oz)	120	1	1	0

FOOD	PORTION	CAL	FAT	CARB	SUG
Wraps Chicken Caesar	1 (9.9 oz)	630	31	46	4
Wraps Southwestern Tuna	1 (14.4 oz)	950	64	53	9
Wraps Summer Turkey	1 (11.7 oz)	340	9	36	12
soups					
Beef Barley	1 serv (8 oz)	75	2	11	2
Beef Stew	1 serv (8 oz)	140	7	14	3
Bohemian Cabbage	1 serv (8 oz)	70	3	11	2
Bread Bowl	1 (9 oz)	640	4	131	4
Broccoli & Cheddar	1 serv (8 oz)	260	22	13	5
Caribbean Black Bean	1 serv (8 oz)	120	1	22	3
Chicken Chili	1 serv (8 oz)	240	12	21	3
Chicken Noodle	1 serv (8 oz)	80	2	10	1
Chili	1 serv (12 oz)	340	14	32	7
Chili	1 serv (8 oz)	230	10	22	4
Clam Chowder	1 serv (8 oz)	270	19	16	5
Corn Chowder	1 serv (8 oz)	260	16	29	7
Cream Of Broccoli	1 serv (8 oz)	220	18	14	6
French Onion	1 serv (8 oz)	80	4	12	7
In A Bread Bowl Beef Barley	1 serv (21 oz)	760	7	147	7
In A Bread Bowl Carribean Black Bean	1 serv (21 oz)	830	5	163	8
In A Bread Bowl Chicken Chili	1 serv (21 oz)	990	22	162	9
In A Bread Bowl Chicken Noodle	1 serv (21 oz)	760	6	146	6
In A Bread Bowl Clam Chowder	1 serv (21 oz)	1050	32	155	12
In A Bread Bowl Cream of Broccoli	1 serv (21 oz)	970	31	152	13

FOOD	PORTION	CAL	FAT	CARB	SUG
In A Bread Bowl French Onion	1 serv (21 oz)	760	8	148	15
In A Bread Bowl New England Potato & Cheese w/ Ham	1 serv (21 oz)	860	15	152	6
In A Bread Bowl Tomato Florentine	1 serv (21 oz)	760	5	150	6
In A Bread Bowl Vegetarian Chili	1 serv (21 oz)	870	7	171	6
Louisiana Beans & Rice	1 serv (8 oz)	180	5	25	1
New England Potato & Cheese w/ Ham	1 serv (8 oz)	150	8	14	1
Potato Leek	1 serv (8 oz)	200	13	18	2
Sante Fe Chicken Tortilla	1 serv (8 oz)	150	7	21	3
Seafood Gumbo	1 serv (8 oz)	130	6	14	1
Tomato Florentine	1 serv (8 oz)	61	1	13	1
Tomato Tortellini	1 serv (8 oz)	60	1	11	2
Vegetable Stew	1 serv (8 oz)	60	1	11	4
Vegetarian Lentil	1 serv (8 oz)	130	0	24	1
Vegetarian Chili	1 serv (8 oz)	139	3	27	1
Vegetarian Corn & Green Chili Bisque	1 serv (8 oz)	190	10	21	5

AUNTIE ANNE'S

FOOD	PORTION	CAL	FAT	CARB	SUG
Caramel Dip	1 serv (1.5 oz)	135	3	27	21
Cheese Sauce	1 serv (1 oz)	70	5	2	2
Chocolate Dip	1 serv (1.25 oz)	130	4	24	12
Cream Cheese Light	1 serv (.75 oz)	45	4	1	1
Cream Cheese Pineapple	1 serv (.75 oz)	70	6	3	3
Cream Cheese Strawberry	1 serv (.75 oz)	70	6	3	3

FOOD	PORTION	CAL	FAT	CARB	SUG
Dutch Ice Kiwi Banana	1 (12 oz)	160	0	38	35
Dutch Ice Kiwi Banana	1 (18 oz)	250	0	57	53
Dutch Ice Lemonade	1 (12 oz)	270	0	66	66
Dutch Ice Mocha	1 (12 oz)	340	9	63	45
Dutch Ice Orange Creme	1 (12 oz)	240	0	55	51
Dutch Ice Raspberry	1 (12 oz)	150	0	34	32
Dutch Ice Strawberry	1 (12 oz)	190	0	43	41
Marinara Sauce	1 serv (1 oz)	10	0	3	2
Pretzel Almond w/ Butter	1	400	8	72	15
Pretzel Almond w/o Butter	1	350	2	72	1
Pretzel Cinnamon Raisin w/o Butter	1	350	2	74	16
Pretzel Cinnamon Sugar w/ Butter	1	450	9	83	26
Pretzel Garlic w/ Butter	1	350	5	68	9
Pretzel Garlic w/o Butter	1	320	1	66	9
Pretzel Glazein' Raisin w/ Butter	1	510	4	107	38
Pretzel Glazin' Raisin w/o Butter	1	470	1	104	37
Pretzel Jalapeno w/ Butter	1	310	5	59	9
Pretzel Jalapeno w/o Butter	1	270	1	58	8
Pretzel Original w/ Butter	1	370	4	72	10
Pretzel Original w/o Butter	1	340	1	72	10
Pretzel Sesame w/ Butter	1	410	12	64	9

FOOD	PORTION	CAL	FAT	CARB	SUG
Pretzel Sesame w/o Butter	1	350	6	63	9
Pretzel Sour Cream & Onion w/ Butter	1	340	5	66	10
Pretzel Sour Cream & Onion w/o Butter	1	310	1	66	9
Pretzel Whole Wheat w/ Butter	1	370	5	72	10
Pretzel Whole Wheat w/o Butter	1	350	2	72	10
Sweet Mustard	1 serv (1 oz)	60	2	8	8

BASKIN-ROBBINS

frozen yogurt

FOOD	PORTION	CAL	FAT	CARB	SUG
Maui Brownie Madness	½ cup	140	3	26	23
Perils Of Pauline	½ cup	140	3	25	23

ice cream

FOOD	PORTION	CAL	FAT	CARB	SUG
Banana Strawberry	½ cup	130	7	17	16
Baseball Nut	½ cup	160	9	18	17
Black Walnut	½ cup	160	11	13	12
Cherries Jubilee	½ cup	140	7	16	14
Chocolate	½ cup	150	9	18	16
Chocolate Almond	½ cup	180	11	17	15
Chocolate Chip	½ cup	150	10	15	14
Chocolate Chip Cookie Dough	½ cup	170	9	20	16
Chocolate Fudge	½ cup	160	9	21	19
Chocolate Mousse Royale	½ cup	170	10	20	18
Chocolate Raspberry Truffle	½ cup	180	9	23	21
Chunky Heath Bar	½ cup	170	10	19	18
Cookies N Cream	½ cup	170	11	16	14

FOOD	PORTION	CAL	FAT	CARB	SUG
Dirt 'N Worms	½ cup	160	8	22	19
Egg Nog	½ cup	150	8	16	16
Everybody's Favorite Candy Bar	½ cup	170	9	20	19
French Vanilla	½ cup	160	10	14	14
Fudge Brownie	½ cup	170	11	19	17
German Chocolate Cake	½ cup	180	10	20	19
Gold Medal Ribbon	½ cup	150	8	20	19
Jamoca	½ cup	140	9	14	14
Jamoca Almond Fudge	½ cup	140	9	17	16
Lemon Custard	½ cup	150	8	16	16
Lowfat Carmel Apple Ala Mode	½ cup	100	2	20	19
Lowfat Espresso 'N Cream	½ cup	100	3	18	16
Mint Chocolate Chip	½ cup	150	10	15	14
No Sugar Added Call Me Nuts	½ cup	110	2	21	6
No Sugar Added Cherry Cordial	½ cup	100	2	18	5
No Sugar Added Mad About Chocolate	½ cup	100	2	19	4
No Sugar Added Pineapple Coconut	½ cup	90	2	16	5
No Sugar Added Thin Mint	½ cup	100	3	16	4
Nonfat Berry Innocent Cheese	½ cup	110	0	24	21
Nonfat Check-It-Out Cherry	½ cup	100	0	22	20

FOOD	PORTION	CAL	FAT	CARB	SUG
Nonfat Jamoca Swirl	½ cup	110	0	23	22
Ocean Commotion	½ cup	150	7	20	18
Old Fashion Butter Pecan	½ cup	160	11	13	12
Oregon Blueberry	½ cup	140	8	16	14
Peanut Butter N Chocolate	½ cup	180	12	16	15
Pink Bubblegum	½ cup	150	8	19	15
Pistachio Almond	½ cup	170	12	13	12
Pralines N Cream	½ cup	160	9	19	18
Pumpkin Pie	½ cup	130	7	16	15
Quarterback Crunch	½ cup	160	10	18	17
Reeses Peanut Butter	½ cup	180	11	17	16
Rocky Road	½ cup	170	10	19	17
Rum Raisin	½ cup	140	7	18	18
Strawberry Cheesecake	½ cup	150	9	17	16
Triple Chocolate Passion	½ cup	180	11	21	18
Vanilla	½ cup	140	8	14	14
Very Berry Strawberry	½ cup	130	7	16	15
Winter White Chocolate	½ cup	150	9	18	16
World Class Chocolate	½ cup	160	9	18	17
ices and ice pops					
Daiquiri Ice	½ cup	110	0	28	27
Sherbet Blue Raspberry	½ cup	120	2	25	25
Sherbet Orange	½ cup	120	2	26	22
Sherbet Rainbow	½ cup	120	2	26	23
Sorbet Pink Raspberry Lemon	½ cup	120	0	29	27

FOOD	PORTION	CAL	FAT	CARB	SUG
The Mask Ice	½ cup	120	0	29	28
Watermelon Ice	½ cup	110	0	28	28

BEN & JERRY'S

Sugar Cone	1	48	tr	10	3

frozen yogurt

Cherry Garcia	½ cup (3.3 oz)	150	3	29	23
Chocolate Cherry Garcia	½ cup (3.3 oz)	170	4	37	25
Chocolate Fudge Brownie	½ cup (3.3 oz)	180	3	32	27
No Fat Black Raspberry	½ cup (3.4 oz)	140	0	30	25
No Fat Coffee Fudge	½ cup (3.4 oz)	140	0	30	24
No Fat Vanilla	½ cup (3.4 oz)	140	0	28	23
No Fat Vanilla Fudge Swirl	½ cup (3.4 oz)	130	0	29	24

Ice cream

Bovinity Divinity	½ cup (3.1 oz)	240	14	24	22
Butter Pecan	½ cup (3.1 oz)	270	21	17	15
Cherry Garcia	½ cup (3.1 oz)	210	12	20	19
Chocolate Chip Cookie Dough	½ cup (3.1 oz)	180	11	17	16
Chocolate Fudge Brownie	½ cup (3.1 oz)	230	11	28	24
Chubby Hubby	½ cup (3.1 oz)	280	17	26	20
Chunky Monkey	½ cup (3.1 oz)	220	13	25	23
Coconut Almond Fudge Chip	½ cup (3.1 oz)	250	18	19	16
Coffee Coffee Buzz Buzz	½ cup (3.1 oz)	240	16	23	20
Coffee Ole	½ cup (3.1 oz)	200	13	18	16

FOOD	PORTION	CAL	FAT	CARB	SUG
Coffee w/ Heath Bar Crunch	½ cup (3.1 oz)	250	16	25	23
Deep Dark Chocolate	½ cup (3.1 oz)	210	12	22	19
Dilbert's World Totally Nuts	½ cup (3.1 oz)	260	18	21	21
Low Fat Blackberry Cobbler	½ cup (3.2 oz)	160	2	32	26
Low Fat Chocolate Comfort	½ cup (3.2 oz)	150	2	27	23
Low Fat Coconut Creme Pie	½ cup (3.2 oz)	160	3	29	23
Low Fat Mocha Latte	½ cup (3.2 oz)	150	2	27	23
Low Fat Rockin Road	½ cup (3.2 oz)	180	3	34	25
Low Fat Smore's	½ cup (3.2 oz)	180	2	34	25
Low Fat Vanilla & Chocolate Mint Patty	½ cup (3.2 oz)	170	3	32	27
Maple Walnut	½ cup (3.1 oz)	240	13	19	17
Mint Chocolate Chunk	½ cup (3.1 oz)	240	16	24	21
Mint Chocolate Cookie	½ cup (3.1 oz)	230	14	24	19
New York Super Fudge Chunk	½ cup (3.1 oz)	250	16	25	21
Peanut Butter Cup	½ cup (3.1 oz)	270	18	21	18
Phish Food	½ cup (3.1 oz)	230	12	30	23
Pistachio Pistachio	½ cup (3.1 oz)	190	13	17	15
Praline Pecan	½ cup (3.1 oz)	230	14	24	21
Southern Pecan Pie	½ cup (3.1 oz)	240	16	21	18
Strawberry	½ cup (3.1 oz)	180	10	20	17
Sweet Cream Cookie	½ cup (3.1 oz)	230	14	23	19
Triple Caramel Chunk	½ cup (3.1 oz)	240	13	28	24
Vanilla Caramel Fudge	½ cup (3.1 oz)	230	13	25	21
Vanilla Chocolate Chunk	½ cup (3.1 oz)	240	16	23	21

FOOD	PORTION	CAL	FAT	CARB	SUG
Vanilla World's Best	½ cup (3.1 oz)	200	13	17	16
Vanilla w/ Heath Toffee Crunch	½ cup (3.1 oz)	250	16	25	23
Wavy Gravy	½ cup (3.1 oz)	260	17	24	21
White Russian	½ cup (3.1 oz)	200	13	18	16
sorbets					
Doonesberry	½ cup (3.2 oz)	100	0	27	24
Lemon Swirl	½ cup (3.2 oz)	100	0	25	22
Purple Passion Fruit	½ cup (3.2 oz)	100	0	27	24
Strawberry Kiwi	½ cup (3.2 oz)	110	0	27	25
BIG BOY					
desserts					
Frozen Yogurt Fat Free	1 serv	118	0	27	—
Frozen Yogurt Shake	1	156	1	33	—
main menu selections					
Baked Cod w/ Salad Baked Potato Roll & Margarine	1 meal	744	21	82	—
Baked Potato	1	163	2	37	—
Breast of Chicken Pita w/ Mozzarella & Ranch Dressing	1	361	11	23	—
Breast of Chicken w/ Mozzarella Salad Baked Potato Roll & Margarine	1 meal	697	20	80	—
Cabbage Soup	1 cup	34	4	6	—
Cajun Cod w/ Salad Baked Potato Roll & Margarine	1 meal	736	21	80	—
Chicken & Pasta Primavera w/ Salad Roll & Margarine	1 meal	676	14	83	—

FOOD	PORTION	CAL	FAT	CARB	SUG
Chicken 'n Vegetable Stir Fry w/ Salad Baked Potato Roll & Margarine	1 meal	795	18	109	—
Dinner Roll	1	210	5	36	—
Plain Egg Beaters Omelette w/ Whole Wheat Bread & Margarine	1 meal	305	10	36	—
Promise Margarine	1 pat	25	3	0	—
Rice Pilaf	1 serv	153	4	25	—
Scrambled Egg Beaters w/ Whole Wheat Bread & Margarine	1 meal	305	10	36	—
Southwest Chicken w/ Salad Baked Potato Roll & Margarine	1 meal	702	18	85	—
Spaghetti Marinara w/ Salad Roll & Margarine	1 meal	754	11	105	—
Turkey Pita w/ Ranch Dressing	1	245	6	23	—
Vegetable Stir Fry w/ Salad Baked Potato Roll & Margarine	1 meal	616	14	109	—
Vegetarian Egg Beaters Omelette w/ Whole Wheat Bread & Margarine	1 meal	330	10	40	—
salad dressings					
Italian Fat Free	1 oz	11	0	3	—
Lo Cal Oriental	1 oz	20	2	4	—
Lo Cal Ranch	1 oz	41	3	3	—

FOOD	PORTION	CAL	FAT	CARB	SUG
salads and salad bars					
Chicken Breast Salad w/ Roll & Margarine	1 serv	523	16	50	—
Oriental Chicken Breast Salad w/ Dinner Roll & Margarine	1 serv	660	20	73	—
Tossed Salad	1	35	2	7	—
BLIMPIE					
6 inch sub					
5 Meatball	1 (7.8 oz)	500	22	52	6
Blimpie Best	1 (8.5 oz)	410	13	47	3
Cheese Trio	1 (8.2 oz)	510	23	51	3
Club	1 (9.8 oz)	450	13	53	4
Grilled Chicken	1 (9.1 oz)	400	9	52	2
Ham & Swiss	1 (8.2 oz)	400	13	47	2
Ham Salami Provolone	1 (9.8 oz)	590	28	52	3
Roast Beef	1 (8.5 oz)	340	5	47	3
Steak & Cheese	1 (7.1 oz)	550	26	51	3
Tuna	1 (10.2 oz)	570	32	50	5
Turkey	1 (8.2 oz)	320	5	51	3
salads and salad bars					
Grilled Chicken Salad	1 serv (16.2 oz)	350	12	13	3
BOJANGLES					
baked selections					
Biscuit	1	243	12	29	—
Multi-Grain Roll	1	150	3	26	—
Sweet Biscuit Apple Cinnamon	1	330	13	48	—
Sweet Biscuit Bo*Berry	1	220	10	29	—

FOOD	PORTION	CAL	FAT	CARB	SUG
Sweet Biscuit Cinnamon	1	320	18	37	—
main menu selections					
Biscuit Sandwich Bacon	1	290	17	26	—
Biscuit Sandwich Bacon Egg & Cheese	1	550	42	27	—
Biscuit Sandwich Cajun Filet	1	454	21	46	—
Biscuit Sandwich Country Ham	1	270	15	26	—
Biscuit Sandwich Egg	1	400	30	26	—
Biscuit Sandwich Sausage	1	350	23	26	—
Biscuit Sandwich Smoked Sausage	1	380	26	27	—
Biscuit Sandwich Steak	1	649	49	13	—
Bo Rounds	1 serv	235	11	31	—
Buffalo Bites	1 serv	180	5	5	—
Cajun Pintos	1 serv	110	0	18	—
Cajun Roast Skinfree Breast	1 serv	143	5	tr	—
Cajun Roast Skinfree Leg	1 serv	161	8	tr	—
Cajun Roast Skinfree Thigh	1 serv	215	15	tr	—
Cajun Roast Wing	1 serv	231	15	3	—
Cajun Spiced Breast	1 serv	278	17	12	—
Cajun Spiced Leg	1 serv	310	23	11	—
Cajun Spiced Thigh	1 serv	264	16	11	—
Cajun Spiced Wing	1 serv	355	25	11	—
Chicken Supremes	1 serv	337	16	26	—

FOOD	PORTION	CAL	FAT	CARB	SUG
Corn On The Cob	1 serv	140	2	34	—
Dirty Rice	1 serv	166	6	24	—
Green Beans	1 serv	25	0	25	—
Macaroni & Cheese	1 serv	198	14	12	—
Marinated Cole Slaw	1 serv	136	3	26	—
Potatoes w/o Gravy	1 serv	80	1	16	—
Sandwich Cajun Filet w/ Mayonnaise	1	437	22	41	—
Sandwich Cajun Filet w/o Mayonnaise	1	337	11	41	—
Sandwich Cajun Steak w/ Horseradish Sauce & Pickles	1	434	26	39	—
Sandwich Grilled Filet w/ Mayonnaise	1	335	16	25	—
Sandwich Grilled Filet w/o Mayonnaise	1 serv (5.2 oz)	329	7	37	—
Seasoned Fries	1 serv	344	19	39	—
Southern Style Breast	1 serv	261	16	12	—
Southern Style Leg	1 serv	254	15	11	—
Southern Style Thigh	1 serv	308	21	14	—
Southern Style Wing	1 serv	307	21	19	—

BOSTON MARKET

baked selections

FOOD	PORTION	CAL	FAT	CARB	SUG
Brownie	1 (3.3 oz)	450	27	47	32
Cinnamon Apple Pie	⅛ pie (4.8 oz)	390	23	46	—
Cookie Chocolate Chip	1 (2.8 oz)	340	17	48	29

main menu selections

FOOD	PORTION	CAL	FAT	CARB	SUG
½ Chicken w/ Skin	1 serv (9.7 oz)	590	33	4	4
¼ Dark Meat Chicken No Skin	1 serv (3.3 oz)	190	10	1	—

FOOD	PORTION	CAL	FAT	CARB	SUG
¼ Dark Meat Chicken w/ Skin	1 serv (4.4 oz)	320	21	2	2
¼ White Meat Chicken No Skin Or Wing	1 serv (4.9 oz)	170	4	2	1
¼ White Meat Chicken w/ Skin And Wing	1 serv (5.3 oz)	280	12	2	2
BBQ Baked Beans	¾ cup (7.1 oz)	270	5	48	20
BBQ Chicken Sandwich	1 (9.9 oz)	540	9	84	33
Baked Sweet Potato Low Fat	1 (12.5 oz)	460	7	94	49
Black Beans And Rice	1 cup (8 oz)	300	10	45	3
Boston Hearth Ham Lean	1 serv (5 oz)	210	9	9	7
Broccoli Cauliflower Au Gratin	¾ cup (6.1 oz)	200	11	14	4
Broccoli Rice Casserole	¾ cup (6 oz)	240	12	26	2
Broccoli With Red Peppers	¾ cup (3.4 oz)	60	4	5	1
Butternut Squash Low Fat	¾ cup (6.8 oz)	160	6	25	13
Chicken Gravy	1 serv (1 oz)	15	1	2	0
Chicken Salad Sandwich	1 (11.5 oz)	680	30	63	12
Chicken Sandwich w/ Cheese & Sauce	1 (12.4 oz)	750	33	72	13
Chicken Sandwich w/o Cheese & Sauce Low Fat	1 (10 oz)	430	5	62	12
Chunky Chicken Salad	¾ cup (5.5 oz)	370	27	3	1
Chunky Cinnamon Apple Sauce No Fat	¾ cup (6.4 oz)	250	0	62	55
Cole Slaw	¾ cup (6.5 oz)	300	19	30	26

FOOD	PORTION	CAL	FAT	CARB	SUG
Corn Bread	1 (2.4 oz)	200	6	33	13
Coyote Bean Salad	¾ cup (5.3 oz)	190	9	24	2
Cranberry Relish Low Fat	¾ cup (7.9 oz)	370	5	84	72
Creamed Spinach	¾ cup (6.4 oz)	260	20	11	2
Fruit Salad Low Fat	¾ cup (5.5 oz)	70	1	15	14
Green Bean Casserole	¾ cup (6 oz)	130	9	10	3
Green Beans	¾ cup (3 oz)	80	6	5	2
Ham Sandwich w/ Cheese & Sauce	1 (11.8 oz)	760	34	72	20
Ham Sandwich w/o Cheese & Sauce	1 (9.3 oz)	440	8	66	16
Homestyle Mashed Potatoes & Gravy	¾ cup (6.6 oz)	210	10	26	4
Honey Glazed Carrots	¾ cup (5.4 oz)	280	15	35	9
Hot Cinnamon Apples	¾ cup (6.4 oz)	250	5	56	48
Macaroni & Cheese	¾ cup (6.7 oz)	280	11	32	8
Mashed Potatoes	⅔ cup (5.6 oz)	190	9	24	4
Meat Loaf & Brown Gravy	1 serv (7 oz)	390	22	19	4
Meat Loaf & Chunky Tomato Sauce	1 serv (8 oz)	370	18	22	5
Meat Loaf Sandwich w/ Cheese	1 (13.8 oz)	860	33	95	21
Meat Loaf Sandwich w/o Cheese	1 (12.3 oz)	690	21	86	21
New Potatoes Low Fat	¾ cup (4.6 oz)	130	3	25	2
Old Fashioned Potato Salad	¾ cup (6.2 oz)	340	24	30	8
Open Face Turkey Sandwich	1 (13.4 oz)	500	12	61	13
Original Chicken Pot Pie	1 pie (14.9 oz)	780	46	61	5

FOOD	PORTION	CAL	FAT	CARB	SUG
Oven Roasted Potato Planks Low Fat	5 pieces (5.8 oz)	180	5	32	3
Pastry Sandwich BBQ Chicken	1 (7.2 oz)	640	39	56	13
Pastry Sandwich Broccoli Chicken Cheddar	1 (7.2 oz)	690	47	45	2
Pastry Sandwich Ham & Cheddar	1 (6.6 oz)	640	41	47	5
Pastry Sandwich Italian Chicken	1 (7.2 oz)	630	41	43	3
Red Beans And Rice Low Fat	1 cup (8 oz)	260	5	45	2
Rice Pilaf	⅔ cup (5.1 oz)	180	5	32	0
Rotisserie Turkey Breast Skinless Low Fat	1 serv (5 oz)	170	1	1	0
Savory Stuffing	¾ cup (6.1 oz)	310	12	44	3
Southwest Savory Chicken	1 serv (9.6 oz)	400	15	26	4
Squash Casserole	¾ cup (6.6 oz)	330	24	20	8
Steamed Vegetables Low Fat	⅔ cup (3.7 oz)	35	1	7	3
Sweet Potato Casserole	¾ cup (6.4 oz)	280	18	39	23
Tabasco BBQ Drumstick	1 (2.4 oz)	130	6	4	4
Tabasco BBQ Wing	1 (1.8 oz)	110	7	4	4
Teriyaki Chicken ¼ White w/ Skin	1 serv (6.8 oz)	340	12	17	14
Teriyaki Chicken ¼ w/ Skin	1 serv (5.9 oz)	380	21	17	15
Tossed Salad w/ Caesar Dressing	1 serv (8 oz)	380	31	18	—

FOOD	PORTION	CAL	FAT	CARB	SUG
Triple Topped Chicken	1 serv (9.2 oz)	470	22	20	5
Turkey Club Sandwich	1 (11.1 oz)	650	26	64	16
Turkey Sandwich w/ Cheese & Sauce	1 (11.8 oz)	710	28	68	17
Turkey Sandwich w/o Cheese & Sauce	1 (9.3 oz)	400	4	61	12
Whole Kernel Corn	¾ cup (5.8 oz)	180	4	30	13
Zucchini Marinara Low Fat	¾ cup (6.6 oz)	60	3	7	3

salads and salad bars

FOOD	PORTION	CAL	FAT	CARB	SUG
Caesar Salad Entree	1 serv (10 oz)	510	42	17	5
Caesar Salad w/o Dressing	1 serv (8 oz)	230	12	14	4
Caesar Side Salad	1 (4 oz)	200	17	7	2
Chicken Caesar Salad	1 serv (13 oz)	650	45	17	5
Tossed Salad w/ Fat Free Ranch	1 serv (8 oz)	160	3	29	9
Tossed Salad w/ Old Venice Dressing	1 serv (8 oz)	340	27	20	6

soups

FOOD	PORTION	CAL	FAT	CARB	SUG
Chicken Chili	1 cup (8.7 oz)	220	7	21	4
Chicken Noodle	1 cup (8.4 oz)	130	5	12	2
Chicken Tortilla	1 cup (8.4 oz)	220	11	19	2
Potato	1 cup (8 oz)	270	16	24	5
Tomato Bisque	1 cup (8 oz)	280	23	16	12

BROWN'S CHICKEN

FOOD	PORTION	CAL	FAT	CARB	SUG
Breadsticks w/ Garlic Butter	1	199	4	36	—
Breast	3.5 oz	284	15	12	—
Coleslaw	3.5 oz	131	10	9	—
Corn Fritters	3.5 oz	415	25	42	—

FOOD	PORTION	CAL	FAT	CARB	SUG
Corn On Cob	1 ear (3 inch)	126	3	22	—
Fettucini Alfredo	1 serv (12 oz)	1507	64	173	—
French Fries	3.5 oz	503	22	44	—
Gizzard	3.5 oz	387	20	26	—
Leg	3.5 oz	287	16	9	—
Liver	3.5 oz	341	19	19	—
Mostaccioli w/ Meat	1 serv (12 oz)	835	14	44	—
Mostaccioli w/o Meat	1 serv (12 oz)	792	10	146	—
Mushrooms	3.5 oz	289	16	30	—
Potato Salad	3.5 oz	94	4	13	—
Ravioli w/ Meat	1 serv (12 oz)	865	20	138	—
Ravioli w/o Meat	1 serv (12 oz)	822	16	140	—
Shrimp	3.5 oz	277	10	34	—
Thigh	3.5 oz	355	24	13	—
Wing	3.5 oz	385	25	17	—

BRUEGGER'S BAGELS

FOOD	PORTION	CAL	FAT	CARB	SUG
Blueberry	1 (3.5 oz)	300	2	60	10
Cinnamon Raisin	1 (3.5 oz)	290	2	60	9
Egg	1 (3.5 oz)	280	1	67	6
Everything	1 (3.6 oz)	290	2	55	5
Garlic	1 (3.6 oz)	280	2	57	4
Honey Grain	1 (3.6 oz)	300	3	58	7
Onion	1 (3.6 oz)	280	2	57	4
Orange Cranberry	1 (3.5 oz)	290	1	61	10
Pesto	1 (3.5 oz)	280	2	55	4
Plain	1 (3.5 oz)	280	2	56	5
Poppy Seed	1 (3.6 oz)	280	2	57	6
Pumpernickel	1 (3.5 oz)	280	2	56	4
Salt	1 (3.6 oz)	270	2	55	5
Sesame	1 (3.6 oz)	290	3	57	5

FOOD	PORTION	CAL	FAT	CARB	SUG
Spinach	1 (3.5 oz)	280	1	56	2
Sun Dried Tomato	1 (3.5 oz)	280	2	58	5
Wheat Bran	1 (3.5 oz)	280	2	55	7

BURGER KING
beverages

FOOD	PORTION	CAL	FAT	CARB	SUG
Cocoa Cola Classic	1 med (22 fl oz)	280	0	70	70
Coffee	1 serv (12 oz)	5	0	1	0
Diet Coke	1 med (22 fl oz)	1	0	tr	tr
Milk 2%	1 (8 oz)	130	5	12	12
Shake Chocolate	1 med (13.9 oz)	440	10	75	—
Shake Chocolate	1 sm (10.7 oz)	330	7	58	51
Shake Vanilla	1 sm (10.7 oz)	330	7	56	51
Sprite	1 med (22 fl oz)	260	0	66	66
Tropicana Orange Juice	1 serv (10 oz)	140	0	33	28

breakfast selections

FOOD	PORTION	CAL	FAT	CARB	SUG
AM Express Grape Jam	1 serv (0.4 oz)	30	0	7	—
AM Express Strawberry Jam	1 serv (0.4 oz)	30	0	8	—
AM Express Dip	1 serv (1 oz)	80	0	21	—
Bacon	3 strips (0.3 oz)	40	3	0	—
Biscuit	1 (3.3 oz)	300	15	35	3
Biscuit w/ Bacon Egg & Cheese	1 (6.6 oz)	620	43	37	4
Biscuit w/ Egg	1 (4.6 oz)	380	21	37	3
Biscuit w/ Sausage	1 (4.6 oz)	490	33	36	3
Cini-minis w/o Icing	4 (3.8 oz)	440	23	51	—
Croissan'wich Sausage Egg & Cheese	1 (5.3 oz)	530	41	23	4

FOOD	PORTION	CAL	FAT	CARB	SUG
Croissan'wich w/ Sausage & Cheese	1 (3.7 oz)	450	35	21	3
French Toast Sticks	5 sticks (4 oz)	440	23	51	12
Ham	1 serv (1.2 oz)	35	1	0	—
Hash Browns	1 sm (2.6 oz)	240	15	25	0
Land O'Lakes Whipped Blend	1 serv (0.4 oz)	65	7	0	—
Vanilla Icing Cini-Minis	1 serv (1 oz)	110	3	20	—
main menu selections					
American Cheese	2 slices (0.9 oz)	90	8	0	—
BK Big Fish Sandwich	1 (8.8 oz)	720	43	59	4
BK Broiler Chicken Breast Patty	1 (3.5 oz)	140	4	4	—
BK Broiler Chicken Sandwich	1 (8.7 oz)	530	16	45	5
BK Broiler Chicken Sandwich w/o Mayo	1 (8.7 oz)	370	9	45	5
Bacon Cheeseburger	1 (4.9 oz)	400	22	27	4
Bacon Double Cheeseburger	1 (7.2 oz)	630	38	28	5
Big King Sandwich	1 (7.6 oz)	640	42	28	4
Bull's Eye Barbecue Sauce	1 serv (0.5 oz)	20	0	5	5
Cheeseburger	1 (4.7 oz)	360	19	27	4
Chick'N Crisp Sandwich	1 (4.9 oz)	460	27	37	3
Chick'N Crisp Sandwich w/o Mayo	1 (4.9 oz)	360	16	37	3
Chicken Sandwich	1 (8 oz)	710	43	54	4
Chicken Sandwich w/o Mayo	1 (8 oz)	500	20	54	4

FOOD	PORTION	CAL	FAT	CARB	SUG
Chicken Tenders	4 (2.2 oz)	180	11	9	0
Dipping Sauce Barbecue	1 serv (1 oz)	35	0	9	—
Dipping Sauce Honey	1 serv (1 oz)	90	0	23	—
Dipping Sauce Honey Mustard	1 serv (1 oz)	90	6	10	—
Dipping Sauce Ranch	1 serv (1 oz)	170	17	2	—
Dipping Sauce Sweet & Sour	1 serv (1 oz)	45	0	11	—
Double Cheeseburger	1 (6.9 oz)	580	36	27	5
Double Whopper	1 (12.2 oz)	920	59	47	8
Double Whopper w/ Cheese	1 (13.1 oz)	1010	67	47	8
Double Whopper w/o Mayo	1 (12.2 oz)	760	42	47	8
Double Whopper w/o Mayo	1 (13.1 oz)	850	50	47	8
Dutch Apple Pie	1 serv (4 oz)	300	15	39	22
French Fries Salted	1 sm (2.6 oz)	250	13	32	0
Hamburger	1 (4.2 oz)	320	15	27	4
Hamburger Bun	1 (4.6 oz)	130	2	24	—
Hamburger Patty	1 (1.9 oz)	170	13	0	—
Hash Browns	1 lg (4.5 oz)	410	26	42	0
Ketchup	1 serv (0.5 oz)	15	0	4	—
King Sauce	1 serv (0.5 oz)	70	7	2	—
Lettuce	1 leaf (0.7 oz)	0	0	0	—
Mustard	1 serv (3 g)	0	0	0	—
Onion	1 serv (0.5 oz)	5	0	1	—
Onion Rings	1 med serv (3.3 oz)	380	19	46	4
Pickles	4 slices (0.5 oz)	0	0	0	—
Tartar Sauce	1 serv (1.5 oz)	260	29	0	—

FOOD	PORTION	CAL	FAT	CARB	SUG
Tomato	2 slices (1 oz)	5	0	1	—
Whopper	1 (9.5 oz)	660	40	47	8
Whopper Bun	1 (2.7 oz)	220	4	39	—
Whopper Jr.	1 (5.5 oz)	400	24	28	5
Whopper Jr. w/ Cheese	1 (6 oz)	450	28	28	5
Whopper Jr. w/ Cheese w/o Mayo	1 (6 oz)	370	19	28	5
Whopper Jr. w/o Mayo	1 (5.5 oz)	320	15	28	5
Whopper Patty	1 (2.8 oz)	250	19	0	—
Whopper w/ Cheese	1 (10.4 oz)	760	48	47	8
Whopper w/ Cheese w/o Mayo	1 (10.4 oz)	600	31	47	8
Whopper w/o Mayo	1 (9.5 oz)	510	23	47	8

CARVEL

frozen yogurt

FOOD	PORTION	CAL	FAT	CARB	SUG
Vanilla Low Fat No Sugar Added	4 fl oz	110	2	22	—

ice cream

FOOD	PORTION	CAL	FAT	CARB	SUG
Brown Bonnet Cone	1 (4.7 oz)	380	21	43	32
Brown Bonnet Cone No Fat Vanilla	1 (4.7 oz)	300	11	47	36
Cake	1 pkg (7 oz)	450	23	54	38
Cake	1 pkg (4 oz)	270	14	33	23
Cake Cheesecake	1 serv (4 oz)	280	14	34	26
Cake Chocolate Vanilla Chocolate Crunchies	1/15 cake (3.4 oz)	230	12	27	20
Cake Cookies & Cream	1 serv (4 oz)	270	14	32	24
Cake Fudge Drizzle	1/8 cake (4 oz)	310	17	35	25
Cake Fudgie The Whale	1/14 cake (3.6 oz)	290	16	33	23

FOOD	PORTION	CAL	FAT	CARB	SUG
Cake Holiday	⅟₁₅ cake (3.4 oz)	240	12	30	21
Cake S'mores	1 serv (4 oz)	270	14	33	26
Cake Sinfully Chocolate	1 serv (4 oz)	280	14	34	25
Cake Strawberries & Cream	⅛ cake (3.8 oz)	240	12	31	23
Chocolate	4 fl oz	190	10	22	19
Chocolate No Fat	4 fl oz	120	0	28	25
Flying Saucer Chocolate	1 (4 oz)	230	9	33	19
Flying Saucer Chocolate w/ Sprinkles	1 (4 oz)	330	14	49	23
Flying Saucer Low Fat Chocolate	1 (4 oz)	190	3	38	23
Flying Saucer Low Fat Vanilla	1 (4 oz)	180	3	36	22
Flying Saucer Vanilla	1 (4 oz)	240	10	33	19
Flying Saucer Vanilla w/ Sprinkles	1 (4 oz)	340	14	49	23
Lil'Love Cake All Vanilla	1 piece (4.4 oz)	330	16	41	27
Lil'Love Cake Chocolate & Vanilla	1 piece (4 oz)	260	13	31	22
Nature's Crunch	1 (4.2 g)	450	25	55	35
Olde Fashion Sundae Butterscotch	1 (8 oz)	500	17	80	57
Olde Fashion Sundae Chocolate	1 (8 oz)	470	19	71	55
Olde Fashion Sundae Strawberry	1 (8 oz)	420	15	64	53
Sheet Cake Chocolate Vanilla Chocolate Crunchies	⅟₂₆ cake (3.3 oz)	230	12	27	—

FOOD	PORTION	CAL	FAT	CARB	SUG
Sinful Love Bar	1 (4.2 oz)	460	29	48	30
Thick Shake Chocolate	1 (16 oz)	719	31	96	—
Thick Shake Low Fat Chocolate	1 (16 oz)	490	1	108	68
Thick Shake Low Fat Strawberry	1 (16 oz)	460	1	96	68
Thick Shake Low Fat Vanilla	1 (16 oz)	460	1	98	83
Thick Shake No Fat Chocolate	1 (16 oz)	524	8	100	72
Thick Shake No Fat Strawberry	1 (16 oz)	453	7	82	70
Thick Shake No Fat Vanilla	1 (16 oz)	462	7	84	74
Thick Shake Strawberry	1 (16 oz)	648	30	77	52
Thick Shake Vanilla	1 (16 oz)	657	30	79	73
Vanilla	4 fl oz	200	10	21	19
Vanilla No Fat	4 fl oz	120	0	25	22
sherbet					
Black Raspberry	½ cup (3.4 oz)	150	1	33	26
Blueberry	½ cup (3.4 oz)	150	1	33	24
Lemon	½ cup (3.5 oz)	150	1	31	23
Lime	½ cup (3.5 oz)	150	1	31	23
Mango	½ cup (3.5 oz)	140	1	30	23
Orange	½ cup (3.5 oz)	150	1	31	23
Peach	½ cup (3.4 oz)	150	1	32	24
Pineapple	½ cup (3.5 oz)	150	1	33	25
Strawberry	½ cup (3.5 oz)	150	1	32	25

CHICK-FIL-A

beverages

FOOD	PORTION	CAL	FAT	CARB	SUG
Coca-Cola Classic	1 serv (9 oz)	110	0	28	28
Diet Coke	1 serv (9 oz)	0	0	0	0

FOOD	PORTION	CAL	FAT	CARB	SUG
Diet Lemonade	1 serv (9 oz)	5	0	2	1
Ice Tea Sweetened	1 serv (9 oz)	150	0	38	38
Iced Tea Unsweetened	1 serv (9 oz)	0	0	0	0
Lemonade	1 sm (9 oz)	90	0	23	22
desserts					
Cheesecake + One Side	1 slice (3.1 oz)	300	21	23	20
Fudge Nut Brownie	1 (2.6 oz)	350	16	41	37
Icedream Cone	1 sm (4.5 oz)	140	4	16	16
Lemon Pie	1 slice (3.5 oz)	280	22	19	15
main menu selections					
Barbecue Sauce	1 serv (1 oz)	45	0	11	9
Carrot & Raisin Salad	1 sm (2.7 oz)	150	2	28	3
Chargrilled Chicken Club Sandwich	1 (8.2 oz)	390	12	38	1
Chargrilled Chicken Garden Salad	1 serv (9.8 oz)	190	5	12	3
Chargrilled Chicken Sandwich	1 (5.3 oz)	280	3	36	1
Chick-n-Strips	4 (4.2 oz)	230	8	10	1
Chick-n-Strips Salad	1 serv (11.7 oz)	370	17	21	7
Chicken Sandwich	1 (5.9 oz)	290	9	29	0
Chicken Caesar Salad	1 serv (8.1 oz)	230	10	5	1
Chicken Salad Sandwich	1 (5.9 oz)	320	5	42	3
Cole Slaw	1 sm (2.8 oz)	130	6	11	0
Dijon Honey Sauce	1 serv (0.4 oz)	60	1	2	2
Hearty Breast of Chicken Soup	1 cup (7.6 oz)	110	1	10	0
Honey Mustard Sauce	1 serv (1 oz)	45	0	11	10
Nuggets	8 (3.9 oz)	290	14	12	0
Polynesian Sauce	1 serv (1 oz)	110	6	13	12

FOOD	PORTION	CAL	FAT	CARB	SUG
Side Salad	1 serv (4.6 oz)	70	0	13	0
Waffle Potato Fries	1 sm (3 oz)	290	10	49	1
salad dressings					
Basil Vinaigrette	1 serv (1.5 oz)	250	26	5	5
Blue Cheese	1 serv (1.5 oz)	230	24	2	2
Buttermilk Ranch	1 serv (1.5 oz)	220	24	2	2
Fat Free Dijon Honey Mustard	1 serv (1.5 oz)	70	1	17	14
House	1 serv (1.6 oz)	190	17	9	7
Light Italian	1 serv (1.5 oz)	20	1	2	2
Spicy	1 serv (1.2 oz)	210	22	2	1
Thousand Island	1 serv (1.5 oz)	210	20	6	6
CHILI'S					
desserts					
Diet By Chocolate Cake	1 serv	370	2	79	43
Diet By Chocolate Cake w/ Yogurt	1 serv	465	2	99	59
Diet By Chocolate Cake w/ Yogurt & Fudge Topping	1 serv	534	3	116	74
main menu selections					
Guiltless Grill Chicken Fajitas	1 serv	726	13	108	8
Guiltless Grill Chicken Platter	1 serv	563	7	83	5
Guiltless Grill Chicken Salad w/ Dressing	1 serv	254	3	27	20
Guiltless Grill Chicken Sandwich	1	527	7	70	7
Guiltless Grill Veggie Pasta	1 serv	590	11	98	3
Guiltless Grill Veggie Pasta w/ Chicken	1 serv	696	13	102	6

FOOD	PORTION	CAL	FAT	CARB	SUG
CHURCH'S CHICKEN					
Apple Pie	1 serv (3.1 oz)	280	12	41	13
Biscuit	1 (2.1 oz)	250	16	26	3
Breast	1 serv (2.8 oz)	200	12	4	0
Cajun Rice	1 serv (3.1 oz)	130	7	16	0
Cole Slaw	1 serv (3 oz)	92	6	8	6
Corn On The Cob	1 serv (5.7 oz)	139	3	24	2
French Fries	1 serv (2.7 oz)	210	11	29	0
Leg	1 serv (2 oz)	140	9	2	0
Okra	1 serv (2.8 oz)	210	16	19	tr
Potatoes & Gravy	1 serv (3.7 oz)	90	3	14	2
Tender Strip	1 (1.1 oz)	80	4	5	0
Thigh	1 serv (2.8 oz)	230	16	5	0
Wing	1 serv (3.1 oz)	250	16	8	0
COLOMBO FROZEN YOGURT					
Alpine Strawberry Nonfat	4 fl oz	100	0	22	—
Banana Strawberry Nonfat	4 fl oz	50	0	12	—
Brazlian Banana Nonfat	4 fl oz	100	0	22	—
Butter Pecan Nonfat	4 fl oz	100	0	22	—
Cappuccino Nonfat	4 fl oz	100	0	22	—
Cherry Amaretto Nonfat	4 fl oz	50	0	12	—
Cherry Vanilla Nonfat	4 fl oz	100	0	22	—
Chocolate Nonfat	4 fl oz	50	0	12	—
Coconut Cooler Nonfat	4 fl oz	100	0	22	—
Cool Berry Blue Nonfat	4 fl oz	100	0	22	—
Country Pumpkin Nonfat	4 fl oz	100	0	22	—

FOOD	PORTION	CAL	FAT	CARB	SUG
Double Dutch Chocolate Nonfat	4 fl oz	100	0	22	—
Egg Nog Nonfat	4 fl oz	100	0	22	—
French Vanilla Lowfat	4 fl oz	110	2	22	—
French Vanilla Nonfat	4 fl oz	100	0	22	—
Georgia Peach Nonfat	4 fl oz	100	0	22	—
German Fudge Chocolate Nonfat	4 fl oz	100	0	22	—
Hawaiian Pineapple Nonfat	4 fl oz	100	0	22	—
Hazelnut Amaretto Nonfat	4 fl oz	100	0	22	—
Honey Almond Nonfat	4 fl oz	100	0	22	—
Irish Cream Nonfat	4 fl oz	100	0	22	—
New York Cheesecake Nonfat	4 fl oz	100	0	22	—
Old World Chocolate Lowfat	4 fl oz	110	2	22	—
Orange Bavarian Creme Nonfat	4 fl oz	100	0	22	—
Peanut Butter Lowfat	4 fl oz	110	2	22	—
Pecan Praline Nonfat	4 fl oz	100	0	22	—
Pina Colada Nonfat	4 fl oz	100	0	22	—
Raspberry Nonfat	4 fl oz	50	0	12	—
Rockin' Raspberry Nonfat	4 fl oz	100	0	22	—
Simply Vanilla Lowfat	4 fl oz	110	2	22	—
Simply Vanilla Nonfat	4 fl oz	100	0	22	—
Strawberry Nonfat	4 fl oz	50	0	12	—
Tropical Tango Nonfat	4 fl oz	100	0	22	—
Vanilla Nonfat	4 fl oz	50	0	12	—

FOOD	PORTION	CAL	FAT	CARB	SUG
White Chocolate Almond Nonfat	4 fl oz	100	0	22	—
Wild Strawberry Lowfat	4 fl oz	110	2	22	—

DAIRY QUEEN

food selections

FOOD	PORTION	CAL	FAT	CARB	SUG
Chicken Breast Fillet Sandwich	1 (6.7 oz)	430	20	37	5
Chicken Strip Basket	1 serv (14.5 oz)	1000	50	102	3
Chili 'n' Cheese Dog	1 (5 oz)	330	21	22	4
DQ Homestyle Bacon Double Cheeseburger	1 (8.9 oz)	610	36	31	6
DQ Homestyle Cheeseburger	1 (5.3 oz)	340	17	29	5
DQ Homestyle Double Cheeseburger	1 (7.7 oz)	540	31	30	5
DQ Homestyle Hamburger	1 (4.8 oz)	290	12	29	5
DQ Ultimate Burger	1 (9.4 oz)	670	43	29	6
French Fries	1 sm (4 oz)	350	18	42	tr
Grilled Chicken Sandwich	1 (6.5 oz)	310	10	30	5
Hot Dog	1 (3.5 oz)	240	14	19	4
Onion Rings	1 serv (4 oz)	320	16	39	4
The Great Steakmelt Basket	1 serv (13.2 oz)	770	38	72	7

ice cream

FOOD	PORTION	CAL	FAT	CARB	SUG
Banana Split	1 (12.9 oz)	510	12	96	82
Blizzard Chocolate Sandwich Cookie	1 sm (12 oz)	520	18	79	61

FOOD	PORTION	CAL	FAT	CARB	SUG
Blizzard Chocolate Chip Cookie Dough	1 sm (12 oz)	660	24	99	74
Breeze Heath	1 sm (10.2 oz)	470	10	85	70
Breeze Strawberry	1 sm (12 oz)	320	1	68	54
Buster Bar	1 (5.2 oz)	450	28	41	33
Chocolate Malt	1 sm (14.7 oz)	650	16	111	95
Cone Chocolate	1 sm (5 oz)	240	8	37	25
Cone Vanilla	1 sm (5 oz)	230	7	38	27
Cone Yogurt	1 med (6.9 oz)	260	1	56	36
Cone Dipped	1 sm (5.5 oz)	340	17	42	31
Cup Of Yogurt	1 med (6.7 oz)	230	1	48	36
DQ 8 Inch Round Cake Undecorated	⅛ of cake (6.2 oz)	340	13	56	42
DQ Fudge Bar No Sugar Added	1 (2.3 oz)	50	0	13	3
DQ Lemon Freez'r	½ cup (3.2 oz)	80	0	20	20
DQ Nonfat Frozen Yogurt	½ cup (3 oz)	100	0	21	16
DQ Sandwich	1 (2.1 oz)	200	6	31	18
DQ Soft Serve Chocolate	½ cup (3.3 oz)	150	5	22	17
DQ Soft Serve Vanilla	½ cup (3.3 oz)	140	5	22	19
DQ Treatzza Pizza Heath	⅛ of pie (2.3 oz)	180	7	28	18
DQ Treatzza Pizza M&M	⅛ of pie (2.4 oz)	190	7	29	20
DQ Vanilla Orange Bar No Sugar Added	1 (2.3 oz)	60	0	17	2
Dilly Bar Chocolate	1 (3 oz)	210	13	21	17
Frozen Hot Chocolate	1 (20.9 oz)	860	35	127	109
Misty Slush	1 sm (15.9 oz)	220	0	56	56
Peanut Buster Parfait	1 (10.7 oz)	730	31	99	85

FOOD	PORTION	CAL	FAT	CARB	SUG
Pecan Mudslide Treat	1 (4.6 oz)	650	30	85	70
S'more Galore Parfait	1 (10.7 oz)	730	30	111	86
Shake Chocolate	1 sm (13.9 oz)	560	15	94	81
Starkiss	1 (3 oz)	80	0	21	21
Strawberry Shortcake	1 (8.5 oz)	430	14	70	57
Sundae Chocolate	1 sm (5.7 oz)	280	7	49	42
Yogurt Sundae Strawberry	1 med (8.2 oz)	280	1	61	49

D'ANGELO'S SANDWICH SHOP

salads and salad bars

FOOD	PORTION	CAL	FAT	CARB	SUG
Antipasto Salad w/o Dressing	1	420	14	56	—
Caesar Salad w/ Dressing	1	740	45	61	—
Caesar Salad w/o Dressing	1	490	20	60	—
Chicken Caesar Salad w/ Dressing	1	860	48	62	—
Chicken Caesar Salad w/o Dressing	1	600	23	60	—
Chicken Salad D'Lite	1	325	4	34	—
Chicken Salad w/o Dressing	1	390	5	50	—
Greek Salad w/ Dressing	1	940	71	63	—
Greek Salad w/ Tuna & Dressing	1	1010	72	63	—
Greek Salad w/ Tuna w/o Dressing	1	490	15	58	—
Greek Salad w/o Dressing	1	420	15	58	—
Roast Beef Salad D'Lite	1	350	5	33	—

FOOD	PORTION	CAL	FAT	CARB	SUG
Roast Beef Salad w/o Dressing	1	400	6	55	—
Tossed Garden Salad w/o Dressing	1	270	2	55	—
Tuna Salad D'Lite	1	305	2	33	—
Tuna Salad w/o Dressing	1	330	3	55	—
Turkey Salad w/o Dressing	1	400	3	55	—
sandwiches					
BLT w/ Cheese Medium Sub	1	870	47	64	—
BLT w/ Cheese Pokket	1	570	31	41	—
Barbecue Curls	1	480	19	45	—
Buffalo Chicken Wrap w/ Blue Cheese Dressing	1	621	28	51	—
Buffalo Chicken Wrap w/o Dressing	1	417	13	48	—
Caesar Salad w/ Dressing Pokket	1	590	26	68	—
Caesar Salad w/o Dressing Pokket	1	460	13	68	—
Caesar Salad w/ Chicken w/ Dressing Pokket	1	570	16	68	—
Caesar Salad w/ Chicken w/ Dressing Pokket	1	700	28	69	—
Caesar Wrap w/ Dressing	1	484	15	66	—
Caesar Wrap w/ Fat Free Dressing	1	484	15	66	—

FOOD	PORTION	CAL	FAT	CARB	SUG
Capicola Ham & Cheese Pokket	1	350	11	41	—
Capicola Ham & Cheese Small Sub	1	390	13	45	—
Cheeseburger Pokket	1	490	23	40	—
Cheeseburger Small Sub	1	530	25	44	—
Chicken Salad Pokket	1	650	38	41	—
Chicken Salad Small Sub	1	690	39	44	—
Chicken Stir Fry D'Lite Pokket	1	360	5	46	—
Chicken Stir Fry D'Lite Sub	1	280	6	47	—
Chicken Stir Fry Pokket	1	360	5	46	—
Chicken Stir Fry Small Sub	1	380	6	47	—
Classic Vegetable D'Lite Pokket	1	340	10	48	—
Classic Vegetable Pokket	1	400	15	48	—
Classic Vegetable Small Sub	1	400	16	52	—
Crunchy Vegetable D'Lite Pokket	1	350	10	52	—
Crunchy Vegetable D'Lite Small Sub	1	385	11	56	—
Crunchy Vegetable Pokket	1	410	15	50	—
Crunchy Vegetables Small Sub	1	440	16	53	—
Ginger Chicken Stir Fry D'Lite Pokket	1	400	5	55	—

FOOD	PORTION	CAL	FAT	CARB	SUG
Greek Pokket	1	910	71	57	—
Grilled Spicy Steak D'Lite Pokket	1	425	11	59	—
Grilled Steak Cheese Pokket	1	550	26	40	—
Grilled Steak Cheese Small Sub	1	580	28	44	—
Grilled Steak Combo Pokket	1	550	26	43	—
Grilled Steak Combo Small Sub	1	590	28	46	—
Grilled Steak D'Lite Pokket	1	390	11	51	—
Grilled Steak Mushrooms Pokket	1	450	18	41	—
Grilled Steak Mushrooms Small Sub	1	480	19	45	—
Grilled Steak Onions Small Sub	1	480	19	45	—
Grilled Steak Onions Pokket	1	450	17	42	—
Grilled Steak Peppers	1	690	27	65	—
Grilled Steak Peppers Pokket	1	540	17	42	—
Grilled Steak Pokket	1	440	17	40	—
Grilled Steak Small Sub	1	470	19	43	—
Ham & Cheese Pokket	1	370	13	40	—
Ham & Cheese Small Sub	1	400	14	44	—
Ham Salami & Cheese Pokket	1	420	18	41	—

FOOD	PORTION	CAL	FAT	CARB	SUG
Ham Salami & Cheese Small Sub	1	450	20	44	—
Hamburger Pokket	1	430	18	40	—
Hamburger Small Sub	1	460	19	43	—
Italian Cold Cut Pokket	1	550	30	42	—
Italian Cold Cut Small Sub	1	580	32	46	—
Meatball Pokket	1	480	20	50	—
Meatball Small Sub	1	520	21	54	—
Meatball w/ Cheese Pokket	1	580	28	51	—
Meatball w/ Cheese Small Sub	1	620	29	54	—
Pastrami Pokket	1	550	30	40	—
Pastrami Small Sub	1	580	31	44	—
Pastrami w/ Cheese Pokket	1	780	49	41	—
Pastrami w/ Cheese Small Sub	1	820	51	45	—
Roast Beef D'Lite Pokket	1	330	6	42	—
Roast Beef D'Lite Small Sub	1	365	7	45	—
Seafood Salad Pokket	1	570	33	56	—
Seafood Salad Small Sub	1	610	34	59	—
Stuffed Turkey D'Lite Pokket	1	510	8	71	—
Stuffed Turkey D'Lite Small Sub	1	545	9	75	—
Tuna Salad Pokket	1	720	50	41	—
Turkey D'Lite Pokket	1	330	2	40	—
Turkey D'Lite Small Sub	1	365	4	43	—

FOOD	PORTION	CAL	FAT	CARB	SUG
Turkey Club Pokket	1	400	9	40	—
Turkey Club Small Sub	1	430	10	43	—

DELTACO
beverages

FOOD	PORTION	CAL	FAT	CARB	SUG
Coffee	1 serv (8 oz)	0	0	1	0
Coke Classic	1 sm (10 oz)	120	0	29	29
Diet Coke	1 sm (10 oz)	0	0	0	0
Iced Tea	1 sm (10 oz)	0	0	0	0
Milk 1% Lowfat	1 serv (11 oz)	130	3	15	15
Mr Pibb	1 sm (10 oz)	120	0	29	29
Orange Juice	1 serv (11 oz)	140	0	34	33
Shake Chocolate	1 sm (11.4 oz)	520	12	89	77
Shake Strawberry	1 sm (11.4 oz)	410	6	76	65
Shake Vanilla	1 sm (11.4 oz)	420	7	75	62
Sprite	1 sm (10 oz)	110	0	29	29

breakfast selections

FOOD	PORTION	CAL	FAT	CARB	SUG
Burrito Breakfast	1 (3.8 oz)	250	11	24	2
Burrito Egg & Cheese	1 (7.5 oz)	450	24	39	2
Burrito Macho Bacon & Egg	1 (15.9 oz)	1030	60	82	6
Burrito Steak & Egg	1 (9 oz)	580	34	41	2
Quesadilla Bacon & Egg	1 (6.1 oz)	450	23	40	2
Side of Bacon	2 strips (0.3 oz)	50	4	0	0

main menu selections

FOOD	PORTION	CAL	FAT	CARB	SUG
Beans 'n Cheese Cup	1 serv (7.7 oz)	260	3	44	4
Burrito Combo	1 (8.2 oz)	490	21	53	3
Burrito Del Beef	1 (8 oz)	550	30	42	2
Burrito Del Classic Chicken	1 (8.5 oz)	580	38	42	4
Burrito Deluxe Combo	1 (10.7 oz)	530	25	56	5

FOOD	PORTION	CAL	FAT	CARB	SUG
Burrito Deluxe Del Beef	1 (10.5 oz)	590	33	45	4
Burrito Green	1 (5 oz)	280	8	38	2
Burrito Macho Beef	1 (18.9 oz)	1170	62	89	8
Burrito Macho Combo	1 (19.4 oz)	1050	44	113	9
Burrito Red	1 (5 oz)	270	8	38	2
Burrito Red Regular	1 (7.5 oz)	390	12	59	3
Burrito Regular Green	1 (7.5 oz)	400	12	59	3
Burrito Spicy Chicken	1 (8.7 oz)	480	16	65	3
Burrito The Works	1 (10.2 oz)	480	18	69	5
Cheeseburger	1 (4.6 oz)	330	13	37	4
Del Cheeseburger	1 (5.6 oz)	430	25	35	3
Double Del Cheeseburger	1 (7.1 oz)	560	35	35	4
Fries	1 sm (3 oz)	210	14	20	0
Fries Chili Cheese	1 serv (10.5 oz)	670	46	51	2
Fries Deluxe Chili Cheese	1 serv (11.9 oz)	710	49	53	4
Get A Lot Meals #1 Combo Burrito Fries Drink	1 meal	980	44	124	41
Get A Lot Meals #2 Del Classic Chicken Burrito Fries Drink	1 meal	1080	61	113	42
Get A Lot Meals #3 Regular Red Burrito Fries Drink	1 meal	890	35	130	41
Get A Lot Meals #4 Two Chicken Soft Tacos Fries Drink	1 meal	910	46	102	39

FOOD	PORTION	CAL	FAT	CARB	SUG
Get A Lot Meals #5 Taco Combo Burrito Drink	1 meal	790	31	101	40
Get A Lot Meals #6 Two Tacos Quesadilla Drink	1 meal	960	47	98	40
Get A Lot Meals #7 Macho Combo Burrito Fries Drink	1 meal	1530	67	183	47
Get A Lot Meals #8 Two Big Fat Tacos Fries Drink	1 meal	802	45	148	44
Get A Lot Meals #9 Double Del Cheeseburger Fries Drink	1 meal	1050	58	106	41
Nachos	1 serv (4 oz)	380	24	40	1
Nachos Macho	1 serv (17 oz)	1200	66	130	7
Quesadilla Chicken	1 (6.8 oz)	580	31	41	2
Quesadilla Regular	1 (5.3 oz)	500	27	39	2
Quesadilla Spicy Jack Chicken	1 (6.8 oz)	570	30	40	1
Quesadilla Spicy Jack Regular	1 (5.3 oz)	490	26	38	1
Rice Cup	1 serv (4 oz)	150	2	28	2
Soft Taco	1 (2.8 oz)	160	8	16	1
Soft Taco Chicken	1 (3.3 oz)	210	12	16	1
Taco	1 (2.2 oz)	160	10	11	1
Taco Big Fat	1 (5.4 oz)	320	11	39	3
Taco Big Fat Chicken	1 (5.4 oz)	340	13	38	3
Taco Big Fat Steak	1 (5.4 oz)	390	19	38	3
Taco Salad Deluxe	1 (18.8 oz)	760	37	76	10
Tostada Salad	1 (4.5 oz)	210	9	24	2

FOOD	PORTION	CAL	FAT	CARB	SUG
DENNY'S					
beverages					
2% Milk	1 serv (10 oz)	151	6	15	14
Chocolate Milk	1 serv (10 oz)	235	9	30	24
Coffee French Vanilla	1 serv (8 oz)	76	1	16	15
Coffee Hazelnut	1 serv (8 oz)	66	1	14	13
Coffee Irish Cream	1 serv (8 oz)	73	1	16	15
Grapefruit Juice	1 serv (10 oz)	115	0	29	29
Hot Chocolate	1 serv (8 oz)	90	2	18	16
Lemonade	1 serv (16 oz)	150	0	35	35
Orange Juice	1 serv (10 oz)	126	0	31	24
Raspberry Ice Tea	1 serv (16 oz)	78	0	21	21
Tomato Juice	1 serv (10 oz)	56	0	11	0
breakfast selections					
All American Slam	1 serv (15 oz)	1028	87	24	5
Applesauce	1 serv (3 oz)	60	0	15	15
Bacon	4 strips (1 oz)	162	18	1	1
Bagel Dry	1 (3 oz)	235	1	46	0
Banana	1 (4 oz)	110	0	29	21
Banana Strawberry Medley	1 serv (4 oz)	108	1	27	13
Biscuit Plain	1 (3 oz)	375	22	40	0
Biscuit w/ Sausage Gravy	1 serv (7 oz)	570	38	45	1
Blueberry Topping	1 serv (3 oz)	106	0	26	11
Canadian Bacon	1 serv (3 oz)	110	5	1	1
Cantaloup	1 serv (3 oz)	32	0	8	7
Cheddar Cheese Omelette	1 serv (13 oz)	770	62	24	2
Cherry Topping	1 serv (3 oz)	86	0	21	9

FOOD	PORTION	CAL	FAT	CARB	SUG
Chicken Fried Steak & Eggs	1 serv (14 oz)	723	56	31	—
Country Scramble	1 serv (16 oz)	795	50	67	2
Cream Cheese	1 oz	100	10	1	1
Egg	1 (2 oz)	134	12	1	1
Egg Beaters	1 serv (2.3 oz)	71	5	1	0
Eggs Benedict	1 serv (19 oz)	860	56	55	2
English Muffin Dry	1 (4 oz)	125	1	24	0
Farmer's Omelette	1 serv (18 oz)	912	69	38	6
French Slam	1 serv (14 oz)	1029	71	58	10
French Toast	2 pieces (8 oz)	510	25	51	4
Fresh Fruit Mix	1 serv (3 oz)	36	0	9	9
Grapefruit	½ (5 oz)	60	0	16	10
Grapes	1 serv (3 oz)	55	1	15	14
Grits	1 serv (4 oz)	80	0	18	0
Ham	1 serv (3 oz)	94	3	2	0
Ham'n'Cheddar Omelette	1 serv (14 oz)	743	55	24	2
Hashed Browns	1 serv (4 oz)	218	14	20	0
Hashed Browns Covered	1 serv (6 oz)	318	23	21	0
Hashed Browns Covered & Smothered	1 serv (8 oz)	359	26	26	1
Honeydew	1 serv (3 oz)	31	0	8	7
Junior Meals Basic Breakfast2	1 serv (9 oz)	558	39	38	3
Junior Meals Junior French Slam	1 serv (7 oz)	461	35	18	2
Junior Meals Junior Grand Slam	1 serv (5 oz)	397	25	33	2
Junior Meals Junior Waffle Supreme	1 serv (4 oz)	190	11	20	15

FOOD	PORTION	CAL	FAT	CARB	SUG
Meat Lover's Sampler	1 serv (14 oz)	806	62	24	4
Moon Over My Hammy	1 serv (12 oz)	807	48	46	4
Muffin Blueberry	1 (3 oz)	309	14	42	—
Oatmeal	1 serv (4 oz)	100	2	18	0
Original Grand Slam	1 serv (10 oz)	795	50	65	4
Pancakes	3 (5 oz)	491	7	95	3
Pork Chop & Eggs	1 serv (12 oz)	555	36	21	2
Porterhouse Steak & Eggs	1 serv (18 oz)	1223	95	21	2
Ready To Eat Cereal	1 serv (1 oz)	100	0	23	5
Sausage	4 links (3 oz)	354	32	0	0
Sausage Cheddar Omelette	1 serv (16 oz)	1036	86	24	5
Scram Slam	1 serv (18 oz)	974	80	30	7
Senior Belgian Waffle Slam	1 serv (6 oz)	399	33	12	2
Senior Omelette	1 serv (12 oz)	623	47	27	4
Senior Starter	1 serv (7 oz)	336	24	38	—
Senior Triple Play	1 serv (8 oz)	537	25	64	1
Sirloin Steak & Eggs	1 serv (13 oz)	808	64	21	2
Slim Slam	1 serv (14 oz)	638	12	08	26
Southern Slam	1 serv (13 oz)	1065	84	47	4
Strawberries w/ Sugar	1 serv (3 oz)	115	1	26	19
Strawberry Topping	1 serv (3 oz)	115	1	26	19
Sunshine Slam	1 serv (8 oz)	537	25	64	1
Super Play It Again Slam	1 serv (15 oz)	1192	75	98	51
Syrup	3 tbsp (1.5 oz)	143	0	36	36
Syrup Reduced Calorie	1 serv (1.5 oz)	25	0	6	0
T-Bone Steak & Eggs	1 serv (16 oz)	1045	82	21	2
Toast Dry	1 slice (1 oz)	92	1	17	1

FOOD	PORTION	CAL	FAT	CARB	SUG
Ultimate Omelette	1 serv (17 oz)	780	62	29	5
Vegggie Cheese Omelette	1 serv (16 oz)	714	53	29	5
Waffle	1 (6 oz)	304	21	23	3
Whipped Margarine	1 serv (0.5 oz)	87	10	0	0
Whipped Cream	1 serv (2 oz)	23	2	2	0
desserts					
Apple Pie	1 serv (7 oz)	430	20	59	30
Apple Pie w/ Equal	1 serv (7 oz)	370	20	43	13
Banana Split	1 serv (19 oz)	894	43	121	29
Blueberry Topping	1 serv (3 oz)	106	0	26	11
Cheesecake Pie	1 serv (4 oz)	470	27	48	31
Cherry Topping	1 serv (3 oz)	86	0	21	9
Cherry Pie	1 serv (7 oz)	540	21	83	51
Chocolate Topping	1 serv (2 oz)	317	25	27	27
Chocolate Cake	1 serv (4 oz)	370	17	53	26
Chocolate Pecan Pie	1 serv (6 oz)	790	37	107	54
Chocolate Shake	1 serv (10 oz)	579	27	77	66
Coconut Cream Pie	1 serv (7 oz)	480	26	58	35
Double Scoop Sundae	1 serv (6 oz)	375	27	29	8
Dutch Apple Pie	1 serv (7 oz)	440	19	65	35
French Silk Pie	1 serv (6 oz)	650	43	60	45
Fudge Topping	1 serv (2 oz)	201	10	30	27
German Chocolate Pie	1 serv (7 oz)	580	33	66	42
Hot Fudge Cake Sundae	1 serv (8 oz)	687	38	83	45
Ice Cream Float	1 serv (12 oz)	280	10	47	33
Key Lime Pie	1 serv (6 oz)	600	27	79	61
Lemon Meringue Pie	1 serv (7 oz)	460	17	71	47
Pecan Pie	1 serv (6 oz)	600	28	81	46

FOOD	PORTION	CAL	FAT	CARB	SUG
Single Scoop Sundae	1 serv (3 oz)	188	14	14	4
Strawberry Topping	1 serv (3 oz)	115	1	26	19
Vanilla Shake	1 serv (11 oz)	581	27	77	65
main menu selections					
BBQ Sauce	1 serv (1.5 oz)	47	1	11	5
Bacon Cheddar Burger	1 (14 oz)	935	63	43	8
Bacon Lettuce & Tomato Sandwich	1 (6 oz)	634	46	37	4
Baked Potato Plain	1 (6 oz)	186	0	43	0
Battered Cod Dinner w/ Tartar Sauce	1 serv (9 oz)	732	47	48	6
Broccoli In Butter Sauce	2 serv (4 oz)	50	2	7	3
Brown Gravy	1 serv (1 oz)	13	0	2	1
Buffalo Chicken Strips	1 serv (10 oz)	734	42	43	0
Buffalo Wings	12 pieces (15 oz)	856	54	1	0
Carrots In Honey Glaze	2 serv (4 oz)	80	3	12	7
Charleston Chicken Sandwich	1 (11 oz)	632	32	53	6
Chicken Quesadilla	1 serv (16 oz)	827	55	43	7
Chicken Fried Chicken	1 serv (6 oz)	327	18	16	0
Chicken Fried Steak w/ Gravy	1 serv (4 oz)	265	17	14	0
Chicken Gravy	1 serv (1 oz)	14	1	2	1
Chicken Melt Sandwich	1 (7 oz)	520	29	43	4
Chicken Strips w/ Dressing	1 serv (10 oz)	635	25	55	13
Chicken Strips	5 pieces (10 oz)	720	33	56	14
Classic Burger	1 (11 oz)	673	40	42	7
Classic Burger w/ Cheese	1 (13 oz)	836	53	43	7

FOOD	PORTION	CAL	FAT	CARB	SUG
Club Sandwich	1	485	35	40	—
Corn In Butter Sauce	2 serv (4 oz)	120	4	19	4
Cornbread Stuffing Plain	1 serv (2 oz)	182	9	20	0
Cottage Cheese	1 serv (3 oz)	72	3	2	0
Country Gravy	1 serv (1 oz)	17	1	2	0
Delidinger Sandwich	1 (14 oz)	852	45	62	—
Deluxe Grilled Cheese Sandwich	1 (7 oz)	482	26	44	4
Dinner Roll	1 (1.5 oz)	132	2	26	3
French Fries Unsalted	1 serv (4 oz)	323	14	44	0
Fried Fish Sandwich	1 (11 oz)	905	56	74	10
Gardenburger Patty	1 patty (3.4 oz)	160	3	22	2
Gardenburger Patty w/ Bun & Fat Free Honey Mustard Dressing	1 serv (11.1 oz)	653	32	72	11
Green Beans w/ Bacon	2 serv (4 oz)	60	4	6	2
Green Peas In Butter Sauce	2 serv (4 oz)	100	2	14	6
Grilled Mushrooms	1 serv (2 oz)	14	0	2	0
Grilled Alaskan Salmon	1 serv (7 oz)	296	14	1	1
Grilled Chicken Breast	1 serv (4 oz)	130	4	0	0
Grilled Chicken Dinner	1 serv (4 oz)	130	4	0	0
Grilled Chicken Sandwich	1 (11 oz)	509	19	52	—
Grilled Chopped Steak w/ Gravy	1 serv (10 oz)	400	26	12	4
Ham & Swiss On Rye	1 (9 oz)	533	31	40	9
Hashed Browns	1 serv (4 oz)	218	14	20	0
Herb Toast	1 serv (2 oz)	200	11	21	2

FOOD	PORTION	CAL	FAT	CARB	SUG
Horseradish Sauce	1 serv (1.5 oz)	170	20	3	1
Junior Meals Junior Burger	1 serv (3 oz)	261	15	16	0
Junior Meals Junior Chicken Strips	1 serv (5 oz)	318	12	28	6
Junior Meals Junior Fried Fish	1 serv (5 oz)	465	34	25	4
Junior Meals Junior Grilled Cheese	1 serv (4 oz)	375	22	35	2
Junior Meals Junior Shrimp Basket	1 serv (4 oz)	291	16	27	4
Lunch Basket Charleston Chicken Ranch Melt	1 serv (14 oz)	975	59	68	7
Lunch Basket Chicken Strips	1 serv (8 oz)	568	26	45	14
Lunch Basket Classic Burger	1 serv (12 oz)	674	39	42	7
Lunch Basket Delidinger	1 serv (14 oz)	852	45	62	6
Lunch Basket Five Star Philly	1 serv (10 oz)	657	29	55	7
Lunch Basket Patty Melt	1 serv (8 oz)	696	42	39	1
Mashed Potatoes Plain	1 serv (6 oz)	105	1	21	1
Mayonnaise	2 tbsp (1 oz)	200	22	1	0
Mozzarella Sticks w/ Sauce	8 pieces (10 oz)	756	43	56	5
Onion Ring Basket	1 serv (5 oz)	439	27	44	2
Onion Rings	1 serv (3 oz)	264	16	27	1
Patty Melt Sandwich	1 (8 oz)	695	44	39	1
Pork Chop Dinner w/ Gravy	1 serv (8 oz)	386	24	0	0
Porterhouse Steak	1 (14 oz)	708	54	0	0

FOOD	PORTION	CAL	FAT	CARB	SUG
Pot Roast Dinner w/ Gravy	1 serv (7 oz)	260	11	5	2
Rice Pilaf	1 serv (3 oz)	112	2	21	2
Roast Turkey & Stuffing	1 serv (12 oz)	701	27	63	9
Sampler	1 serv (15 oz)	1120	59	104	7
Seasoned Fries	1 serv (4 oz)	261	12	35	0
Senior Battered Cod	1 serv (5 oz)	465	34	25	4
Senior Chicken Fried Steak	1 serv (8 oz)	341	18	29	1
Senior Grilled Cheese Sandwich	1 serv	360	25	21	—
Senior Grilled Chicken Breast	1 serv (6 oz)	219	6	16	0
Senior Liver w/ Bacon & Onions	1 serv (8 oz)	322	19	20	2
Senior Pork Chop	1 serv (4 oz)	193	12	0	0
Senior Pot Roast	1 serv (5 oz)	149	6	6	3
Senior Roast Turkey & Stuffing	1 serv (8 oz)	596	25	61	8
Senior Turkey Sandwich	1	340	27	26	—
Senior Sandwich Ham & Swiss	1 serv (9 oz)	497	30	34	7
Shrimp Dinner	1 serv (8 oz)	558	32	49	5
Sirloin Steak Dinner	1 serv (5.5 oz)	271	21	0	0
Sliced Tomatoes	3 slices (2 oz)	13	0	3	2
Sour Cream	1 serv (1.5 oz)	91	9	2	0
Steak & Shrimp Dinner w/ Gravy	1 serv (9 oz)	645	42	31	4
Super Bird Sandwich	1 (9 oz)	620	32	48	4
T-Bone Steak Dinner	1 serv (10 oz)	530	40	0	0
Turkey Breast On Multigrain	1 (9 oz)	476	26	39	5

FOOD	PORTION	CAL	FAT	CARB	SUG
salad dressings					
Bleu Cheese	1 oz	124	12	4	4
Caesar	1 oz	142	15	1	1
Creamy Italian	1 oz	106	10	4	3
Fat Free Honey Mustard	1 oz	38	0	9	9
French	1 oz	106	10	3	3
Oriental Peanut Dressing	1 serv (1 oz)	106	8	6	5
Ranch	1 oz	101	11	1	1
Reduced Calorie French	1 oz	76	5	8	7
Reduced Calorie Italian	1 oz	32	1	3	3
Thousand Island	1 oz	104	10	2	2
salads and salad bars					
Buffalo Chicken Salad	1 serv (17 oz)	615	37	36	5
Fried Chicken Salad	1 serv (13 oz)	506	31	30	5
Garden Chicken Delight Salad	1 serv (16 oz)	277	5	30	8
Grilled Chicken Caesar Salad w/ Dressing	1 serv (13 oz)	655	47	23	3
Oriental Chicken Salad w/ Dressing	1 serv (20 oz)	568	26	40	10
Side Caesar w/ Dressing	1 serv (6 oz)	338	25	20	2
Side Garden Salad w/ Dressing	1 serv (7 oz)	113	4	16	4
soups					
Cheese	1 serv (8 oz)	293	23	13	2
Chicken Noodle	1 serv (8 oz)	60	2	8	0
Clam Chowder	1 serv (8 oz)	214	11	22	1
Cream Of Broccoli	1 serv (8 oz)	193	12	15	3
Cream of Potato	1 serv (8 oz)	222	12	23	3

FOOD	PORTION	CAL	FAT	CARB	SUG
Split Pea	1 serv (8 oz)	146	6	18	3
Vegetable Beef	1 serv (8 oz)	79	1	11	2

DOMINO'S PIZZA
12 inch medium pizzas

FOOD	PORTION	CAL	FAT	CARB	SUG
Add A Topping Anchovies	1 topping serv	23	1	0	0
Add A Topping Bacon	1 topping serv	81	7	tr	tr
Add A Topping Banana Peppers	1 topping serv	3	tr	1	—
Add A Topping Canned Mushrooms	1 topping serv	4	tr	1	tr
Add A Topping Cheddar Cheese	1 topping serv	57	5	tr	—
Add A Topping Cooked Beef	1 topping serv	56	5	tr	tr
Add A Topping Extra Cheese	1 topping serv	48	4	1	tr
Add A Topping Fresh Mushrooms	1 topping serv	4	tr	1	tr
Add A Topping Green Olives	1 topping serv	12	1	tr	tr
Add A Topping Green Peppers	1 topping serv	3	tr	1	—
Add A Topping Ham	1 topping serv	18	1	tr	tr
Add A Topping Italian Sausage	1 topping serv	55	4	2	tr
Add A Topping Onion	1 topping serv	4	tr	1	—
Add A Topping Pepperoni	1 topping serv	62	6	tr	tr
Add A Topping Pineapple Tidbits	1 topping serv	10	0	2	2
Add A Topping Ripe Olives	1 topping serv	14	1	1	tr

FOOD	PORTION	CAL	FAT	CARB	SUG
Deep Dish Cheese	2 slices (6.3 oz)	477	22	50	5
Hand Tossed Cheese	2 slices (5.2 oz)	347	11	49	3
Thin Crust Cheese	¼ pie (3.7 oz)	271	12	31	3
14 inch large pizzas					
Add A Topping Anchovies	1 topping serv	23	1	0	0
Add A Topping Bacon	1 topping serv	75	6	tr	tr
Add A Topping Banana Peppers	1 topping serv	3	tr	1	—
Add A Topping Canned Mushrooms	1 topping serv	3	tr	1	tr
Add A Topping Cheddar Cheese	1 topping serv	48	4	tr	tr
Add A Topping Cooked Beef	1 topping serv	44	4	tr	tr
Add A Topping Extra Cheese	1 topping serv	45	4	1	tr
Add A Topping Fresh Mushrooms	1 topping serv	3	tr	1	tr
Add A Topping Green Olives	1 topping serv	11	1	tr	tr
Add A Topping Green Peppers	1 topping serv	2	tr	1	—
Add A Topping Ham	1 topping serv	17	1	tr	tr
Add A Topping Italian Sausage	1 topping serv	44	3	1	tr
Add A Topping Onion	1 topping serv	3	tr	1	—
Add A Topping Pepperoni	1 topping serv	55	5	tr	tr
Add A Topping Pineapple Tidbits	1 topping serv	8	0	tr	2
Add A Topping Ripe Olives	1 topping serv	12	1	1	tr

FOOD	PORTION	CAL	FAT	CARB	SUG
Deep Dish Cheese	2 slices (6.1 oz)	455	20	54	5
Hand-Tossed Cheese	2 slices (4.8 oz)	317	10	45	3
Thin Crust Cheese	⅛ pie (3.5 oz)	253	11	29	2
6 inch deep dish pizzas					
Add A Topping Anchovies	1 topping serv	45	2	0	0
Add A Topping Bacon	1 topping serv	82	7	tr	tr
Add A Topping Banana Peppers	1 topping serv	3	tr	tr	—
Add A Topping Canned Mushrooms	1 topping serv	2	tr	tr	tr
Add A Topping Cheddar Cheese	1 topping serv	86	7	tr	tr
Add A Topping Cooked Beef	1 topping serv	44	4	tr	tr
Add A Topping Extra Cheese	1 topping serv	57	5	1	1
Add A Topping Fresh Mushrooms	1 topping serv	2	tr	tr	tr
Add A Topping Green Olives	1 topping serv	10	1	tr	tr
Add A Topping Green Peppers	1 topping serv	2	tr	tr	—
Add A Topping Ham	1 topping serv	17	1	tr	tr
Add A Topping Italian Sausage	1 topping serv	44	3	1	tr
Add A Topping Onion	1 topping serv	3	tr	1	—
Add A Topping Pepperoni	1 topping serv	50	5	tr	tr
Add A Topping Pineapple Tidbits	1 topping serv	5	0	1	1

FOOD	PORTION	CAL	FAT	CARB	SUG
Add A Topping Ripe Olives	1 topping serv	11	1	tr	tr
Cheese	1 pie (7.6 oz)	595	27	68	6

main menu selections

FOOD	PORTION	CAL	FAT	CARB	SUG
Breadstick	1 (0.8 oz)	78	3	11	tr
Buffalo Wings Barbeque	1 piece (0.9 oz)	50	2	2	1
Buffalo Wings Hot	1 piece (0.9 oz)	45	2	1	tr
Cheesy Bread	1 piece (1 oz)	103	5	11	tr
Garden Salad	1 sm (4.3 oz)	22	tr	4	3

salad dressings

FOOD	PORTION	CAL	FAT	CARB	SUG
Marzetti Blue Cheese	1 serv (1.5 oz)	220	24	2	2
Marzetti Creamy Caesar	1 serv (1.5 oz)	200	22	2	1
Marzetti Fat Free Ranch	1 serv (1.5 oz)	40	0	10	3
Marzetti Honey French	1 serv (1.5 oz)	210	18	14	14
Marzetti House Italian	1 serv (1.5 oz)	220	24	1	1
Marzetti Light Italian	1 serv (1.5 oz)	20	1	2	2
Marzetti Ranch	1 serv (1.5 oz)	260	29	1	1
Marzetti Thousand Island	1 serv (1.5 oz)	200	20	5	—

DUNKIN' DONUTS
bagels and cream cheese

FOOD	PORTION	CAL	FAT	CARB	SUG
Bagel Blueberry	1	340	1	75	7
Bagel Cinnamon Raisin	1	340	1	74	11
Bagel Egg	1	350	2	72	3
Bagel Everything	1	360	2	74	3
Bagel Garlic	1	360	1	76	4

FOOD	PORTION	CAL	FAT	CARB	SUG
Bagel Onion	1	330	1	70	3
Bagel Plain	1	340	1	73	3
Bagel Poppyseed	1	360	3	74	3
Bagel Pumpernickel	1	350	2	75	6
Bagel Salt	1	340	1	73	3
Bagel Sesame	1	380	5	74	3
Bagel Wheat	1	330	2	73	6
Cream Cheese Chive	1 pkg	190	19	3	3
Cream Cheese Garden Vegetable	1 pkg	180	17	3	2
Cream Cheese Lite	1 pkg	130	11	3	2
Cream Cheese Plain	1 pkg	200	19	3	2
Cream Cheese Salmon	1 pkg	180	17	2	2
baked selections					
Bow Tie Donut	1	300	17	34	10
Cake Donut Blueberry	1	290	16	35	16
Cake Donut Butternut	1	300	16	36	16
Cake Donut Chocolate Coconut	1	300	19	31	12
Cake Donut Chocolate Frosted	1	300	16	38	18
Cake Donut Chocolate Glazed	1	290	16	33	14
Cake Donut Cinnamon	1	270	15	31	12
Cake Donut Coconut	1	290	17	33	13
Cake Donut Double Chocolate	1	310	17	37	18
Cake Donut Glazed	1	270	15	33	14
Cake Donut Old Fashioned	1	250	15	26	7

FOOD	PORTION	CAL	FAT	CARB	SUG
Cake Donut Powdered	1	270	15	32	13
Cake Donut Toasted Coconut	1	300	17	35	16
Cake Donut Whole Wheat Glazed	1	310	19	32	14
Chocolate Frosted Donut	1	200	9	29	10
Chocolate Kreme Filled Donut	1	270	13	35	16
Cinnamon Bun	1	510	15	85	42
Coffee Roll	1	270	14	33	10
Coffee Roll Chocolate Frosted	1	290	15	36	12
Coffee Roll Maple Frosted	1	290	14	36	13
Coffee Roll Vanilla Frosted	1	290	14	36	13
Cookie Chocolate Chocolate Chunk	1	210	11	26	16
Cookie Chocolate Chunk	1	220	11	28	17
Cookie Chocolate Chunk w/ Nut	1	230	12	27	16
Cookie Chocolate White Chocolate Chunk	1	230	12	28	19
Cookie Oatmeal Raisin Pecan	1	220	10	29	18
Cookie Peanut Butter Chocolate Chunk w/ Nuts	1	240	14	24	16
Cookie Peanut Butter w/ Nuts	1	240	14	24	15

FOOD	PORTION	CAL	FAT	CARB	SUG
Croissant Almond	1	350	22	34	13
Croissant Chocolate	1	400	25	37	15
Croissant Plain	1	290	18	26	3
Cruller Glazed	1	290	15	37	18
Cruller Glazed Chocolate	1	280	15	35	16
Cruller Plain	1	240	15	25	6
Cruller Powdered	1	270	15	30	11
Cruller Sugar	1	250	15	27	8
Donut Apple Crumb	1	230	10	34	12
Donut Apple N' Spice	1	200	8	29	7
Donut Bavarian Kreme	1	210	9	30	9
Donut Black Raspberry	1	210	8	32	10
Donut Blueberry Crumb	1	240	10	36	15
Donut Boston Kreme	1	240	9	36	14
Donut Chocolate Iced Bismark	1	340	15	50	31
Dunkin' Donut	1	240	15	25	6
Eclair Donut	1	270	11	39	17
Fritter Glazed	1	260	14	31	7
Glazed Donut	1	180	8	25	6
Jelly Filled Donut	1	210	8	32	14
Jelly Stick	1	290	12	44	24
Lemon Donut	1	200	9	28	8
Maple Frosted Donut	1	210	9	30	12
Marble Frosted Donut	1	200	9	29	11
Muffin Apple Cinnamon Pecan	1	510	21	74	41
Muffin Apple N'Spice	1	350	12	57	29
Muffin Banana Nut	1	360	15	52	29
Muffin Blueberry	1 (4 oz)	320	12	49	41

FOOD	PORTION	CAL	FAT	CARB	SUG
Muffin Blueberry	1 (6 oz)	490	17	78	—
Muffin Bran	1	390	12	60	34
Muffin Cherry	1	340	12	53	29
Muffin Chocolate Hazelnut	1	610	26	87	52
Muffin Chocolate Chip	1 (6 oz)	590	24	88	50
Muffin Chocolate Chip	1 (4 oz)	400	17	58	36
Muffin Corn	1 (4 oz)	390	15	57	22
Muffin Corn	1 (6 oz)	500	16	78	34
Muffin Cranberry Orange	1	470	15	76	41
Muffin Cranberry Orange Nut	1	350	15	52	27
Muffin Honey Raisin Bran	1 (3.3 oz)	330	10	57	27
Muffin Lemon Poppyseed	1	360	13	56	27
Muffin Oat Bran	1	370	13	55	29
Muffin Lowfat Apple & Spice	1	240	2	54	32
Muffin Lowfat Banana	1	250	2	57	35
Muffin Lowfat Blueberry	1	250	2	55	33
Muffin Lowfat Bran	1	240	1	57	32
Muffin Lowfat Cherry	1	250	2	56	34
Muffin Lowfat Chocolate	1	250	3	53	29
Muffin Lowfat Corn	1	240	3	52	20
Muffin Lowfat Cranberry Orange	1	240	2	55	32
Muffin Reduced Fat Blueberry	1	450	12	77	42
Muffin Reduced Fat Corn	1	460	11	79	35

FOOD	PORTION	CAL	FAT	CARB	SUG
Munchkins Chocolate Cake Glazed	3	200	10	26	13
Munchkins Cake Butternut	3	200	11	25	12
Munchkins Cake Cinnamon	4	250	14	29	13
Munchkins Cake Coconut	3	200	12	23	10
Munchkins Cake Glazed	3	200	10	27	14
Munchkins Cake Plain	4	220	14	22	6
Munchkins Cake Powdered	4	250	14	29	12
Munchkins Cake Sugared	4	240	14	28	12
Munchkins Cake Toasted Coconut	3	200	11	24	11
Munchkins Yeast Glazed	5	200	9	27	12
Munchkins Yeast Jelly Filled	5	210	9	30	15
Munchkins Yeast Lemon Filled	4	170	8	23	9
Munchkins Yeast Sugar Raised	7	220	12	26	5
Strawberry Frosted Donut	1	210	9	30	12
Strawberry Donut	1	210	8	32	11
Sugar Raised Donut	1	170	8	22	4
Sugared Cake Donut	1	250	15	27	9
Vanilla Frosted Donut	1	210	9	30	12
Vanilla Kreme Filled Donut	1	270	13	36	17

FOOD	PORTION	CAL	FAT	CARB	SUG
beverages					
Coffee Coolatta w/ Skim Milk	1 (16 oz)	230	0	52	51
Collatta Orange Mango Fruit	1 (16 oz)	290	0	71	63
Collatta Pink Lemonade Fruit	1 (16 oz)	350	0	88	63
Collatta Raspberry Lemonade	1 (16 oz)	280	0	68	64
Collatta Vanilla	1 (16 oz)	450	7	94	80
Coolatta Strawberry Fruit	1 (16 oz)	280	0	70	63
Cream	1 serv (1 oz)	60	5	1	1
Dark Roast Coffee	1 serv (10 oz)	5	0	1	0
Decaf Coffee	1 serv (10 oz)	0	0	0	0
Dunkaccino	1 (10 oz)	250	11	34	25
French Vanilla Coffee	1 serv (10 oz)	5	0	1	0
Hazelnut Coffee	1 serv (10 oz)	5	0	1	0
Hot Cocoa	1 (10 oz)	230	8	38	29
Regular Coffee	1 serv (10 oz)	5	0	1	0
sandwiches					
Breakfast Sandwich Ham Egg Cheese	1	320	12	31	3
Omwich Bagel Bacon Cheddar	1	600	21	79	5
Omwich Bagel Spanish Cheese	1	570	18	79	5
Omwich Bagel Three Cheese	1	610	22	78	5
Omwich Croissant Bacon Cheddar	1	560	38	33	5
Omwich Croissant Spanish Cheese	1	530	36	33	5

FOOD	PORTION	CAL	FAT	CARB	SUG
Omwich Croissant Three Cheese	1	560	39	33	5
Omwich English Muffin Bacon Cheddar	1	400	21	33	4
Omwich English Muffin Spanish Cheese	1	370	18	34	4
Omwich English Muffin Three Cheese	1	400	22	33	4

EINSTEIN BROS BAGELS

bagels

FOOD	PORTION	CAL	FAT	CARB	SUG
Bagel Chips Cinnamon Raisin Swirl	1 serv (1 oz)	90	1	19	3
Bagel Chips Plain	1 serv (1 oz)	90	0	18	1
Bagel Chips Sourdough Dill	1 serv (1 oz)	90	1	18	1
Bagel Chips Sun Dried Tomato	1 serv (1 oz)	90	1	17	0
Bagel Chips Sunflower	1 serv (1 oz)	100	2	8	1
Bagel Chips Wild Blueberry	1 serv (1 oz)	90	1	19	3
Chocolate Chip	1 (4 oz)	380	3	78	11
Chopped Garlic	1 (4.2 oz)	377	4	81	3
Chopped Onion	1 (4 oz)	340	3	72	3
Cinnamon Raisin Swirl	1 (4 oz)	360	1	78	13
Cinnamon Sugar	1	330	0	72	6
Dark Pumpernickel	1 (3.8 oz)	330	1	72	3
Everything	1 (4 oz)	342	2	74	5
Honey 8 Grain	1 (4 oz)	320	1	71	6
Nutty Banana	1 (4 oz)	370	3	77	8
Plain	1 (3.7 oz)	330	1	72	3
Poppy Dip'd	1 (3.9 oz)	346	2	73	3
Salt	1 (3.9 oz)	330	1	72	3

FOOD	PORTION	CAL	FAT	CARB	SUG
Sesame Dip'd	1 (4.1 oz)	381	5	74	3
Spinach Herb	1 (3.8 oz)	320	1	71	1
Sun Dried Tomato	1 (3.8 oz)	320	1	70	3
Veggie Confetti	1 (3.8 oz)	330	1	71	4
Wild Blueberry	1 (4 oz)	360	1	79	10
sandwiches and fillings					
Butter & Margarine Blend	1 serv (0.4 oz)	60	7	0	0
Capers	1 tbsp	0	0	0	0
Cheddar Cheese	1 serv (0.75 oz)	110	9	1	0
Classic New York Lox & Bagel	1 (11.4 oz)	560	24	31	7
Cream Cheese Cheddarpeno	1 serv (1 oz)	90	8	2	1
Cream Cheese Chive	1 serv (1 oz)	90	9	2	2
Cream Cheese Maple Walnut Raisin	1 serv (1 oz)	100	8	7	6
Cream Cheese Plain	1 serv (1 oz)	100	9	2	2
Cream Cheese Smoked Salmon	1 serv (1 oz)	90	8	2	1
Cream Cheese Strawberry	1 serv (1 oz)	90	8	4	4
Cream Cheese Sun Dried Tomato	1 serv (1 oz)	90	8	3	2
Cucumbers	1 serv (1 oz)	0	0	1	1
Fruit Spreads	1 tbsp	40	0	10	9
Ham	1 serv (2.5 oz)	75	2	1	1
Ham & Cheese Sandwich	1 (9.9 oz)	520	15	63	8
Honey	1 tbsp	64	0	18	18
Hummus	2 tbsp	60	3	4	0

FOOD	PORTION	CAL	FAT	CARB	SUG
Hummus Sandwich	1 (6 oz)	440	7	62	4
Lettuce	1 leaf	0	0	0	0
Lite Cream Cheese Plain	1 serv (1 oz)	60	5	2	2
Lite Cream Cheese Spinach Dill	1 serv (1 oz)	60	5	2	2
Lite Cream Cheese Veggie	1 serv (1 oz)	60	5	3	3
Lite Cream Cheese Wildberry	1 serv (1 oz)	70	4	7	7
Lowfat Chicken Salad Sandwich	1 (11.6 oz)	440	9	63	8
Lowfat Tuna Salad Sandwich	1 (11.6 oz)	440	8	62	7
Marshall's Loz	1 serv (2 oz)	90	4	2	1
Mayonnaise Lite Reduced Calorie	1 serv (0.5 oz)	50	5	1	0
Peanut Butter	1 serv (1.1 oz)	190	16	8	3
Peanut Butter & Jelly Sandwich	1 (6 oz)	595	17	99	6
Scrambled Egg Sandwich	1 (7.7 oz)	480	17	56	4
Scrambled Egg Sandwich w/ Meat & Cheese	1 (8.9 oz)	520	31	57	4
Smoked Turkey	1 serv (2.5 oz)	75	1	0	0
Smoked Turkey Sandwich	1 (9.9 oz)	480	14	59	5
Spouts Alfalfa	1 serv (0.5 oz)	0	0	3	2
Sweet Onions	1 serv (1 oz)	0	0	2	1
Swiss Cheese	1 serv (0.75 oz)	100	8	0	0
Tasty Turkey Sandwich	1 (10 oz)	530	22	61	8

FOOD	PORTION	CAL	FAT	CARB	SUG
Tomato	1 serv (1.5 oz)	0	0	2	1
Turkey Pastrami 99% Fat Free	1 serv (2.5 oz)	75	6	2	1
Turkey Pastrami Sandwich	1 (9.7 oz)	460	12	60	5
Veg Out Sandwich	1 (8.9 oz)	350	17	62	9
Whitefish Salad Sandwich	1 (9.2 oz)	630	23	59	6

EL POLLO LOCO
main menu selections

FOOD	PORTION	CAL	FAT	CARB	SUG
Broccoli Slaw	1 serv (5 oz)	203	17	14	2
Burrito BRC	1 (9.3 oz)	482	15	72	1
Burrito Classic Chicken	1 (9.3 oz)	556	22	61	2
Burrito Grilled Steak	1 (11.3 oz)	705	32	68	1
Burrito Loco Grande	1 (13.1 oz)	632	26	67	3
Burrito Smokey Black Bean	1 (9.3 oz)	566	22	78	10
Burrito Spicy Hot Chicken	1 (9.8 oz)	559	22	61	2
Burrito Whole Wheat Chicken	1 (10.8 oz)	592	26	60	1
Chicken Breast	1 piece (3 oz)	160	6	0	0
Chicken Leg	1 piece (1.75 oz)	90	5	0	0
Chicken Soft Taco	1 (4 oz)	224	12	15	1
Chicken Thigh	1 piece (2 oz)	180	12	0	0
Chicken Wing	1 (1.5 oz)	110	6	0	0
Chicken Tamale	1 (3.5 oz)	190	8	23	0
Cole Slaw	1 serv (5 oz)	206	16	12	5
Corn-On-Cob	1 ear (5.5 oz)	146	2	33	7
Cornbread Stuffing	1 serv (6 oz)	281	12	40	4
Crispy Green Beans	1 serv (5 oz)	41	2	6	3

FOOD	PORTION	CAL	FAT	CARB	SUG
Cucumber Salad	1 serv (4.2 oz)	34	0	7	1
Fiesta Corn	1 serv (5 oz)	152	6	25	2
Flame Broiled Chicken Salad	1 serv (14.9 oz)	167	5	11	4
French Fries	1 serv (4.4 oz)	323	14	44	0
Garden Salad	1 serv (6.4 oz)	29	0	6	2
Gravy	1 serv (1 oz)	14	0	2	1
Honey Glazed Carrots	1 serv (5 oz)	104	6	14	9
Lime Parfait	1 serv (5 oz)	125	3	25	24
Macaroni & Cheese	1 serv (6 oz)	238	12	22	2
Mashed Potatoes	1 serv (5 oz)	97	1	21	1
Pinto Beans	1 serv (6 oz)	185	4	29	0
Polo Bowl	1 serv (19 oz)	504	13	69	3
Potato Salad	1 serv (6 oz)	256	14	30	6
Rainbow Pasta Salad	1 serv (5 oz)	157	1	30	3
Salad Shell	1 (5.6 oz)	440	27	42	0
Smokey Black Beans	1 serv (5 oz)	255	13	29	16
Southwest Cole Slaw	1 serv (5 oz)	178	13	15	5
Spanish Rice	1 serv (4 oz)	130	3	24	1
Spiced Apples	1 serv (5 oz)	146	0	39	19
Steak Bowl	1 serv (15.2 oz)	616	26	62	2
Taco Al Carbon Chicken	1 serv (4.4 oz)	265	12	30	1
Taco Al Carbon Steak	1 (4.4 oz)	394	22	30	1
Taquito	1 serv (5 oz)	370	17	43	2
Tortilla Corn	1 (1.1 oz)	70	1	14	0
Tortilla Flour	1 (1 oz)	90	3	13	0
Tortilla Wrap Chicken Caesar	1 (10.47 oz)	518	19	59	4
Tortilla Wrap Southwest	1 (11.97 oz)	632	27	69	6
Tostada Salad Chicken	1 serv (14.7 oz)	332	14	26	2
Tostado Salad Steak	1 serv (13.2 oz)	525	31	26	1

FOOD	PORTION	CAL	FAT	CARB	SUG
salad dressings					
Blue Cheese	1 serv (2 oz)	300	32	2	2
Light Italian	1 serv (2 oz)	25	1	3	3
Ranch	1 serv (2 oz)	350	39	2	1
Thousand Island	1 serv (2 oz)	270	27	9	9
FAZOLI'S					
desserts					
Cheesecake Plain	1 slice	339	26	20	—
Cheesecake Turtle	1 slice	373	27	28	—
Cookie Milk Chocolate Chunk	1	300	15	54	33
Lemon Ice	1 serv (12 oz)	142	0	36	—
Strawberry Topping	1 serv (1 oz)	33	0	8	8
main menu selections					
Baked Spaghetti Parmesan	1 serv	697	26	76	8
Baked Ziti	1 sm	486	17	56	7
Breadstick	1	173	8	19	—
Breadstick Dry	1	100	1	18	—
Broccoli Fettuccine Alfredo	1 sm	563	15	85	5
Broccoli Lasagna	1 serv	423	18	45	—
Cheese Ravioli w/ Meat Sauce	1 serv	511	17	65	8
Cheese Ravioli w/ Tomato Sauce	1 serv	476	15	65	9
Chicken Parmesan	1 serv	468	9	47	—
Fettuccine Alfredo	1 sm	535	15	80	3
Lasagna	1 serv	437	19	41	—
Minestrone Soup	1 serv	123	1	23	8
Pizza Cheese Double Slice	1 serv	465	15	58	6

FOOD	PORTION	CAL	FAT	CARB	SUG
Pizza Combination Double Slice	1 serv	572	25	63	7
Pizza Pepperoni Double Slice	1 serv	526	22	61	6
Sampler Platter	1 serv	708	21	97	—
Shrimp & Scallop Fettuccine	1 serv	649	20	80	—
Spaghetti w/ Meat Sauce	1 sm	372	8	60	—
Spaghetti w/ Meatballs	1 sm	718	31	80	9
Spaghetti w/ Tomato Sauce	1 sm	358	8	62	—
salad dressings					
Honey French	1 serv	146	12	9	9
House Italian	1 serv	106	9	5	5
Ranch	1 serv	155	17	1	1
Reduced Calorie Italian	1 serv	55	5	3	2
Thousand Island	1 serv	129	13	4	4
salads and salad bars					
Garden Salad	1	30	tr	6	—
Italian Chef Salad	1	262	21	13	3
Pasta Salad	1 serv	599	26	69	—

FRIENDLY'S

ice cream

FOOD	PORTION	CAL	FAT	CARB	SUG
Heath English Toffee	½ cup (2.7 oz)	190	10	24	19
Purely Pistachio	½ cup	160	10	16	15
Vanilla	½ cup	150	8	16	11

FOOD	PORTION	CAL	FAT	CARB	SUG
GODFATHER'S PIZZA					
Golden Crust Cheese	1/10 lg (3.5 oz)	242	9	28	—
Golden Crust Cheese	1/8 med (3.1 oz)	212	8	26	—
Golden Crust Combo	1/10 lg (4.9 oz)	305	14	31	—
Golden Crust Combo	1/8 med (4.4 oz)	271	12	28	—
Original Crust Cheese	1/4 mini (1.9 oz)	131	3	19	—
Original Crust Cheese	1/10 lg (4 oz)	258	6	36	—
Original Crust Cheese	1/8 med (3.5 oz)	231	5	24	—
Original Crust Cheese	1/10 jumbo (5.8 oz)	382	9	53	—
Original Crust Combo	1/8 med (5.1 oz)	306	11	36	—
Original Crust Combo	1/10 lg (5.6 oz)	338	12	38	—
Original Crust Combo	1/10 jumbo (8.3 oz)	503	18	56	—
Original Crust Combo	1/4 mini (2.9 oz)	176	7	21	—
GODIVA					
Almond Butter Dome	3 pieces (1.5 oz)	240	17	19	14
Bouchee Au Chocolat	1 piece (1.5 oz)	210	11	25	10
Bouchee Ivory Raspberry	1 piece (1 oz)	160	9	17	11
Chocolatier Dark Chocolate w/ Raspberry	1 bar (1.5 oz)	220	11	28	—
Chocolatier Milk Chocolate	1 bar (1.5 oz)	230	13	26	25
Gold Ballotin	3 pieces (1.5 oz)	210	10	27	21
Mochaccino Mousse	2 pieces (1.25 oz)	210	15	17	14
Truffle Amaretto Di Saronno	2 pieces (1.5 oz)	210	12	24	17
Truffle Assorted	2 pieces (1.5 oz)	220	13	24	20

FOOD	PORTION	CAL	FAT	CARB	SUG
HAAGEN-DAZS					
frozen yogurt					
Pinapple Coconut	½ cup	230	13	25	—
Soft Serve Nonfat Chocolate	½ cup	110	0	23	20
Soft Serve Nonfat Chocolate Mousse	½ cup	80	0	24	7
Soft Serve Nonfat Coffee	½ cup	110	0	22	21
Soft Serve Nonfat Strawberry	½ cup	110	0	24	23
Soft Serve Nonfat Vanilla	½ cup	110	0	22	21
Soft Serve Nonfat Vanilla Mousse	½ cup	70	0	23	7
Soft Serve Nonfat White Chocolate	½ cup	110	0	22	21
Vanilla Fudge	½ cup	160	0	34	—
Vanilla Raspberry Swirl	½ cup	130	0	29	20
ice cream					
Bailey's Irish Cream	½ cup	270	17	23	—
Bar Chocolate	1 (2.7 oz)	200	12	16	15
Bar Chocolate & Dark Chocolate	1 (3.6 oz)	350	24	28	24
Bar Coffee	1 (2.7 oz)	190	13	15	15
Bar Coffee & Almond Crunch	1 (3.7 oz)	370	27	27	26
Bar Vanilla	1 (2.7 oz)	190	13	15	15
Bar Vanilla & Almonds	1 (3.7 oz)	380	28	26	24
Bar Vanilla & Milk Chocolate	1 (3.5 oz)	340	24	25	24
Belgian Chocolate Chocolate	½ cup	330	21	29	26

FOOD	PORTION	CAL	FAT	CARB	SUG
Brownies A La Mode	½ cup	280	16	28	23
Butter Pecan	½ cup	300	22	20	17
Cappuccino Commotion	½ cup	310	21	25	23
Chocolate	½ cup	269	17	21	20
Chocolate Chocolate Chip	½ cup	300	19	26	23
Chocolate Chocolate Mint	½ cup	300	20	25	22
Chocolate Swiss Almond	½ cup	300	20	24	21
Coffee	½ cup	250	17	20	20
Coffee Mocha Chip	½ cup	270	19	24	21
Cookie Dough Dynamo	½ cup	310	20	29	24
Cookies & Cream	½ cup	270	17	23	21
Cookies & Fudge	½ cup	180	3	33	20
Deep Chocolate Peanut Butter	½ cup	350	24	26	21
Dulce De Leche Caramel	½ cup	270	16	27	27
Lowfat Coffee Fudge	½ cup	170	3	32	22
Macadamia Brittle	½ cup	280	19	24	23
Macadamia Nut	½ cup	320	24	20	19
Mint Chip	½ cup	280	18	25	22
Pistachio	½ cup	280	19	21	18
Pralines & Cream	½ cup	280	17	28	26
Rum Raisin	½ cup	260	17	21	20
Strawberry	½ cup	250	16	22	21
Vanilla	½ cup	250	17	20	20
Vanilla Chocolate Chip	½ cup	290	19	25	22
Vanilla Swiss Almond	½ cup	290	20	23	20

FOOD	PORTION	CAL	FAT	CARB	SUG
sorbet					
Bar Raspberry & Vanilla	1 (2.5 oz)	90	0	21	15
Mango	½ cup	120	0	31	29
Orange	½ cup	120	0	30	24
Raspberry	½ cup	120	0	30	—
Soft Serve Raspberry	½ cup	110	0	28	25
Strawberry	½ cup	120	0	30	27
Zesty Lemon	½ cup	120	0	31	27
HARDEE'S					
beverages					
Orange Juice	1 serv (11 oz)	140	tr	34	—
Shake Chocolate	1 (12.2 oz)	370	5	67	—
Shake Peach	1 (12.1 oz)	390	4	77	—
Shake Strawberry	1 (12.7 oz)	420	4	83	—
Shake Vanilla	1 (12.2 oz)	350	5	65	—
breakfast selections					
Apple Cinnamon 'N' Raisin Biscuit	1 (2.18 oz)	200	8	30	—
Bacon & Egg Biscuit	1 (5.5 oz)	570	33	45	—
Bacon Egg & Cheese Biscuit	1 (5.9 oz)	610	37	45	—
Big Country Breakfast Bacon	1 serv (9.4 oz)	820	49	62	—
Big Country Breakfast Sausage	1 serv (11.4 oz)	1000	66	62	—
Biscuit 'N' Gravy	1 (7.8 oz)	510	28	55	—
Country Ham Biscuit	1 (3.8 oz)	430	22	45	—
Frisco Breakfast Sandwich Ham	1 (7.4 oz)	500	25	46	—
Ham Biscuit	1 (4 oz)	400	20	47	—

FOOD	PORTION	CAL	FAT	CARB	SUG
Ham Egg & Cheese Biscuit	1 (6.5 oz)	540	30	48	—
Hash Rounds	1 serv (2.8 oz)	230	14	24	—
Jelly Biscuit	1 (3.5 oz)	440	21	57	—
Rise 'N' Shine Biscuit	1 (2.9 oz)	390	21	44	—
Sausage Biscuit	1 (4.1 oz)	510	31	44	—
Sausage & Egg Biscuit	1 (6.3 oz)	630	40	45	—
Three Pancakes	1 serv (4.8 oz)	280	2	56	—
Ultimate Omelet Biscuit	1 (5.8 oz)	570	33	45	—
desserts					
Big Cookie	1 (2.0 oz)	280	12	41	—
Cone Chocolate	1 (4.1 oz)	180	2	34	—
Cone Vanilla	1 (4.1 oz)	170	2	34	—
Cool Twist Cone Vanilla / Chocolate	1 (4.1 oz)	180	2	34	—
Peach Cobbler	1 serv (6 oz)	310	7	60	—
Sundae Hot Fudge	1 (5.5 oz)	290	6	51	—
Sundae Strawberry	1 (5.8 oz)	210	2	43	—
main menu selections					
Baked Beans	1 serv (5 oz)	170	1	32	—
Big Roast Beef Sandwich	1 (6.5 oz)	460	24	35	—
Cheeseburger	1 (4.3 oz)	310	14	30	—
Chicken Fillet Sandwich	1 (7.5 oz)	480	18	54	—
Cole Slaw	1 serv (4 oz)	240	20	13	—
Cravin' Bacon Cheeseburger	1 (8.1 oz)	690	46	38	—
Fisherman's Fillet	1 (8.3 oz)	560	27	54	—
French Fries	1 sm (3.4 oz)	240	10	33	—
Fried Chicken Breast	1 piece (5.2 oz)	370	15	29	—

FOOD	PORTION	CAL	FAT	CARB	SUG
Fried Chicken Leg	1 piece (2.4 oz)	170	7	15	—
Fried Chicken Thigh	1 piece (4.2 oz)	330	15	30	—
Fried Chicken Wing	1 piece (2.3 oz)	200	8	23	—
Frisco Burger	1 (8.1 oz)	720	46	43	—
Gravy	1 serv (1.5 oz)	20	tr	3	—
Grilled Chicken Sandwich	1 (7.1 oz)	350	11	38	—
Hamburger	1 (3.9 oz)	270	11	29	—
Hot Ham 'N' Cheese	1 (5.1 oz)	310	12	34	—
Mashed Potatoes	1 serv (4 oz)	70	tr	14	—
Mesquite Bacon Cheeseburger	1 (4.5 oz)	370	18	32	—
Mushroom 'N' Swiss Burger	1 (6.8 oz)	490	25	39	—
Quarter Pound Double Cheeseburger	1 (6 oz)	470	27	31	—
Regular Roast Beef	1 (4.3 oz)	320	16	26	—
The Boss	1 (7 oz)	570	33	42	—
The Works Burger	1 (8.1 oz)	530	30	41	—
salad dressings					
French Fat Free	1 serv (2 oz)	70	0	18	—
Ranch	1 serv (2 oz)	290	29	6	—
Thousand Island	1 serv (2 oz)	250	23	9	—
salads and salad bars					
Garden Salad	1 (10.2 oz)	220	13	11	—
Grilled Chicken Salad	1 (11.5 oz)	150	3	11	—
Side Salad	1 (4.6 oz)	25	tr	4	—
HOT SAM'S PRETZELS					
Bavarian	1 reg (2.5 oz)	200	0	42	2
Sweet Dough	1 (4.5 oz)	360	3	73	4
Sweet Dough Blueberry	1 (4.5 oz)	400	4	81	18

FOOD	PORTION	CAL	FAT	CARB	SUG
IHOP					
Pancake Buckwheat	1 (2.5 oz)	134	5	19	—
Pancake Buttermilk	1 (2 oz)	108	3	17	—
Pancake Country Griddle	1 (2.25 oz)	134	4	22	—
Pancake Egg	1 (2 oz)	102	5	12	—
Pancake Harvest Grain 'N Nut	1 (2.25 oz)	160	8	18	—
Waffle	1 (4 oz)	305	15	37	—
Waffle Belgian	1 (6 oz)	408	20	49	—
Waffle Belgian Harvest Grain 'N Nut	1 (6 oz)	445	28	40	—
JACK IN THE BOX					
beverages					
2% Milk	1 serv (8 fl oz)	130	5	14	14
Barq's Root Beer	1 reg (20 fl oz)	180	0	50	50
Classic Ice Cream Shake Cappuccino	1 reg (11 oz)	630	29	80	58
Classic Ice Cream Shake Chocolate	1 reg (11 fl oz)	630	27	85	67
Classic Ice Cream Shake Oreo Cookie	1 reg (12 oz)	740	36	91	45
Classic Ice Cream Shake Strawberry	1 reg (10 fl oz)	640	28	85	67
Classic Ice Cream Shake Vanilla	1 reg (11 oz)	610	31	73	62
Coca-Cola Classic	1 reg (20 fl oz)	170	0	46	46
Coffee	1 reg (12 fl oz)	5	0	1	0
Diet Coke	1 reg (20 fl oz)	0	0	0	0
Dr Pepper	1 reg (20 fl oz)	190	0	49	—
Iced Tea	1 reg (20 fl oz)	0	0	0	0

FOOD	PORTION	CAL	FAT	CARB	SUG
Minute Maid Lemonade	1 reg (20 fl oz)	190	0	48	48
Orange Juice	1 serv (10 oz)	150	0	34	28
Sprite	1 reg (20 fl oz)	160	0	41	41
breakfast selections					
Breakfast Jack	1 (4.2 oz)	300	12	30	5
Country Crock Spread	1 pat (5 g)	25	3	0	0
Grape Jelly	1 serv (0.5 oz)	40	0	9	6
Hash Browns	1 serv (2 oz)	160	11	14	0
Pancake Syrup	1 serv (1.5 oz)	120	0	30	20
Pancakes w/ Bacon	1 serv (5.6 oz)	400	12	59	12
Sausage Croissant	1 (6.4 oz)	670	48	39	4
Sourdough Breakfast Sandwich	1 (5.2 oz)	380	21	31	2
Supreme Croissant	1 (6 oz)	570	20	39	4
Ultimate Breakfast Sandwich	1 (8.5 oz)	620	36	39	4
desserts					
Carrot Cake	1 serv (3.5 oz)	370	16	54	28
Cheesecake	1 serv (3.5 oz)	310	18	29	22
Double Fudge Cake	1 serv (3 oz)	300	10	50	25
Hot Apple Turnover	1 (3.8 oz)	340	18	41	12
main menu selections					
¼ lb Burger	1 (6 oz)	510	27	39	8
American Cheese	1 slice (0.4 oz)	45	4	0	0
Bacon & Cheddar Potato Wedges	1 serv (9.3 oz)	800	58	49	2
Bacon Ultimate Cheeseburger	1 (10.4 oz)	1150	89	31	6
Barbeque Dipping Sauce	1 serv (1 fl oz)	45	0	11	7
Cheeseburger	1 (4 oz)	330	15	32	7

FOOD	PORTION	CAL	FAT	CARB	SUG
Chicken & Fries	1 serv (9.3 oz)	730	34	79	0
Chicken Caesar Sandwich	1 (8.3 oz)	520	26	44	5
Chicken Fajita Pita	1 (6.6 oz)	280	9	25	5
Chicken Sandwich	1 (5.9 oz)	450	26	38	6
Chicken Strips Breaded	5 pieces (5.3 oz)	360	17	24	0
Chicken Supreme Sandwich	1 (8.2 oz)	680	45	46	8
Chili Cheese Curly Fries	1 serv (8.1 oz)	650	41	60	4
Double Cheeseburger	1 (5.3 oz)	450	24	35	6
Egg Rolls	3 pieces (6 oz)	440	24	40	5
Fish & Chips	1 serv (9 oz)	720	35	81	2
French Fries	1 reg (4.1 oz)	360	17	48	0
Grilled Chicken Fillet Sandwich	1 (8.1 oz)	520	26	42	9
Hamburger	1 (3.6 oz)	280	12	32	6
Jumbo Jack	1 (7.8 oz)	560	36	31	5
Jumbo Jack w/ Cheese	1 (8.6 oz)	650	43	32	5
Ketchup	1 pkg (0.3 oz)	10	0	3	2
Monster Taco	1 (4 oz)	290	18	21	2
Onion Rings	1 serv (4.2 oz)	460	25	50	3
Philly Cheesesteak Sandwich	1 (7.6 oz)	520	25	41	7
Salsa	1 serv (1 oz)	10	0	2	1
Seasoned Curly Fries	1 serv (4.5 oz)	420	24	46	0
Sour Cream	1 serv (1 oz)	60	6	1	1
Sourdough Jack	1 (7.8 oz)	670	43	39	4
Soy Sauce	1 serv (0.3 oz)	5	0	tr	tr
Spicy Crispy Chicken Sandwich	1 (7.9 oz)	560	27	55	5

FOOD	PORTION	CAL	FAT	CARB	SUG
Stuffed Jalapenos	7 pieces (5.3 oz)	470	28	41	4
Sweet & Sour Dipping Sauce	1 serv (1 oz)	40	0	11	10
Swiss-Style Cheese	1 slice (0.4 oz)	40	3	0	0
Taco	1 (2.7 oz)	190	11	15	0
Tartar Dipping Sauce	1 pkg (1.5 oz)	220	23	2	1
Teriyaki Bowl Chicken	1 serv (17.6 oz)	670	4	128	24
Ultimate Cheeseburger	1 (9.8 oz)	1030	79	30	6
salad dressings					
Blue Cheese	1 serv (2 fl oz)	210	18	11	3
Buttermilk House	1 serv (2 fl oz)	290	30	6	2
Buttermilk House Dipping Sauce	1 serv (0.9 oz)	130	13	3	tr
Low Calorie Italian	1 serv (2 fl oz)	25	2	2	2
Thousand Island	1 serv (2 fl oz)	250	24	10	8
salads and salad bars					
Croutons	1 serv (0.4 oz)	50	2	8	0
Garden Chicken Salad	1 serv (8.9 oz)	200	9	8	4
Side Salad	1 (3 oz)	50	3	3	2
KFC					
BBQ Baked Beans	1 serv (5.5 oz)	190	3	33	13
Biscuit	1 (2 oz)	180	10	20	2
Chicken Pot Pie	1 (13 oz)	770	42	69	8
Chicken Twister	1 (8.7 oz)	550	32	40	8
Cole Slaw	1 serv (5 oz)	180	9	21	20
Corn On The Cob	1 ear (5.7 oz)	150	2	35	8
Cornbread	1 (2 oz)	228	13	25	10
Crispy Strips Colonel's	3 (3.25 oz)	261	16	10	0

FOOD	PORTION	CAL	FAT	CARB	SUG
Extra Tasty Crispy Breast	1 (5.9 oz)	470	28	25	0
Extra Tasty Crispy Drumstick	1 (2.4 oz)	190	11	8	0
Extra Tasty Crispy Thigh	1 (4.2 oz)	370	25	18	0
Extra Tasty Crispy Whole Wing	1 (1.9 oz)	200	13	10	0
Green Beans	1 serv (4.7 oz)	45	2	7	3
Hot & Spicy Breast	1 (6.5 oz)	530	35	23	0
Hot & Spicy Drumstick	1 (2.3 oz)	190	11	10	0
Hot & Spicy Thigh	1 (3.8 oz)	370	27	13	0
Hot & Spicy Whole Wing	1 (1.9 oz)	210	15	9	0
Hot Wings	6 (4.8 oz)	471	33	18	0
Macaroni & Cheese	1 serv (5.4 oz)	180	8	21	2
Mashed Potatoes With Gravy	1 serv (4.8 oz)	120	6	17	0
Mean Greens	1 serv (5.4 oz)	70	3	11	1
Original Recipe Breast	1 (5.4 oz)	400	24	16	0
Original Recipe Chicken Sandwich	1 (7.3 oz)	497	22	46	2
Original Recipe Drumstick	1 (2.2 oz)	140	9	4	0
Original Recipe Thigh	1 (3.2 oz)	250	18	6	0
Original Recipe Whole Wing	1 (1.6 oz)	140	10	5	0
Potato Salad	1 serv (5.6 oz)	230	14	23	9
Potato Wedges	1 serv (4.8 oz)	280	13	28	1
Tender Roast Breast w/ Skin	1 (4.9 oz)	251	11	1	tr

FOOD	PORTION	CAL	FAT	CARB	SUG
Tender Roast Breast w/o Skin	1 (4.2 oz)	169	4	1	0
Tender Roast Drumstick w/ Skin	1 (1.9 oz)	97	4	tr	tr
Tender Roast Drumstick w/o Skin	1 (1.2 oz)	67	2	tr	0
Tender Roast Thigh w/ Skin	1 (3.2 oz)	207	12	<2	tr
Tender Roast Thigh w/o Skin	1 (2.1 oz)	106	6	tr	tr
Tender Roast Wing w/ Skin	1 (1.8 oz)	121	8	1	tr
Value BBQ Chicken Sandwich	1 (5.3 oz)	256	8	28	18

KRISPY KREME

FOOD	PORTION	CAL	FAT	CARB	SUG
Chocolate Iced	1 (2 oz)	260	14	30	24
Chocolate Iced Cake	1 (2 oz)	230	12	28	11
Chocolate Iced Creme Filled	1 (2.3 oz)	270	14	32	19
Chocolate Iced Cruller	1 (1.7 oz)	240	14	26	8
Chocolate Iced Custard Filled	1 (2.7 oz)	250	9	38	26
Chocolated Iced w/ Sprinkles	1 (2 oz)	220	10	31	19
Cinnamon Apple Filled	1 (2.3 oz)	210	9	29	11
Cinnamon Bun	1 (2.1 oz)	220	11	26	7
Glazed Blueberry	1 (2.4 oz)	300	15	37	29
Glazed Creme Filled	1 (2.3 oz)	270	14	32	19
Glazed Cruller	1 (1.5 oz)	220	14	22	5
Glazed Devil's Food	1 (1.9 oz)	240	13	29	20
Lemon Filled	1 (2.2 oz)	210	10	28	14
Maple Iced	1 (1.8 oz)	200	9	28	18

FOOD	PORTION	CAL	FAT	CARB	SUG
Original Glazed	1 (1.3 oz)	180	10	17	7
Powdered Blueberry Filled	1 (2.1 oz)	200	9	26	9
Powdered Cake	1 (1.8 oz)	220	11	26	10
Raspberry Filled	1 (2 oz)	210	10	27	16
Traditional Cake	1 (1.7 oz)	200	11	22	7
MANHATTAN BAGEL					
Blueberry	1 (4 oz)	260	tr	54	4
Cheddar Cheese	1 (4 oz)	270	4	48	3
Chocolate Chip	1 (4 oz)	290	3	56	3
Cinnamon Raisin	1 (4 oz)	280	tr	57	9
Egg	1 (4 oz)	270	2	53	3
Everything	1 (4 oz)	290	3	54	3
Jalapeno Cheddar	1 (4 oz)	260	2	53	2
Marble	1 (4 oz)	260	tr	52	3
Oat Bran	1 (4 oz)	260	1	53	3
Oat Bran Raisin Walnut	1 (4 oz)	270	3	54	5
Onion	1 (4 oz)	270	tr	55	3
Plain	1 (4 oz)	260	tr	52	3
Poppy	1 (4 oz)	300	4	54	3
Pumpernickel	1 (4 oz)	250	1	52	3
Rye	1 (4 oz)	260	1	52	3
Salt	1 (4 oz)	260	tr	53	3
Sesame	1 (4 oz)	310	5	55	3
Spinach	1 (4 oz)	270	tr	54	3
Sun-Dried Tomato	1 (4 oz)	260	1	53	3
Whole Wheat	1 (4 oz)	260	tr	52	3

FOOD	PORTION	CAL	FAT	CARB	SUG

MCDONALD'S

baked selections

FOOD	PORTION	CAL	FAT	CARB	SUG
Apple Pie Baked	1 (2.7 oz)	260	13	34	13
Chocolate Chip Cookie	1 (1.2 oz)	170	10	22	13
Cinnamon Roll	1	390	18	50	—
Danish Apple	1	340	15	47	—
Danish Cheese	1	400	21	45	—
Lowfat Muffin Apple Bran	1 (4 oz)	300	3	61	32
McDonaldland Cookies	1 pkg (1.5 oz)	180	5	32	12

beverages

FOOD	PORTION	CAL	FAT	CARB	SUG
Coca-Cola Classic	1 sm (16 oz)	150	0	40	40
Cocoa-Cola Classic	1 child serv (12 oz)	110	0	29	29
Diet Coke	1 sm (16 oz)	1	0	0	0
Diet Coke	1 child serv (12 oz)	0	0	0	0
Hi-C Orange	1 sm (16 oz)	160	0	44	44
Hi-C Orange	1 child serv (12 oz)	120	0	32	32
Milk 1%	1 serv (8 oz)	100	3	13	13
Orange Juice	1 serv (6 oz)	80	0	20	18
Shake Chocolate	1 sm (14.5 oz)	360	9	60	54
Shake Strawberry	1 sm (14.5 oz)	360	9	60	55
Shake Vanilla	1 sm (14.5 oz)	360	9	59	55
Sprite	1 sm (16 fl oz)	150	0	39	39
Sprite	1 child serv (12 oz)	110	0	28	28

breakfast selections

FOOD	PORTION	CAL	FAT	CARB	SUG
Bacon Egg & Cheese Biscuit	1	540	34	36	—
Bagel Ham & Egg Cheese	1	550	23	58	—
Bagel Steak & Egg Cheese	1	660	31	59	—

FOOD	PORTION	CAL	FAT	CARB	SUG
Biscuit	1 (2.9 oz)	290	15	34	2
Breakfast Burrito	1 (4.1 oz)	320	20	21	—
Egg McMuffin	1 (4.8 oz)	290	14	27	3
English Muffin	1 (1.9 oz)	140	2	25	1
Hash Browns	1 serv (1.9 oz)	130	8	14	0
Hotcakes Margarine & Syrup	1 serv	600	17	104	—
Hotcakes Plain	1 serv	340	8	58	—
Sausage	1 (1.5 oz)	170	16	0	0
Sausage Biscuit	1 (4.5 oz)	470	31	35	3
Sausage Biscuit w/ Egg	1 (6.2 oz)	550	37	35	3
Sausage McMuffin	1 (3.9 oz)	360	23	26	2
Sausage McMuffin w/ Egg	1 (5.7 oz)	440	28	27	3
Scrambled Eggs	2 (3.6 oz)	160	11	1	1
desserts					
McFlurry Butterfinger	1	620	22	90	—
MoFlurry M&M	1	630	23	90	—
McFlurry Nestle Crunch	1	630	24	89	—
McFlurry Oreo	1	570	20	82	—
Nuts For Sundaes	1 serv (7 g)	40	4	2	0
Reduced Fat Ice Cream Cone Vanilla	1 (3.2 oz)	150	5	23	17
Sundae Hot Caramel	1 (6.4 oz)	360	10	61	47
Sundae Hot Fudge	1 (6.3 oz)	340	12	52	47
Sundae Strawberry	1 (6.2 oz)	290	7	50	46
main menu selections					
Bagel Spanish Omelet	1	690	38	59	—
Barbeque Sauce	1 pkg (1 oz)	45	0	10	10
Big Mac	1	570	32	45	8

FOOD	PORTION	CAL	FAT	CARB	SUG
Big Xtra!	1	710	46	51	—
Big Xtra! w/ Cheese	1	810	55	52	—
Cheeseburger	1 (4.2 oz)	320	13	35	7
Chicken McNuggets	4 pieces (2.5 oz)	190	11	13	—
Crispy Chicken Deluxe	1 (7.8 oz)	500	25	43	5
Filet-O-Fish	1	470	26	45	—
French Fries	1 sm (2.4 oz)	210	10	26	0
Grilled Chicken Deluxe	1 (7.8 oz)	440	20	38	6
Grilled Chicken Deluxe Plain w/o Mayonnaise	1 (7.2 oz)	300	5	38	6
Grilled Chicken Salad Deluxe	1 serv (9 oz)	120	2	7	3
Hamburger	1	270	9	35	—
Honey	1 pkg (0.5 oz)	45	0	12	11
Honey Mustard	1 pkg (0.5 oz)	50	5	3	3
Hot Mustard	1 pkg (1 oz)	60	4	7	6
Light Mayonnaise	1 pkg (0.4 oz)	40	4	tr	0
Quarter Pounder	1	430	21	37	8
Quarter Pounder w/ Cheese	1 (7 oz)	530	30	38	9
Sweet 'N Sour Sauce	1 pkg (1 oz)	50	0	11	10
salad dressings					
Caesar	1 pkg (2.1 oz)	160	14	7	0
Fat Free Herb Vinaigrette	1 pkg (2.1 oz)	50	0	11	9
Ranch	1 pkg (2.1 oz)	230	21	10	6
Reduced Calorie Red French	1 pkg (2.1 oz)	160	8	23	15
salads and salad bars					
Croutons	1 pkg	50	1	9	—
Garden Salad	1 serv (6.2 oz)	35	0	7	3

FOOD	PORTION	CAL	FAT	CARB	SUG
MRS. FIELDS					
Brownie Double Fudge	1 (3.1 oz)	420	20	56	38
Brownie Fudge Walnut	1 (3.4 oz)	500	29	54	27
Brownie Pecan Fudge	1 (2.8 oz)	390	21	48	28
Brownie Pecan Pie	1 (3 oz)	400	21	48	22
Cookie Chewy Fudge	1 (1.7 oz)	230	12	32	22
Cookie Coconut Macadamia	1 (1.7 oz)	250	15	28	16
Cookie Milk Chocolate Chip	1 (1.7 oz)	240	12	32	21
Cookie Milk Chocolate Macadamia	1 (1.7 oz)	250	14	29	19
Cookie Milk Chocolate w/ Walnuts	1 (1.7 oz)	250	13	30	20
Cookie Oatmeal Raisin	1 (1.7 oz)	220	10	31	19
Cookie Peanut Butter	1 (1.7 oz)	240	13	27	15
Cookie Semi-Sweet Chocolate	1 (1.7 oz)	230	12	32	21
Cookie Semi-Sweet Chocolate w/ Walnuts	1 (1.8 oz)	240	13	30	20
Cookie Triple Chocolate	1 (1.7 oz)	230	12	31	23
Cookie White Chunk Macadamia	1 (1.7 oz)	260	15	29	19
Muffin Banana Walnut	1 (3.9 oz)	460	24	53	19
Muffin Blueberry	1 (4 oz)	390	15	58	24
Muffin Chocolate Chip	1 (4 oz)	450	19	65	26
Muffin Mandarin Orange	1 (4 oz)	420	17	59	24
Peanut Butter Dream Bar	1 (5 oz)	750	40	85	44

FOOD	PORTION	CAL	FAT	CARB	SUG
Stokabunga Energy Cookie	1 (5 oz)	750	48	74	46

NATHAN'S
main menu selections

FOOD	PORTION	CAL	FAT	CARB	SUG
Frankfurter	1 (3.2 oz)	310	19	22	—
French Fries	1 serv (8.6 oz)	514	26	62	—
Knish	1 (5.9 oz)	318	7	53	—

NEWPORT CREAMERY
ice cream

FOOD	PORTION	CAL	FAT	CARB	SUG
Reduced Fat No Sugar Added Chocolate	½ cup (2.6 oz)	110	3	22	5
Reduced Fat No Sugar Added Coffee	½ cup (2.6 oz)	100	4	18	6

OLIVE GARDEN

FOOD	PORTION	CAL	FAT	CARB	SUG
Garden Fare Apple Carmellina	1 serv (12.2 oz)	560	2	131	—
Garden Fare Dinner Capellini Pomodoro	1 serv (21.1 oz)	610	16	98	—
Garden Fare Dinner Capellini Primavera	1 serv (20.1 oz)	400	7	68	—
Garden Fare Dinner Capellini Primavera w/ Chicken	1 serv (23.8 oz)	560	10	71	—
Garden Fare Dinner Chicken Giardino	1 serv (20.6 oz)	550	11	71	—
Garden Fare Dinner Linguine Alla Marinara	1 serv (16.3 oz)	500	9	89	—

FOOD	PORTION	CAL	FAT	CARB	SUG
Garden Fare Dinner Penne Fra Diavolo	1 serv (14.3 oz)	420	7	77	—
Garden Fare Dinner Shrimp Primavera	1 serv (28.4 oz)	740	15	104	—
Garden Fare Lunch Capellini Pamodoro	1 serv (11.7 oz)	360	9	57	—
Garden Fare Lunch Capellini Primavera	1 serv (11.2 oz)	260	5	42	—
Garden Fare Lunch Capellini Primavera w/ Chicken	1 serv (14.9 oz)	420	8	45	—
Garden Fare Lunch Chicken Giardino	1 serv (12.8 oz)	360	9	47	—
Garden Fare Lunch Linguine Alla Marinara	1 serv (10.2 oz)	310	6	54	—
Garden Fare Lunch Penne Fra Diavolo	1 serv (10.2 oz)	300	5	57	—
Garden Fare Lunch Shrimp Primavera	1 serv (15.2 oz)	410	8	60	—
Minestrone Soup	1 serv (6 oz)	80	1	15	—

PIZZA HUT
desserts

FOOD	PORTION	CAL	FAT	CARB	SUG
Apple Pizza	1 slice (2.8 oz)	250	5	48	—
Cherry Pizza	1 slice (2.8 oz)	250	5	47	—

main menu selections

FOOD	PORTION	CAL	FAT	CARB	SUG
Bread Stick	1 (1.3 oz)	130	4	20	—
Bread Stick Dipping Sauce	1 serv (1.2 oz)	30	1	5	—

FOOD	PORTION	CAL	FAT	CARB	SUG
Buffalo Wings Hot	4 pieces (2.1 oz)	210	12	4	—
Buffalo Wings Mild	5 pieces (2.9 oz)	200	12	tr	—
Cavatini Pasta	1 serv (12.5 oz)	480	14	66	—
Cavatini Supreme Pasta	1 serv (13.9 oz)	560	19	73	—
Garlic Bread	1 slice (1.3 oz)	150	8	16	—
Ham & Cheese Sandwich	1 (9.7 oz)	550	21	57	—
Spaghetti Marinara	1 serv (16.6 oz)	490	6	91	—
Spaghetti Meat Sauce	1 serv (16.4 oz)	600	13	98	—
Spaghetti Meatballs	1 serv (18.8 oz)	850	24	120	—
Supreme Sandwich	1 (10.2 oz)	640	28	62	—
pizza					
Edge Chicken Supreme	1 sq (2.5 oz)	90	4	9	—
Edge Meat Lover's	1 sq (2 oz)	160	11	8	—
Edge The Works	1 sq (2.2 oz)	110	6	9	—
Edge Veggie Lover's	1 sq (1.9 oz)	70	3	9	—
Hand Tossed Beef Topping	1 slice	330	17	29	—
Hand Tossed Cheese	1 slice	240	10	28	—
Hand Tossed Chicken Supreme	1 slice	230	7	29	—
Hand Tossed Ham	1 slice	260	10	28	—
Hand Tossed Italian Sausage	1 slice	340	18	28	—
Hand Tossed Meat Lover's	1 slice	320	17	28	—
Hand Tossed Pepperoni	1 slice	280	13	28	—
Hand Tossed Pepperoni Lover's	1 slice	250	11	27	—

FOOD	PORTION	CAL	FAT	CARB	SUG
Hand Tossed Pork Topping	1 slice	320	16	29	—
Hand Tossed Super Supreme	1 slice	290	14	29	—
Hand Tossed Supreme	1 slice	270	12	29	—
Hand Tossed Veggie Lover's	1 slice	220	8	29	—
Insider Cheese	1 med slice (4.9 oz)	370	16	41	—
Pan Beef Topping	1 med slice (4.3 oz)	330	18	29	—
Pan Cheese	1 med slice (3.9 oz)	290	14	28	—
Pan Chicken Supreme	1 med slice (4.5 oz)	270	12	29	—
Pan Ham	1 med slice (3.8 oz)	260	12	28	—
Pan Italian Sausage	1 med slice (4.3 oz)	340	20	29	—
Pan Meat Lover's	1 med slice (4.7 oz)	360	21	29	—
Pan Pepperoni	1 med slice (3.7 oz)	280	14	28	—
Pan Pepperoni Lover's	1 med slice (4.3 oz)	330	18	29	—
Pan Pork Topping	1 med slice (3.7 oz)	320	17	29	—
Pan Super Supreme	1 med slice (5 oz)	340	18	30	—
Pan Supreme	1 med slice (4.7 oz)	320	17	29	—
Pan Veggie Lover's	1 med slice (4.6 oz)	270	12	30	—
Personal Pan Beef Topping	1 pie (10.2 oz)	710	35	71	—
Personal Pan Cheese	1 pie (9.2 oz)	630	28	71	—
Personal Pan Ham	1 pie (9.1 oz)	580	23	70	—
Personal Pan Italian Sausage	1 pie (10.2 oz)	740	39	71	—
Personal Pan Pepperoni	1 pie (9 oz)	620	28	70	—
Personal Pan Pork Topping	1 pie (10.2 oz)	700	34	71	—
Sicilian Beef Topping	1 slice (4 oz)	260	11	31	—

FOOD	PORTION	CAL	FAT	CARB	SUG
Sicilian Cheese	1 slice (4 oz)	290	13	31	—
Sicilian Chicken Supreme	1 slice (4.6 oz)	270	11	32	—
Sicilian Ham	1 slice (3.8 oz)	257	10	30	—
Sicilian Italian Sausage	1 slice (4.4 oz)	333	18	31	—
Sicilian Meat Lover's	1 slice (4.7 oz)	350	19	31	—
Sicilian Pepperoni	1 slice (3.9 oz)	280	13	31	—
Sicilian Pepperoni Lover's	1 slice (4.4 oz)	320	16	31	—
Sicilian Pork Topping	1 slice (4.4 oz)	320	16	31	—
Sicilian Super Supreme	1 slice (5 oz)	340	18	32	—
Sicilian Supreme	1 slice (4.7 oz)	310	15	32	—
Sicilian Veggies Lover's	1 slice (4.6 oz)	270	11	32	—
Stuffed Crust Beef Topping	1 lg slice (5.8 oz)	390	18	40	—
Stuffed Crust Cheese	1 lg slice (5.5 oz)	360	16	39	—
Stuffed Crust Chicken Supreme	1 lg slice (6.5 oz)	350	13	41	—
Stuffed Crust Ham	1 lg slice (5.5 oz)	330	13	39	—
Stuffed Crust Italian Sausage	1 lg slice (5.8 oz)	400	20	40	—
Stuffed Crust Meat Lover's	1 lg slice (6.7 oz)	470	25	13	—
Stuffed Crust Pepperoni	1 lg slice (5.4 oz)	360	16	39	—
Stuffed Crust Pepperoni Lover's	1 lg slice (6.2 oz)	420	21	40	—
Stuffed Crust Pork Topping	1 lg slice (5.7 oz)	380	18	40	—
Stuffed Crust Super Supreme	1 lg slice (7.2 oz)	430	22	41	—

FOOD	PORTION	CAL	FAT	CARB	SUG
Stuffed Crust Supreme	1 lg slice (6.7 oz)	410	20	41	—
Stuffed Crust Veggie Lover's	1 lg slice (6.6 oz)	340	14	42	—
The Big New Yorker Beef Topping	1 slice (7.2 oz)	480	26	42	—
The Big New Yorker Cheese	1 slice (6.1 oz)	380	17	41	—
The Big New Yorker Ham	1 slice (5.9 oz)	340	13	41	—
The Big New Yorker Pepperoni	1 slice (5.6 oz)	370	16	41	—
The Big New Yorker Pork Topping	1 slice (7.2 oz)	470	25	42	—
The Big New Yorker Sausage	1 slice (8 oz)	570	33	42	—
The Big New Yorker Supreme	1 slice (7.8 oz)	450	23	43	—
The Big New Yorker Veggie Lover's	1 slice (12 oz)	450	22	52	—
Thin'N Crispy Cheese	1 med slice (3 oz)	200	9	22	—
Thin'N Crispy Chicken Supreme	1 med slice (4 oz)	200	7	23	—
Thin'N Crispy Ham	1 med slice (2.9 oz)	170	7	21	—
Thin'N Crispy Italian Sausage	1 med slice (3.7 oz)	290	17	22	—
Thin'N Crispy Meat Lovers	1 med slice (4.1 oz)	310	19	22	—
Thin'N Crispy Pepperoni	1 med slice (2.8 oz)	190	9	21	—
Thin'N Crispy Pepperoni Lover's	1 med slice (3.4 oz)	250	13	22	—
Thin'N Crispy Pork Topping	1 med slice (3.7 oz)	270	14	22	—

FOOD	PORTION	CAL	FAT	CARB	SUG
Thin'N Crispy Super Supreme	1 med slice (4.6 oz)	280	15	23	—
Thin'N Crispy Supreme	1 med slice (4.1 oz)	250	13	23	—
Thin'N Crispy Veggie Lover's	1 med slice (4 oz)	190	7	22	—
Thin'n Crispy Beef Topping	1 med slice (3.7 oz)	270	15	22	—
Twist Crust Cheese	1 lg slice (6.7 oz)	450	16	58	—
Twist Crust Marinara Sauce	1 serv (3 oz)	60	1	12	—
Twist Crust Ranch Sauce	1 serv (3 oz)	440	48	4	—
Twist Crust Supreme	1 lg slice (7.5 oz)	470	18	59	—

POPEYE'S

FOOD	PORTION	CAL	FAT	CARB	SUG
Apple Pie	1 serv (3.1 oz)	290	16	37	13
Biscuit	1 serv (2.3 oz)	250	15	26	1
Breast Mild	1 (3.7 oz)	270	16	9	0
Breast Spicy	1 (3.7 oz)	270	16	9	0
Cajun Rice	1 serv (3.9 oz)	150	5	17	0
Cole Slaw	1 serv (4 oz)	149	11	14	9
Corn On The Cob	1 serv (5.2 oz)	127	3	21	1
French Fries	1 serv (3 oz)	240	12	31	0
Leg Mild	1 (1.7 oz)	120	7	4	0
Leg Spicy	1 (1.7 oz)	120	7	4	0
Nuggets	1 serv (4.2 oz)	410	32	18	1
Nuggets Mild Tender	1 (1.2 oz)	110	7	6	0
Nuggets Spicy Tender	1 (1.2 oz)	110	7	6	1
Onion Rings	1 serv (3.1 oz)	310	19	31	3
Potatoes & Gravy	1 serv (3.8 oz)	100	6	11	2
Red Beans & Rice	1 serv (5.9 oz)	270	17	30	19
Shrimp	1 serv (2.8 oz)	250	16	13	0

FOOD	PORTION	CAL	FAT	CARB	SUG
Thigh Mild	1 (3.1 oz)	300	23	9	0
Thigh Spicy	1 (3.1 oz)	300	23	9	0
Wing Mild	1 (1.6 oz)	160	11	7	0
Wing Spicy	1 (1.6 oz)	160	11	7	0

QUINCY'S
baked selections
Banana Nut Bread	1 serv (2 oz)	165	7	22	—
Biscuit	1 (2.5 oz)	270	15	29	—
Cornbread	1 serv (2 oz)	140	5	19	—
Yeast Roll	1 (2 oz)	160	4	29	—

breakfast selections
Bacon	1 serv (0.25 oz)	35	3	0	—
Corned Beef Hash	1 serv (4.5 oz)	210	15	11	—
Country Ham	1 serv (1.5 oz)	90	6	1	—
Escalloped Apples	1 serv (3.5 oz)	120	2	26	—
Oatmeal	1 serv (1 oz)	175	2	18	—
Pancakes	1 (1.5 oz)	95	3	12	—
Sausage Gravy	1 serv (4 oz)	70	6	3	—
Sausage Links	1 (2 oz)	225	22	0	—
Sausage Patties	1 (2 oz)	230	23	0	—
Scrambled Eggs	1 serv (2 oz)	95	7	1	—
Steak Fingers	1 serv (3.5 oz)	360	25	18	—
Syrup	1 oz	75	0	20	—

desserts
Banana Pudding	1 serv (5 oz)	240	12	30	—
Brownie Pudding Cake	1 serv (4 oz)	310	5	66	—
Caramel Topping	1 serv (1 oz)	105	1	24	—
Chocolate Chip Cookies	1 (0.5 oz)	60	8	8	—
Cobbler Apple	1 serv (6 oz)	255	8	49	—

FOOD	PORTION	CAL	FAT	CARB	SUG
Cobbler Cherry	1 serv (6 oz)	410	8	55	—
Cobbler Peach	1 serv (6 oz)	305	8	50	—
Frozen Yogurt	1 serv (4 oz)	135	2	25	—
Fudge Topping	1 serv (1 oz)	105	4	15	—
Sugar Cookie	1 (0.5 oz)	60	3	8	—
main menu selections					
⅛ Pound Hamburger	1 serv (8 oz)	565	33	32	—
BBQ Beans	1 serv (4 oz)	114	1	21	—
Bacon Cheese Burger	1 (9 oz)	663	41	33	—
Baked Potato	1 (6 oz)	115	0	30	—
Broccoli	1 serv (4 oz)	34	0	5	—
Cheese Sauce	1 serv (1 oz)	58	5	1	—
Chopped Steak Steak	1 serv (8 oz)	499	42	0	—
Cinnamon Apples	1 serv (4 oz)	172	5	34	—
Corn	1 serv (4 oz)	96	1	24	—
Country Steak w/ Gravy	1 serv (8 oz)	530	25	44	—
Cowboy Steak	1 serv (14 oz)	580	33	9	—
Filet w/ Bacon	1 serv (8 oz)	340	17	2	—
Green Beans	1 serv (4 oz)	61	4	6	—
Grilled Chicken	1 reg serv (5 oz)	120	2	1	—
Grilled Chicken Sandwich	1 (9 oz)	324	4	39	—
Grilled Salmon	1 serv (7 oz)	228	4	1	—
Homestyle Chicken Fillet	1 serv (3 oz)	217	9	21	—
Junior Sirloin Steak	1 serv (5.5 oz)	194	10	0	—
Mashed Potatoes	1 serv (4 oz)	54	6	11	—
NY Strip Steak	1 serv (10 oz)	450	26	1	—
Philly Cheese Steak	1 serv (11 oz)	588	30	38	—
Porterhouse Steak	1 serv (17 oz)	683	46	0	—

FOOD	PORTION	CAL	FAT	CARB	SUG
Regular Sirloin Steak	1 serv (8 oz)	285	16	0	—
Ribeye Steak	1 serv (10 oz)	452	29	0	—
Rice Pilaf	1 serv (4 oz)	119	2	23	—
Roasted BBQ Chicken	1 serv (14 oz)	941	65	21	—
Roasted Herb Chicken	1 serv (14 oz)	875	65	4	—
Sirloin Tips w/ Mushroom Gravy	1 serv (6 oz)	196	7	5	—
Sirloin Tips w/ Peppers & Onions	1 serv (5 oz)	203	8	4	—
Smothered Steak Sandwich	1 (9 oz)	429	15	36	—
Smothered Strip Steak	1 serv (10 oz)	622	41	12	—
Southern Breaded Shrimp	1 serv (7 oz)	546	31	47	—
Spicy BBQ Chicken Sandwich	1 (10 oz)	368	1	45	—
Steak & Shrimp	1 serv (9 oz)	677	39	33	—
Steak Fries	1 serv (4 oz)	358	19	45	—
T-Bone Steak	1 serv (13 oz)	521	35	0	—
salad dressings					
Blue Cheese	1 serv (1 oz)	155	16	2	—
French	1 serv (1 oz)	125	12	4	—
Honey Mustard	1 serv (1 oz)	100	6	10	—
Italian	1 serv (1 oz)	135	14	3	—
Light Creamy Italian	1 serv (1 oz)	65	4	8	—
Light French	1 serv (1 oz)	85	4	13	—
Light Italian	1 serv (1 oz)	20	2	2	—
Light Thousand Island	1 serv (1 oz)	65	4	8	—
Parmesan Peppercorn	1 serv (1 oz)	150	14	4	—
Ranch	1 serv (1 oz)	110	11	1	—

FOOD	PORTION	CAL	FAT	CARB	SUG
soups					
Chili With Beans	1 serv (6 oz)	235	11	21	—
Clam Chowder	1 serv (6 oz)	180	9	21	—
Cream Of Broccoli	1 serv (6 oz)	170	10	18	—
Vegetable Beef	1 serv (6 oz)	90	2	14	—
QUIZNO'S					
Sub Honey Burbon Chicken	1 sm	329	6	45	—
Sub Turkey Lite	1 sm	334	6	52	—
Sub Tuscan Chicken Salad	1 sm	326	6	45	—
RALLY'S					
beverages					
Coke	1 serv (16 oz)	132	0	35	—
Diet Coke	1 serv (20 oz)	1	0	0	—
Fanta Orange	1 serv (16 oz)	150	0	38	—
Mr. Pibb	1 serv (16 oz)	113	0	29	—
Root Beer	1 serv (16 oz)	146	0	38	—
Shake Banana	1 serv	399	11	70	—
Shake Chocolate	1 serv	411	12	73	—
Shake Strawberry	1 serv	399	11	70	—
Shake Vanilla	1 serv	320	11	49	—
Sprite	1 serv (16 oz)	132	0	33	—
main menu selections					
Big Buford	1	743	46	35	—
Chicken Fillet Sandwich	1	399	15	43	—
Chili w/ Cheese & Onion	1 serv (13 oz)	669	41	37	—
Chili w/ Cheese & Onion	1 serv (7 oz)	360	22	20	—

FOOD	PORTION	CAL	FAT	CARB	SUG
French Fries	1 reg (4 oz)	211	11	26	—
Onion Rings	1 serv	210	2	45	—
Rallyburger	1	433	22	35	—
Rallyburger w/ Cheese	1	488	35	35	—
Spicy Chicken Sandwich	1	437	18	50	—
Super Barbecue Bacon	1	593	31	49	—
Super Double Cheeseburger	1	762	48	37	—
SBARRO					
Pizza Veggie Slice	1 serv (10 oz)	490	12	75	—
SEE'S CANDIES					
Bridge Mix	14 pieces (1.4 oz)	200	12	24	19
Dark Chocolate Bordeaux	2 (1.4 oz)	170	27	27	25
Dark Chocolates	2 (1.2 oz)	160	10	19	15
Lollypop Butterscotch	1	90	3	17	12
Lollypop Cafe Latte	1	90	3	16	8
Lollypop Chocolate	1	90	5	14	9
Lollypop Peanut Butter	1	90	4	14	8
Marshmints	3 (1.4 oz)	140	4	27	21
Milk Chocolate Bordeaux	2 (1.4 oz)	170	8	27	25
Milk Chocolate Butter	2 (1.4 oz)	190	9	27	24
Milk Chocolate Buttercreams	2 (1.4 oz)	180	8	27	25
Milk Chocolate California Brittle	2 (1.3 oz)	220	16	19	17
Milk Chocolate Nuts & Chews	3 (1.7 oz)	250	16	26	19

FOOD	PORTION	CAL	FAT	CARB	SUG
Milk Chocolate Peanuts	3 (1.5 oz)	230	17	18	14
Milk Chocolate Soft Centers	2 (1.4 oz)	170	9	25	21
Milk Chocolates	2 (1.2 oz)	160	9	20	17
Nuts & Chews	3 (1.6 oz)	240	16	25	18
P-Nut Crunch	2 (1.4 oz)	220	15	21	17
Peanut Brittle	1.5 oz	230	16	21	15
Pecan Buds	3 (1.7 oz)	270	21	22	16
Red Hot Swamp Goo	3 pieces (1.4 oz)	140	4	27	21
Soft Centers	2 (1.4 oz)	170	9	25	21
Truffles Black or Gold	2 (1.4 oz)	180	11	22	13
Truffles Mint	3 (1.6 oz)	200	11	26	22
Victoria Toffee	1.5 oz	250	19	19	15
SMOOTHIE KING					
Activator Banana	1 (20 oz)	429	1	90	—
Activator Chocolate	1 (20 oz)	429	1	90	—
Activator Strawberry	1 (20 oz)	559	1	123	—
Activator Vanilla	1 (20 oz)	429	1	90	—
Angel Food	1 (20 oz)	330	1	79	—
Blackberry Dream	1 (20 oz)	343	tr	86	—
Caribbean Way	1 (20 oz)	392	tr	96	—
Celestial Cherry High	1 (20 oz)	285	tr	69	—
Coconut Surprise	1 (20 oz)	457	6	99	—
Cranberry Supreme	1 (20 oz)	577	1	139	—
Cranberry Cooler	1 (20 oz)	538	tr	132	—
GoGuava	1 (20 oz)	300	0	72	—
Grape Expectations	1 (20 oz)	399	tr	96	—
Grape Expectations II	1 (20 oz)	529	tr	129	—
Hawaiian Cafe Au Lei	1 (20 oz)	286	tr	62	—

FOOD	PORTION	CAL	FAT	CARB	SUG
High Protein Almond Mocha	1 (20 oz)	402	13	45	—
High Protein Banana	1 (20 oz)	412	14	44	—
High Protein Chocolate	1 (20 oz)	401	13	45	—
High Protein Lemon	1 (20 oz)	390	13	41	—
High Protein Pineapple	1 (20 oz)	380	13	41	—
Hulk Chocolate	1 (20 oz)	846	29	129	—
Hulk Strawberry	1 (20 oz)	953	29	156	—
Hulk Vanilla	1 (20 oz)	846	29	129	—
Immune Builder	1 (20 oz)	333	1	80	—
Instant Vigor	1 (20 oz)	359	1	87	—
Island Treat	1 (20 oz)	334	1	81	—
Lemon Twist Banana	1 (20 oz)	339	tr	82	—
Lemon Twist Strawberry	1 (20 oz)	399	tr	97	—
Light & Fluffy	1 (20 oz)	389	tr	98	—
Malt	1 (20 oz)	887	41	119	—
Mangofest	1 (20 oz)	320	0	78	—
Mo'cuccino	1 (20 oz)	440	12	71	—
Muscle Punch	1 (20 oz)	339	1	80	—
Muscle Punch Plus	1 (20 oz)	340	1	80	—
Peach Slice	1 (20 oz)	341	tr	80	—
Peach Slice Plus	1 (20 oz)	471	tr	113	—
Peanut Power	1 (20 oz)	502	21	72	—
Peanut Power Plus Grape	1 (20 oz)	703	21	119	—
Peanut Power Plus Strawberry	1 (20 oz)	632	21	104	—
Pep Upper	1 (20 oz)	334	1	80	—
Pineapple Pleasure	1 (20 oz)	313	tr	76	—
Power Punch	1 (20 oz)	430	1	102	—
Power Punch Plus	1 (20 oz)	499	2	113	—

FOOD	PORTION	CAL	FAT	CARB	SUG
Raspberry Sunrise	1 (20 oz)	335	1	85	—
Shake	1 (20 oz)	875	41	117	—
Slim & Trim Chocolate	1 (20 oz)	270	2	55	—
Slim & Trim Strawberry	1 (20 oz)	357	1	79	—
Slim & Trim Vanilla	1 (20 oz)	227	1	51	—
Super Punch	1 (20 oz)	425	tr	95	—
Super Punch Plus	1 (20 oz)	516	tr	118	—
Yogurt D'Lite	1 (20 oz)	341	4	65	—
Youth Fountain	1 (20 oz)	267	tr	65	—

STARBUCKS

FOOD	PORTION	CAL	FAT	CARB	SUG
Americano Tall	1 serv	5	0	2	—
Cappuccino Tall Lowfat Milk	1 serv	80	3	9	—
Cappuccino Tall Nonfat Milk	1 serv	60	0	9	—
Cappuccino Tall Whole Milk	1 serv	110	6	9	—
Cocoa w/ Whipping Cream Tall Nonfat Milk	1 serv	230	11	26	—
Drip Coffee Tall	1 serv	10	0	1	—
Espresso Solo	1 serv	5	0	1	—
Latte Tall Lowfat Milk	1 serv	140	5	15	—
Latte Tall Nonfat Milk	1 serv	110	1	15	—
Latte Iced Tall Lowfat Milk	1 serv	120	5	13	—
Latte Iced Tall Nonfat Milk	1 serv	90	0	13	—
Mocha w/o Whipping Cream Tall Nonfat Milk	1 serv	140	2	24	—
Steamed Lowfat Milk Tall	1 serv	140	5	14	—

FOOD	PORTION	CAL	FAT	CARB	SUG
Steamed Nonfat Milk Tall	1 serv	100	1	14	—

ice cream

FOOD	PORTION	CAL	FAT	CARB	SUG
Biscotte Bliss	½ cup	240	12	30	—
Caffe Almond Fudge	½ cup	260	13	30	—
Caffe Almond Roast	1 bar	280	18	26	—
Dark Roast Expresso Swirl	½ cup	220	10	29	—
Frappuccino Coffee	1 bar	110	2	20	—
Italian Roast Coffee	½ cup	230	12	26	—
Javachip	½ cup	250	13	29	—
Low Fat Latte	½ cup	170	3	31	—
Low Fat Mocha Mambo	½ cup	170	3	32	—
Vanilla Mochachip	½ cup	270	16	27	—

snacks

FOOD	PORTION	CAL	FAT	CARB	SUG
Crunchy Honey Bar	1 (1.06 oz)	150	7	18	9
Lively Lemon Bar	1 (1.23 oz)	140	4	23	11
Tangy Apple Bar	1 (1.23 oz)	140	4	23	13

SUBWAY

beverages

FOOD	PORTION	CAL	FAT	CARB	SUG
Fruizle Smoothie Berry 'Lishus	1 serv (12 oz)	154	tr	40	—
Fruizle Smoothie Berry Blitz	1 serv (12 oz)	129	0	37	—
Fruizle Smoothie Berry Breeze	1 serv (12 oz)	120	tr	32	—
Fruizle Smoothie Island Berry	1 serv (12 oz)	120	tr	32	—
Fruizle Smoothie Island Fever	1 serv (12 oz)	137	tr	36	—
Fruizle Smoothie Peach Paradise	1 serv (12 oz)	119	tr	32	—

FOOD	PORTION	CAL	FAT	CARB	SUG
Fruizle Smoothie Peach Pizazz	1 serv (12 oz)	142	tr	33	—
Fruizle Smoothie Pineapple Passion	1 serv (12 oz)	140	tr	38	—
Fruizle Smoothie Pineapple Delite	1 serv (12 oz)	142	tr	38	—
Fruizle Smoothie Sunrise Energizer	1 serv (12 oz)	160	tr	42	—
Fruizle Smoothie Tropical Trio	1 serv (12 oz)	138	tr	36	—
Fruizle Smoothie Wild Berries	1 serv (12 oz)	130	tr	36	—
cookies					
Brazil Nut	1 (1.7 oz)	215	10	29	—
Chocolate Chip	1 (1.8 oz)	214	10	29	—
Chocolate Chip M&M	1 (1.8 oz)	212	10	29	—
Chocolate Chunk	1 (1.8 oz)	215	10	29	—
Low Fat Oatmeal Raisin	1 (1.7 oz)	168	3	33	—
Macadamia Nut	1 (1.8 oz)	222	11	28	—
Oatmeal Raisin	1 (1.8 oz)	199	8	29	—
Peanut Butter	1 (1.8 oz)	223	12	27	—
Sugar	1 (1.8 oz)	225	12	28	—
salad dressings					
Creamy Italian	1 tbsp	65	7	3	—
Fat Free French	1 tbsp	15	0	4	—
Fat Free Italian	1 tbsp	5	0	1	—
Fat Free Ranch	1 tbsp	18	0	4	—
French	1 tbsp	70	6	5	—
Ranch	1 tbsp	88	10	2	—
Thousand Island	1 tbsp	65	7	3	—

FOOD	PORTION	CAL	FAT	CARB	SUG
salads and salad bars					
Classic Italian BMT	1 serv (11.6 oz)	269	19	11	—
Cold Cut Trio	1 serv (11.6 oz)	193	12	12	—
Ham	1 serv (11.1 oz)	112	3	11	—
Meatball	1 serv (12.1 oz)	232	13	17	—
Roast Beef	1 serv (11.1 oz)	115	3	11	—
Roasted Chicken Breast	1 serv (11.6 oz)	162	4	13	—
Steak & Cheese	1 serv (12 oz)	182	8	13	—
Subway Club	1 serv (11.6 oz)	123	3	12	—
Subway Melt	1 serv (11.8 oz)	190	9	12	—
Subway Seafood & Crab w/ Light Mayonnaise	1 serv (11.6 oz)	157	7	17	—
Tuna w/ Light Mayonnaise	1 serv (11.6 oz)	198	12	11	—
Turkey & Ham	1 serv (11.1 oz)	107	2	11	—
Turkey Breast	1 serv (11.1 oz)	101	2	12	—
Veggie Delight	1 serv (9.1 oz)	51	1	10	—
sandwiches					
6 Inch Cold Sub Classic Italian BMT	1 (8.9 oz)	450	21	45	—
6 Inch Cold Sub Cold Cut Trio	1 (8.9 oz)	374	14	45	—
6 Inch Cold Sub Ham	1 (8.4 oz)	293	5	45	—
6 Inch Cold Sub Roast Beef	1 (8.4 oz)	296	5	45	—
6 Inch Cold Sub Seafood & Crab w/ Light Mayonniase	1 (8.9 oz)	338	9	51	—
6 Inch Cold Sub Subway Club	1 (8.9 oz)	304	5	46	—

FOOD	PORTION	CAL	FAT	CARB	SUG
6 Inch Cold Sub Tuna w/ Light Mayonnaise	1 (8.9 oz)	378	14	45	—
6 Inch Cold Sub Turkey & Ham	1 (8.4 oz)	288	4	45	—
6 Inch Cold Sub Turkey Breast	1 (8.4 oz)	282	4	45	—
6 Inch Cold Sub Veggie Delight	1 (6.4 oz)	232	3	43	—
6 Inch Hot Sub Meatball	1 (9.4 oz)	413	15	50	—
6 Inch Hot Sub Roasted Chicken Breast	1 (8.9 oz)	342	6	46	—
6 Inch Hot Sub Steak & Cheese	1	363	10	47	—
6 Inch Hot Sub Subway Melt	1	370	11	46	—
Bacon Slices	2 (0.3 oz)	42	3	0	—
Cheese Triangles	2 (0.4 oz)	41	3	0	—
Deli Style Bologna	1	283	10	37	—
Deli Style Ham	1	224	3	37	—
Deli Style Roll	1 (2.1 oz)	170	2	31	—
Deli Style Tuna w/ Light Mayonnaise	1	267	8	37	—
Deli Style Turkey Breast	1	227	3	37	—
Italian Bread	6 Inch (2.5 oz)	190	1	38	—
Lettuce	1 serv (0.9 oz)	4	0	1	—
Mayonnaise	1 tsp (5 g)	37	4	0	—
Mayonnaise Light	1 tsp (5 g)	18	2	0	—
Mustard	2 tsp (0.3 oz)	0	0	1	—
Olive Oil Blend	1 tsp (5 g)	45	5	0	—

FOOD	PORTION	CAL	FAT	CARB	SUG
Olive Rings	2 (1 g)	2	tr	0	—
Onions	1 serv (0.6 oz)	5	0	1	—
Pepper Strips	2 (0.3 oz)	1	0	0	—
Pickle Chips	3 pieces (0.4 oz)	2	0	0	—
Super Subs Classic Italian BMT	1	668	39	47	—
Super Subs Cold Cut Trio	1	517	24	47	—
Super Subs Subway Club	1	377	7	48	—
Tomato Slices	2 (1 oz)	6	0	1	—
Vinegar	1 tsp (5 g)	1	0	0	—
Wheat Sub	6 Inch (2.6 oz)	210	3	39	—
Wheat Sub	12 Inch (5.3 oz)	420	5	78	—
Wrap 10.5 Inches	1 (2.6 oz)	200	2	45	—
Wraps Chicken Parmesan Ranch	1 (9.4 oz)	333	5	56	—
Wraps Steak & Cheese	1 (9.2 oz)	353	9	53	—
Wraps Turkey Breast & Bacon	1 (9 oz)	355	10	10	—

TACO BELL

beverages

FOOD	PORTION	CAL	FAT	CARB	SUG
2% Lowfat Milk	1 serv (8 oz)	110	5	11	10
Coffee Black	1 serv (12 oz)	5	0	1	0
Diet Pepsi	1 serv (16 oz)	0	0	0	0
Dr. Pepper	1 serv (16 oz)	208	0	52	52
Lipton Iced Tea Sweetened	1 serv (16 oz)	140	0	40	40
Lipton Iced Tea Unsweetened	1 serv (16 oz)	0	0	0	0
Mountain Dew	1 serv (16 oz)	227	0	61	61
Orange Juice	1 serv (6 oz)	80	0	18	18

FOOD	PORTION	CAL	FAT	CARB	SUG
Pepsi Cola	1 serv (16 oz)	200	0	51	—
Slice	1 serv (16 oz)	200	0	53	52
breakfast selections					
Breakfast Quesadilla Cheese	1 (5.5 oz)	380	21	33	1
Breakfast Quesadilla w/ Bacon	1 (6 oz)	450	27	33	1
Breakfast Quesadilla w/ Sausage	1 (6 oz)	430	25	33	1
Country Breakfast Burrito	1 (4 oz)	270	14	26	1
Double Bacon & Egg Burrito	1 (6.25 oz)	480	27	39	2
Fiesta Breakfast Burrito	1 (3.5 oz)	280	16	25	1
Grande Breakfast Burrito	1 (6.25 oz)	420	22	43	2
Hash Brown Nuggets	1 serv (3.5 oz)	280	18	29	0
main menu selections					
7-Layer Burrito	1 (10 oz)	530	23	66	4
BLT Soft Taco	1 (4.5 oz)	340	23	22	8
Bacon Cheeseburger Burrito	1 (8.5 oz)	570	31	46	5
Bean Burrito	1 (7 oz)	380	12	55	3
Big Beef Burrito Supreme	1 (10.5 oz)	520	23	54	4
Big Beef MexiMelt	1 (4.75 oz)	290	15	23	2
Big Chicken Burrito Supreme	1 (9 oz)	510	24	52	3
Border Sauce Fire	1 serv (0.3 oz)	0	0	0	0
Border Sauce Hot	1 serv (0.3 oz)	0	0	0	0
Border Sauce Mild	1 serv (0.3 oz)	0	0	0	0
Burger Sauce	1 serv (0.5 oz)	60	5	2	2

FOOD	PORTION	CAL	FAT	CARB	SUG
Burrito Supreme	1 (9 oz)	440	19	51	4
Cheddar Cheese	1 serv (0.25 oz)	30	2	0	0
Cheese Quesadilla	1 (4.25 oz)	350	18	32	1
Chicken Fajita Wrap	1 (8 oz)	470	22	51	3
Chicken Fajita Wrap Supreme	1 (9 oz)	520	25	53	4
Chicken Quesadilla	1 (6 oz)	410	21	34	2
Chicken Club Burrito	1 (8 oz)	540	32	43	5
Chili Cheese Burrito	1 (5 oz)	330	13	37	2
Choco Taco Ice Cream Dessert	1 serv (4 oz)	310	17	37	27
Cinnamon Twists	1 serv (1 oz)	140	6	19	—
Club Sauce	1 serv (0.5 oz)	80	8	1	0
Double Decker Taco	1 (5.75 oz)	340	15	38	2
Double Decker Taco Supreme	1 (7 oz)	390	19	40	3
Fajita Sauce	1 serv (0.5 oz)	70	7	1	0
Green Sauce	1 serv (1 oz)	5	0	1	0
Grilled Chicken Burrito	1 (7 oz)	410	15	50	3
Grilled Chicken Soft Taco	1 (4.5 oz)	240	12	21	2
Grilled Steak Soft Taco	1 (4.5 oz)	230	10	20	1
Grilled Steak Soft Taco Supreme	1 (5.75 oz)	290	14	24	4
Guacamole	1 serv (0.75 oz)	35	3	1	1
Mexican Pizza	1 serv (7.75 oz)	570	35	42	1
Mexican Rice	1 serv (4.75 oz)	190	9	23	1
Nacho Cheese Sauce	2 serv (2 oz)	120	10	5	2
Nachos	1 serv (3.5 oz)	320	18	34	2
Nachos Beef Beef Supreme	1 serv (7 oz)	450	24	45	3

FOOD	PORTION	CAL	FAT	CARB	SUG
Nachos Bellgrande	1 serv (11 oz)	770	39	84	4
Picante Sauce	1 serv (0.3 oz)	0	0	0	0
Pico De Gallo	1 serv (0.75 oz)	5	0	1	1
Pintos 'n Cheese	1 serv (4.5 oz)	190	9	18	1
Red Sauce	1 serv (1 oz)	10	0	2	0
Soft Taco	1 (3.5 oz)	220	10	21	1
Soft Taco Supreme	1 (5 oz)	260	14	23	3
Sour Cream	1 serv (0.75 oz)	40	4	1	0
Steak Fajita Wrap	1 (8 oz)	470	21	50	3
Steak Fajita Wrap Supreme	1 (9 oz)	510	25	52	4
Taco	1 (2.75 oz)	180	10	12	1
Taco Supreme	1 (4 oz)	220	14	14	2
Taco Salad w/ Salsa	1 (19 oz)	850	52	65	9
Taco Salad w/ Salsa w/o Shell	1 (16.5 oz)	420	22	32	9
Three Cheese Blend	1 serv (0.25 oz)	25	2	0	0
Tostada	1 (6.25 oz)	300	15	31	2
Veggie Fajita Wrap	1 (8 oz)	420	19	53	3
Veggie Fajita Wrap Supreme	1 (9 oz)	470	22	55	4

TACO JOHN'S

children's menu selections

Kid's Meal Crispy Taco	1 serv (8 oz)	579	34	54	4
Kid's Meal Softshell Taco	1 serv (8.5 oz)	617	33	64	4

desserts

Choco Taco	1 serv (3.5 oz)	320	17	38	27
Churro	1 serv (1.5 oz)	147	8	17	4
Flauta Apple	1 serv (2 oz)	84	1	19	3
Flauta Cherry	1 serv (2 oz)	143	4	27	3

FOOD	PORTION	CAL	FAT	CARB	SUG
Flauta Cream Cheese	1 serv (2 oz)	181	8	27	3
Italian Ice	1 serv (4 oz)	80	0	19	17
main menu selections					
Bean Burrito	1 (6.5 oz)	387	11	57	2
Beans Refried	1 serv (9.5 oz)	357	9	53	—
Beef Burrito	1 (6.5 oz)	449	20	44	1
Chicken Fajita Burrito	1 (6.25)	370	12	45	1
Chicken Fajita Salad w/o Dressing	1 serv (12.25 oz)	557	33	44	6
Chicken Fajita Softshell	1 (4.5 oz)	200	7	21	1
Chili	1 serv (9.25 oz)	350	21	19	4
Chimichanga Platter	1 serv (18 oz)	979	38	127	7
Combination Burrito	1 (6.5 oz)	418	16	50	1
Crispy Tacos	1 serv (3.25 oz)	182	11	12	1
Double Enchilada Platter	1 serv (18.25 oz)	967	42	106	6
Meat & Potato Burrito	1 (7.75 oz)	503	24	53	2
Mexi Rolls w/ Nacho Cheese	1 serv (9.75 oz)	863	48	72	1
Mexican Rice	1 serv (8 oz)	567	18	40	2
Nacho Cheese	1 serv (2 oz)	300	10	0	—
Nachos	1 serv (3.5 oz)	333	21	27	0
Potato Oles	1 serv (4.63 oz)	363	23	38	tr
Potato Oles w/ Nacho Cheese	1 serv (6.63 oz)	483	33	38	tr
Ranch Burrito	1 (7 oz)	447	23	44	2
Sampler Platter	1 serv (25.5 oz)	1406	61	156	7
Sierra Chicken Fillet Sandwich	1 (8.5 oz)	534	29	40	3
Smothered Burrito Platter	1 serv (19.5 oz)	1031	40	132	6

FOOD	PORTION	CAL	FAT	CARB	SUG
Softshell Tacos	1 serv (4.25 oz)	230	10	23	1
Sour Cream	1 oz	60	5	1	—
Super Burrito	1 (8.5 oz)	465	19	53	3
Super Nachos	1 serv (13 oz)	919	56	72	3
Taco Bravo	1 serv (6.25 oz)	346	14	39	1
Taco Burger	1 (5 oz)	280	12	28	4
Taco Salad w/o Dressing	1 (12.4 oz)	584	38	43	6

TACOTIME

FOOD	PORTION	CAL	FAT	CARB	SUG
Casita Burrito Meat	1 serv (12 oz)	647	31	54	—
Cheddar Cheese	1 serv (0.75 oz)	86	7	0	—
Chicken	1 serv (2.5 oz)	109	6	2	—
Chips	1 serv (2 oz)	266	12	35	—
Crisp Burrito Bean	1 (5.25 oz)	427	18	53	—
Crisp Burrito Chicken	1 (4.75 oz)	422	25	32	—
Crisp Burrito Meat	1 (5.25 oz)	552	30	39	—
Crisp Taco	1 (4 oz)	295	17	16	—
Crustos	1 serv (3.5 oz)	373	15	47	—
Double Soft Bean Burrito	1 (9.5 oz)	506	12	77	—
Double Soft Combination Burrito	1 (9.5 oz)	617	23	66	—
Double Soft Meat Burrito	1 serv (6.5 oz)	726	33	55	—
Empanada Cherry	1 (4 oz)	250	9	37	—
Enchilada Sauce	1 serv (1 oz)	12	0	3	—
Flour Tortilla 10 in	1 (2.75 oz)	213	4	31	—
Flour Tortilla 7 in	1 (1.75 oz)	88	1	16	—
Flour Tortilla 8 in	1 (1.25 oz)	107	3	16	—
Fried Flour Tortilla 10 in	1 (2.75 oz)	318	16	37	—
Fried Flour Tortilla 8 in	1 (1.35 oz)	205	11	24	—

FOOD	PORTION	CAL	FAT	CARB	SUG
Guacamole	1 serv (1 oz)	29	2	2	—
Hot Sauce	1 serv (1 oz)	10	0	2	—
Lettuce	1 serv (0.5 oz)	2	0	0	—
Mexi Fries	1 reg (4 oz)	266	17	27	—
Mexican Dressing No Fat	1 serv (2 oz)	20	0	5	—
Mexican Rice	1 serv (4 oz)	159	2	30	—
Nachos	1 serv (10.5 oz)	680	38	61	—
Nachos Deluxe	1 serv (15.25 oz)	1048	57	91	—
Natural Super Taco Meat	1 (11.25 oz)	627	27	60	—
Olives	1 serv (0.50 oz)	16	2	1	—
Quesadilla Cheese	1 serv (3.25 oz)	205	11	17	—
Ranchero Salsa	1 serv (2 oz)	21	1	3	—
Refritos	1 serv (2.5 oz)	97	0	18	—
Rolled Soft Flour Taco	1 (7 oz)	512	23	46	—
Shredded Beef	1 serv (2.5 oz)	70	7	1	—
Soft Taco Chicken	1 (7 oz)	387	16	41	—
Sour Cream	1 serv (1 oz)	55	5	1	—
Sour Cream Dressing	1 serv (1.5 oz)	137	14	2	—
Super Shredded Beef Soft Taco	1 (8 oz)	368	11	38	—
Taco Cheeseburger	1 (7.5 oz)	633	36	48	—
Taco Meat	1 serv (2.5 oz)	208	11	7	—
Taco Salad Chicken w/o Dressing	1 serv (9 oz)	370	21	27	—
Taco Salad w/o Dressing	1 serv (7.75 oz)	479	28	30	—
Taco Shell 6 in	1 (1.25 oz)	110	6	14	—
Thousand Island Dressing	1 serv (1 oz)	160	16	4	—

FOOD	PORTION	CAL	FAT	CARB	SUG
Tomato	1 serv (0.5 oz)	3	0	1	—
Tostada Delight Salad Meat	1 (9.75 oz)	628	33	48	—
Value Soft Bean Burrito	1 (6.75 oz)	380	10	58	—
Value Soft Meat Burrito	1 (6.75 oz)	491	21	48	—
Value Soft Taco	1 (5.25 oz)	316	15	23	—
Veggie Burrito	1 (11 oz)	491	16	70	—
Wheat Tortilla 11 in	1 (3.5 oz)	175	3	33	—
TCBY					
Hand Dipped All Flavors 96% Fat Free	½ cup (3 oz)	140	3	26	22
Hand Dipped All Flavors Nonfat	½ cup (2.9 oz)	120	0	25	18
Lowfat Ice Cream All Flavors No Sugar Added	½ cup (2.6 oz)	110	3	19	6
Nonfat Ice Cream All Flavors	½ cup (2.9 oz)	120	0	26	19
Soft Serve All Flavors 96% Fat Free	½ cup (3.4 fl oz)	140	3	23	20
Soft Serve All Flavors No Sugar Added Nonfat	½ cup (2.8 oz)	80	0	20	7
Soft Serve All Flavors Nonfat	½ cup (3.4 oz)	110	0	23	20
Sorbet All Flavors Nonfat & Nondairy	½ cup (3.4 oz)	100	0	24	19
WENDY'S					
beverages					
Cola	11 oz	130	0	36	36
Diet Cola	11 oz	0	0	0	0

FOOD	PORTION	CAL	FAT	CARB	SUG
Frosty Junior	6 oz	170	4	26	21
Frosty Small	12 oz	330	8	56	43
Lemon-Lime Soda	11 oz	130	0	34	34
children's menu selections					
French Fries Kid's Meal	1 serv (3.2 oz)	270	13	35	0
Kid's Meal Cheeseburger	1 (4.2 oz)	310	12	33	6
Kid's Meal Hamburger	1 (3.9 oz)	270	9	33	6
Kid's Meal Chicken Nuggets	4 pieces (2.1 oz)	190	13	9	0
main menu selections					
¼ lb Hamburger Patty	1 (2.6 oz)	200	14	0	0
2 oz Hamburger Patty	1 (1.3 oz)	100	7	0	0
American Cheese	1 slice (0.6 oz)	70	6	0	0
American Cheese Jr.	1 slice (0.4 oz)	45	4	0	0
Bacon	1 strip (4 g)	20	2	0	0
Baked Potato Chili & Cheese	1 (15.4 oz)	630	24	83	7
Big Bacon Classic	1 (9.9 oz)	580	30	46	10
Breaded Chicken Fillet	1 (3.5 oz)	230	11	13	0
Cheddar Cheese Shredded	2 tbsp (0.6 oz)	70	6	1	0
Chicken Breast Fillet Sandwich	1 (7.3 oz)	430	16	46	6
Chicken Club Sandwich	1 (7.6 oz)	470	20	47	6
Chicken Nuggets	5 pieces (2.6 oz)	230	16	11	0
Chili	1 sm (8 oz)	210	7	21	5
Classic Single w/ Everything	1 (7.6 oz)	410	19	37	6
French Fries	1 med (5 oz)	420	20	50	0

FOOD	PORTION	CAL	FAT	CARB	SUG
Grilled Chicken Fillet	1 (2.9 oz)	110	3	1	0
Grilled Chicken Sandwich	1 (6.6 oz)	300	7	36	8
Honey Mustard Reduced Calorie	1 tsp (7 g)	25	2	2	2
Hot Stuffed Bake Potato Plain	1 (10 oz)	310	0	72	5
Hot Stuffed Baked Potato Bacon & Cheese	1 (12.6 oz)	530	18	78	5
Hot Stuffed Baked Potato Broccoli & Cheese	1 (14.4 oz)	470	14	80	6
Jr. Bacon Cheeseburger	1 (5.8 oz)	380	19	34	5
Jr. Cheeseburger	1 (4.5 oz)	310	12	34	6
Jr. Cheeseburger Deluxe	1 (6.3 oz)	360	16	36	7
Kaiser Bun	1 (2.5 oz)	200	3	38	6
Ketchup	1 tsp (7 g)	10	0	2	1
Lettuce	1 leaf (0.5 oz)	0	0	0	0
Mayonnaise	1½ tsp (9 g)	30	3	1	0
Mustard	½ tsp (5 g)	5	0	0	0
Nuggets Sauce Barbeque	1 pkg (1 oz)	45	0	10	7
Nuggets Sauce Honey Mustard	1 pkg (1 oz)	130	12	6	5
Nuggets Sauce Sweet & Sour	1 pkg (1 oz)	50	0	12	10
Onion	4 rings (0.5 oz)	5	0	1	1
Pickles	4 slices (0.4 oz)	0	0	0	0
Saltines	2 (0.2 oz)	25	1	4	0
Sandwich Bun	1 (2 oz)	160	2	31	4
Spicy Chicken Fillet	1 (3.6 oz)	210	9	10	0

FOOD	PORTION	CAL	FAT	CARB	SUG
Spicy Chicken Sandwich	1 (7.5 oz)	410	14	43	5
Tomatoes	1 slice (0.9 oz)	5	0	1	1
Whipped Margarine	1 pkg (0.5 oz)	70	7	0	0
salad dressings					
Blue Cheese	1 pkg (2 oz)	360	36	1	0
French	1 pkg (2 oz)	250	21	13	11
Hidden Valley Ranch	1 pkg (2 oz)	200	20	3	1
Hidden Valley Ranch Reduced Fat Reduced Calorie	1 pkg (2 oz)	120	11	4	1
Italian Reduced Fat Reduced Calorie	1 pkg (2 oz)	80	7	6	4
Italian Caesar	1 pkg (1.5 oz)	230	24	1	0
Thousand Island	1 pkg (2 oz)	260	25	7	6
salads and salad bars					
Bacon Bits	2 tbsp (0.5 oz)	45	2	0	0
Caesar Side Salad w/o Dressing	1 (3.2 oz)	110	5	6	1
Chicken Salad	2 tbsp (1.2 oz)	70	5	2	—
Deluxe Garden Salad w/o Dressing	1 (9.5 oz)	110	6	10	5
Grilled Chicken Salad w/o Dressing	1 (11.9 oz)	200	7	10	5
Side Salad w/o Dressing	1 (5.4 oz)	60	3	5	2
Soft Breadstick	1 (1.5 oz)	130	3	23	—
Taco Chips	15 (1.5 oz)	210	9	28	0
Taco Salad w/o Dressing	1 (16.4 oz)	380	19	28	8

FOOD	PORTION	CAL	FAT	CARB	SUG
WHATABURGER					
baked selections					
Biscuit	1	280	13	37	—
Blueberry Muffin	1	239	8	36	—
Cinnamon Roll	1	320	16	39	—
Cookie Chocolate Chunk	1	247	16	28	—
Cookie White Chocolate Macadamia Nut	1	269	16	31	—
Fried Apple Turnover	1	215	11	27	—
beverages					
Cherry Coke	1 reg	227	0	60	—
Coffee	1 sm	5	0	1	—
Coke Classic	1 reg	211	0	56	—
Creamer	1 pkg	10	1	1	—
Diet Coke	1 reg	2	0	1	—
Dr. Pepper	1 reg	207	1	52	—
Iced Tea	1 reg	5	0	2	—
Lemon Juice	1 pkg	1	0	tr	—
Milk 2%	1 serv	113	4	11	—
Orange Juice	1 serv (10 oz)	140	0	33	—
Root Beer	1 reg	237	0	63	—
Shake Chocolate	1 junior	364	9	61	—
Shake Strawberry	1 junior	352	9	60	—
Shake Vanilla	1 junior	325	10	51	—
Sprite	1 reg	211	0	48	—
Sugar	1 pkg	15	0	4	—
Sweet And Low	1 pkg	4	0	1	—
breakfast selections					
Biscuit w/ Bacon	1	359	20	37	—

FOOD	PORTION	CAL	FAT	CARB	SUG
Biscuit w/ Bacon Egg & Cheese	1	511	33	38	—
Biscuit w/ Egg & Cheese	1	434	26	38	—
Biscuit w/ Sausage	1	446	29	37	—
Biscuit w/ Sausage Egg & Cheese	1	601	42	38	—
Biscuit w/ Sausage Gravy	1	479	27	48	—
Breakfast Platter w/ Bacon	1 serv	695	44	54	—
Breakfast Platter w/ Sausage	1 serv	785	53	54	—
Breakfast On A Bun w/ Bacon	1	365	19	29	—
Breakfast On A Bun w/ Sausage	1	455	28	30	—
Butter	1 pkg	36	4	0	—
Egg Omelette Sandwich	1	288	13	29	—
Grape Jelly	1 pkg	45	0	10	—
Hashbrown	1 serv	150	9	16	—
Honey	1 pkg	25	0	7	—
Margarine	1 pkg	25	3	0	—
Pancake Syrup	1 pkg	180	0	42	—
Pancakes	3	259	6	40	—
Pancakes w/ Bacon	1 serv	335	12	40	—
Pancakes w/ Sausage	1 serv	426	21	40	—
Scrambled Eggs	2	189	15	2	—
Strawberry Jam	1 pkg	40	0	9	—
Taquito Bacon & Egg	1	335	16	32	—

FOOD	PORTION	CAL	FAT	CARB	SUG
main menu selections					
Bacon	1 slice	38	3	0	—
Cheese Slice	1 sm	46	4	tr	—
Chicken Strips	2	120	5	10	—
Club Crackers	1 pkg	30	2	4	—
Croutons	1 pkg	30	1	5	—
Fajita Beef	1	326	12	34	—
Fajita Grilled Chicken	1	272	7	35	—
French Fries	1 reg	332	18	37	—
French Fries	1 junior	221	12	25	—
Garden Salad	1	56	1	11	—
Grilled Chicken Salad	1 serv	150	1	14	—
Grilled Chicken Sandwich	1	442	14	48	—
Grilled Chicken Sandwich w/o Bun Oil w/ Mustard	1	300	3	35	—
Grilled Chicken Sandwich w/o Bun Oil & Dressing	1	358	6	46	—
Grilled Chicken Sandwich w/o Dressing	1	385	9	46	—
Jalapeno Pepper	1	3	tr	1	—
Justaburger	1	276	11	30	—
Ketchup	1 pkg	30	0	7	—
Onion Rings	1 reg	329	19	34	—
Peppered Gravy	1 serv (3 oz)	75	5	8	—
Picante Sauce	1 pkg	5	0	1	—
Taquito Potato & Egg	1	446	22	48	—

FOOD	PORTION	CAL	FAT	CARB	SUG
Taquito Sausage & Egg	1	443	26	32	—
Texas Toast	1 slice	147	5	22	—
Whataburger	1	598	26	61	—
Whataburger Double Meat	1	823	42	62	—
Whataburger Jr.	1	300	12	35	—
Whataburger w/o bun oil	1	407	19	34	—
Whatacatch Sandwich	1	467	25	43	—
Whatachick'n Sandwich	1	501	23	51	—
salad dressings					
Low Fat Ranch	1 pkg	66	3	9	—
Low Fat Vinaigrette	1 pkg	37	2	6	—
Ranch	1 pkg	320	33	4	—
Thousand Island	1 pkg	160	12	12	—
WHITE CASTLE					
Cheeseburger	2 (3.6 oz)	310	17	23	0
Hamburger	2 (3.2 oz)	270	14	23	0
WINCHELL'S DONUTS					
Apple Fritter	1 (4.25 oz)	580	37	59	—
Cinnamon Crumb	1 (2 oz)	240	11	34	—
Cinnamon Roll	1 (3 oz)	360	21	39	—
Glazed Jelly	1 (3 oz)	300	13	43	—
Glazed Round	1 (1.75 oz)	210	12	24	—
Glazed Twist	1 (1.75 oz)	210	11	26	—
Iced Chocolate Bar	1 (2 oz)	220	11	28	—
Iced Chocolate Cake	1 (2 oz)	230	10	31	—
Iced Chocolate Devil's Food	1 (2 oz)	240	12	31	—

FOOD	PORTION	CAL	FAT	CARB	SUG
Iced Chocolate French	1 (1.89 oz)	220	13	23	—
Iced Chocolate Raised	1 (1.75 oz)	210	10	26	—
Plain	1 (1.58 oz)	200	11	24	—
Plain Donut Hole	1 (0.4 oz)	50	3	5	—

Index

(q = quiz, t = table)